T0259138

Cardiac Emergencies

Editor

RAN LEE

CARDIOLOGY CLINICS

www.cardiology.theclinics.com

May 2024 • Volume 42 • Number 2

ELSEVIER

1600 John F. Kennedy Boulevard • Suite 1800 • Philadelphia, Pennsylvania, 19103-2899

http://www.theclinics.com

CARDIOLOGY CLINICS Volume 42, Number 2
May 2024 ISSN 0733-8651, ISBN-13: 978-0-443-12955-1

Editor: Joanna Gascoine
Developmental Editor: Shivank Joshi

Cardiology Clinics (ISSN 0733-8651) is published quarterly by Elsevier Inc., 360 Park Avenue South, New York, NY 10010-1710. Months of issue are February, May, August, and November. Business and Editorial Offices: 1600 John F. Kennedy Blvd., Ste. 1800, Philadelphia, PA 19103-2899. Customer Service Office: 3251 Riverport Lane, Maryland Heights, MO 63043. Periodicals postage paid at New York, NY and additional mailing offices. Subscription prices are $396.00 per year for US individuals, $100.00 per year for US students and residents, $472.00 per year for Canadian individuals, $495.00 per year for international individuals, $100.00 per year for Canadian students/residents and $220.00 per year for international students/residents. For institutional access pricing please contact Customer Service via the contact information below. To receive student/resident rate, orders must be accompanied by name of affiliated institution, data of term, and the *signature* of program/residency coordinator on institution letterhead. Orders will be billed at individual rate until proof of status is received. Foreign air speed delivery is included in all *Clinics* subscription prices. All prices are subject to change without notice. **POSTMASTER:** Send address changes to *Cardiology Clinics*, Elsevier Health Sciences Division, Subscription Customer Service, 3251 Riverport Lane, Maryland Heights, MO 63043. **Customer Service: 1-800-654-2452 (U.S. and Canada); 314-447-8871 (outside U.S. and Canada). Fax: 314-447-8029. E-mail: journalscustomerservice-usa@elsevier.com (for print support); journalsonlinesupport-usa@elsevier.com (for online support).**

Reprints. For copies of 100 or more, of articles in this publication, please contact the Commercial Reprints Department, Elsevier Inc., 360 Park Avenue South, New York, NY 10010-1710. Tel.: 212-633-3874; Fax: 212-633-3820; E-mail: reprints@elsevier.com.

Cardiology Clinics is also published in Spanish by McGraw-Hill Interamericana Editores S. A., P.O. Box 5-237, 06500, Mexico D. F., Mexico; in Portuguese by Reichmann and Alfonso Editores Rio de Janeiro, Brazil; and in Greek by Dimitrios P. Lagos, 8 Pondon Street, GR115-28 Ilissia, Greece.

Cardiology Clinics is covered in *MEDLINE/PubMed (Index Medicus), Excerpta Medica, The Cumulative Index to Nursing and Allied Health Literature* (CINAHL).

Contributors

EDITORIAL BOARD

JAMIL A. ABOULHOSN, MD, FACC, FSCAI
Director, Ahmanson/UCLA Adult Congenital
Heart Center, Streisand/American Heart
Association Endowed Chair, Divisions of
Cardiology and Pediatric Cardiology, David
Geffen School of Medicine at UCLA, Los
Angeles, California, USA

DAVID M. SHAVELLE, MD, FACC, FSCAI
Director, Department of Cardiology,
Interventional Cardiology, MemorialCare Heart
and Vascular Institute, Long Beach Medical
Center, Long Beach, California, USA

AUDREY H. WU, MD, MPH
Associate Professor, Advanced Heart Failure
and Transplant Program, Division of
Cardiovascular Medicine, Department of
Medicine, University of Michigan, Ann Arbor,
Michigan, USA

EDITOR

RAN LEE, MD, FACC
Assistant Professor of Medicine, CCLCM of
CWRU, Sydell and Arnold Miller Family Heart
Vascular and Thoracic Institute, Department of
Cardiovascular Medicine, Sections of Critical

Care Cardiology, Advanced Heart Failure, and
Transplant Cardiology, Cleveland Clinic
Foundation Main Campus, Heart, Vascular,
and Thoracic Institute, Cleveland Clinic,
Cleveland, Ohio, USA

AUTHORS

CARLOS L. ALVIAR, MD
Assistant Professor The Leon H. Charney
Division of Cardiovascular Medicine, New York
University School of Medicine, New York, New
York, USA

WILLARD N. APPLEFELD, MD
Clinical Fellow Division of Cardiology,
Department of Internal Medicine, Duke
University School of Medicine, Duke University
Medical Center, Durham, North Carolina, USA

CHRISTOPHER BARNETT, MD, MPH
Assistant Professor, Division of Cardiology,
Department of Medicine, University of
California San Francisco, San Francisco,
California, USA

COURTNEY BENNETT, MD
Assistant Professor, Heart and Vascular
Institute, Leigh Valley Health Network,
Allentown, Pennsylvania, USA

MURTAZA BHARMAL, MD
Fellow Department of Cardiology, University of
California Irvine Medical Center, Irvine,
California, USA

SANJEEB BHATTACHARYA, MD
Clinical Instructor, Section of Heart Failure and
Cardiac Transplantation, Cleveland Clinic,
Cleveland, Ohio, USA

DREW A. BIRRENKOTT, MD, DPhil
Resident Department of Emergency Medicine,
Massachusetts General Hospital, Boston,
Massachusetts, USA

NICHOLE BOSSON, MD, MPH, NRP, FAEMS
Assistant Medical Director, Los Angeles
County Emergency Medical Services Agency,
Sante Fe Spring, California, USA; EMS
Fellowship Director and Faculty, Department of
Emergency Medicine, Harbor-UCLA Medical
Center, Torrance, California, USA; Clinical
Associate Professor of Emergency Medicine,
David Geffen School of Medicine at UCLA, Los
Angeles, California, USA

FRANCESCO CORRADI, MD
Professor Department of Surgical, Medical,
Molecular Pathology and Critical Care
Medicine, University of Pisa, Pisa, Italy

PAUL C. CREMER, MD, MS
Associate Director Department of
Cardiovascular Medicine, Heart, Vascular and
Thoracic Institute, Cleveland Clinic
Foundation, Cleveland, Ohio, USA

KYLE DIGRANDE, MD
Department of Cardiology, University of
California Irvine Medical Center, Irvine,
California, USA

DAVID M. DUDZINSKI, MD
Fellow Center for Vascular Emergencies,
Department of Cardiology, Cardiac Intensive
Care Unit, Massachusetts General Hospital,
Boston, Massachusetts, USA

ANDREA ELLIOTT, MD
Professor Division of Cardiology, University of
Minnesota, Minneapolis, Minnesota, USA

ANN GAGE, MD
Director of the CICU Centennial Heart, Tristar
Centennial Medical Center, Nashville,
Tennessee, USA

RYAN B. GERECHT, MD
Assistant Medical Director, District of
Columbia Fire and EMS Department,
Emergency Physician, MedStar
Washington Hospital Center, Washington,
DC, USA

MEGAN HEENEY, MD
Resident Physician, Alameda Health System,
Highland Hospital Emergency Department,
Oakland, California, USA

ANDREW HIGGINS, MD
Cardiologist Department of Cardiovascular
Medicine, Heart, Vascular, and Thoracic
Institute, Cleveland Clinic Foundation,
Cleveland, Ohio, USA

ZACHARY J. IL'GIOVINE, MD
Department of Cardiovascular Medicine,
Heart, Vascular, and Thoracic Institute,
Cleveland Clinic Foundation, Cleveland, Ohio,
USA

JACOB C. JENTZER, MD
Assistant Professor Department of
Cardiovascular Medicine, Mayo Clinic,
Rochester, Minnesota, USA

CHRISTOPHER KABRHEL, MD
Director Department of Emergency Medicine,
Center for Vascular Emergencies,
Massachusetts General Hospital, Boston,
Massachusetts, USA

RYAN R. KEANE, MD
Cardiologist Department of Cardiovascular
Medicine, Heart, Vascular and Thoracic
Institute, Cleveland Clinic Foundation,
Cleveland, Ohio, USA

BURTON LEE, MD
Adjunct Professor Department of Critical Care
Medicine, National Institutes of Health Clinical
Center, Bethesda, Maryland, USA

RAN LEE, MD, FACC
Assistant Professor of Medicine, CCLCM of
CWRU, Sydell and Arnold Miller Family Heart
Vascular and Thoracic Institute, Department of
Cardiovascular Medicine, Sections of Critical
Care Cardiology, Advanced Heart Failure, and
Transplant Cardiology, Cleveland Clinic
Foundation Main Campus, Heart, Vascular,
and Thoracic Institute, Cleveland Clinic,
Cleveland, Ohio, USA

MIREIA PADILLA LOPEZ, MD
Department of Cardiology, Hospital de la Santa
Creu i Sant Pau, Biomedical Research Institute
IIB Sant Pau, Universitat Autònoma de
Barcelona, Barcelona, Spain

VENU MENON, MD
Professor Department of Cardiovascular
Medicine, Heart, Vascular and Thoracic

Institute, Cleveland Clinic Foundation, Cleveland, Ohio, USA

ELLIOTT MILLER, MD
Assistant Professor Division of Cardiovascular Medicine, Yale University School of Medicine, New Haven, Connecticut, USA

EDUARDO MIRELES-CABODEVILA, MD
Professor of Medicine Respiratory Institute, Cleveland Clinic, Lerner College of Medicine of Case Western Reserve University, Cleveland, Ohio, USA

MARTHA E. MONTGOMERY, MD, MS
Attending Physician, Alameda Health System, Highland Hospital Emergency Department, Oakland, California, USA

JOSE V. NABLE, MD, NRP
Associate Professor of Emergency Medicine, Georgetown University School of Medicine, Medical Director, Georgetown EMS, Emergency Physician, MedStar Georgetown University Hospital, Washington, DC, USA

AKASH PATEL, MD
Cardiologist Department of Cardiology, University of California Irvine Medical Center, Irvine, California, USA

IAN PERSITS, DO
Resident Department of Internal Medicine, Cleveland Clinic, Cleveland, Ohio, USA

NOSHEEN REZA, MD
Assistant Professor Division of Cardiovascular Medicine, Department of Medicine, Perelman School of Medicine at the University of Pennsylvania, Philadelphia, Pennsylvania, USA

DAVID M. SHAVELLE, MD, FACC, FSCAI
Director, Department of Cardiology, Interventional Cardiology, MemorialCare Heart and Vascular Institute, Long Beach Medical Center, Long Beach, California, USA

MEGAN SHEEHAN, MD, MS
Resident Division of Internal Medicine, Department of Medicine, Perelman School of

Medicine at the University of Pennsylvania, Philadelphia, Pennsylvania, USA

AMANDEEP SINGH, MD
Attending Physician, Department of Emergency Medicine, Emergency Medicine Director of STEMI and Cardiac Arrest Receiving Centers, Alameda Health System, Highland Hospital, Oakland, California, USA

ALESSANDRO SIONIS, MD
Associate Professor Department of Cardiology, Hospital de la Santa Creu i Sant Pau, Biomedical Research Institute IIB Sant Pau, Universitat Autònoma de Barcelona, Barcelona, Spain

LARA SOKOLOFF, MD
Resident Physician Division of Internal Medicine, Department of Medicine, Perelman School of Medicine at the University of Pennsylvania, Philadelphia, Pennsylvania, USA

MICHAEL A. SOLOMON, MD, MBA
Head, Cardiology Section Clinical Center and Cardiology Branch, Critical Care Medicine Department, National Heart, Lung, and Blood Institute, National Institutes of Health, Bethesda, Maryland, USA

RAVI W. SUMER, MD, MS
Core Faculty, Assistant Clerkship Director and Simulation Director, Emergency Medicine Residency Program, Department of Emergency Medicine, Kaiser Permanente Central Valley, Modesto, California, USA

GUIDO TAVAZZI, MD, PhD
Assistant Professor Department of Critical Care Medicine, Intensive Care Fondazione IRCCS Policlinico San Matteo, Pavia, Italy

WILLIAM A. WOODS, MD, MS
Associate Professor of Emergency Medicine and Pediatrics, Vice-Chair for Academic Affairs, Department of Emergency Medicine, University of Virginia Health System, Charlottesville, Virginia, USA

Contents

Pericardiocentesis is an important diagnostic and therapeutic procedure. In the setting of cardiac tamponade, pericardiocentesis can rapidly improve hemodynamics, and in cases of diagnostic uncertainty, pericardiocentesis allows for fluid analysis to aid in diagnosis. In contemporary practice, the widespread availability of ultrasonography has made echocardiographic guidance the standard of care. Additional tools such as micropuncture technique, live ultrasonographic guidance, and adjunctive tools including fluoroscopy continue to advance and enhance procedural efficiency and safety. When performed by experienced operators, pericardiocentesis is a safe, effective, and potentially life-saving procedure.

Acute heart failure (AHF) is a frequent cause of hospitalization around the world and is associated with high in-hospital and post-discharge morbidity and mortality. This review summarizes data on diagnosis and management of AHF from the emergency department to the intensive care unit. While more evidence is needed to guide risk stratification and care of patients with AHF, hospitalization is a key opportunity to optimize evidence-based medical therapy for heart failure. Close linkage to outpatient care is essential to improve post-hospitalization outcomes.

Cardiogenic shock is a lethal condition with significant morbidity, characterized by myocardial insults leading to low cardiac output and ensuing systemic hypoperfusion. While mortality rates remain high, we have improved upon our recognition and definition of cardiogenic shock, now with an emphasis on defining stages of shock to help guide effective treatment strategies with either pharmacologic or mechanical circulatory support. In this review, the authors summarize these stages as well as discuss indications, function, selection, and troubleshooting of the various temporary mechanical circulatory support devices.

The acute aortic syndromes (AAS) are life-threatening vascular compromises within the aortic wall. These include aortic dissection (AD), intramural hematoma (IMH), penetrating aortic ulcer (PAU), and blunt traumatic thoracic aortic injury (BTTAI). While patients classically present with chest pain, the presentation may be highly variable. Timely diagnosis is critical to initiate definitive treatment and maximize chances of survival. In high-risk patients, treatment should begin immediately, even while diagnostic evaluation proceeds. The mainstay of medical therapy is acute reduction of heart rate and blood pressure. Surgical intervention is often required but is informed by patient anatomy and extent of vascular compromise.

Contents   ix

CARDIOLOGY CLINICS

SERIES OF RELATED INTEREST

Heart Failure Clinics
Available at: https://www.heartfailure.theclinics.com/
Cardiac Electrophysiology Clinics
Available at: https://www.cardiacep.theclinics.com/
Interventional Cardiology Clinics
Available at: https://www.interventional.theclinics.com/

Preface

Cardiac Emergencies: A Blueprint for Rescue

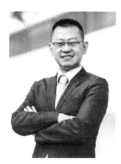

Ran Lee, MD, FACC
Editor

Acute cardiovascular care in the twenty-first century has seen a rapid timeline of focus, evolution, and expansion. Gone are the days when care for the acutely ill patient with a cardiac emergency focused solely on myocardial infarction and its electrical or mechanical sequelae. Now, comprehensive cardiovascular intensive care units are tasked with assessment and management of a multitude of diverse disease entities, such as cardiac tamponade, acute heart failure, cardiogenic shock, pulmonary embolism, valve failure, pulmonary hypertension, and cardiac arrest. Meanwhile, these multidisciplinary units must also combat comorbid cardiac and extracardiac conditions, be facile with new temporary mechanical circulatory support devices, while also be adept at mastering a traditional machine in the mechanical ventilator. Simultaneously, we have seen a significant rise in interest and in dedicated training pathways for dual certification of cardiologists in critical care. While the expectation is not for everyone to be a bona fide certified intensivist, our patients' presenting acute care conditions are mandating that the contemporary cardiologist maintain familiarity and comfort with certain emergent situations. In this vein, we have the privilege of presenting this latest issue of *Cardiology Clinics*, coming into print roughly a decade after our first issue on cardiovascular intensive care in 2013.

Our issue begins with an expert review of cardiac tamponade, its recognition and management, as well as both traditional and certain novel methods on pericardiocentesis. We then follow the acute heart failure patient in their trajectory from the emergency room to the intensive care unit and provide a blueprint on evaluation and management of this increasingly prevalent disease and its ramifications on the health care system. Our next article focuses on probably the defining cardiovascular intensive care disease state of the era—cardiogenic shock—and the multitude of advanced temporary mechanical circulatory support devices available to stabilize and temporize the patient.

We turn our attention thereafter to other extracardiac emergency states that may be seen more in cardiothoracic or medical intensive care units, respectively—the initial triage and management of patients with acute aortic syndromes, such as dissection, and intermediate-/high-risk pulmonary embolism. The contemporary cardiologist will be asked to manage these states, at least in initial triage, and these articles will provide that blueprint for success to not delay prompt care.

The next tranche of review topics focuses on acute valvular emergencies and how best to manage these cardiovascular hemodynamics, complex heart/lung interactions, and emergencies with focus on ventilator management, and emergencies

Cardiol Clin 42 (2024) xi–xii
https://doi.org/10.1016/j.ccl.2024.02.021
0733-8651/24/© 2024 Published by Elsevier Inc.

in pulmonary hypertension states requiring immediate stabilization. I highly recommend these high-yield topics, as often these conditions bring anxiety and uncertainty regarding best practices and troubleshooting.

Our final four articles expertly review certain topics in cardiac arrest, which could have its own special issue dedicated to its best practices and latest evidence. We specifically highlight the impact of the recent coronavirus pandemic on cardiac arrest and emergency care as well as cardiac arrest in special populations.

We hope that this issue on cardiac emergencies will provide familiarity and knowledge to our readers on managing the acutely ill cardiovascular patient, and that these topics serve as a blueprint to the best contemporary cardiovascular intensive care that we can provide today. We would like to thank the authors for their time, dedication, and expertise as well as the editors of *Cardiology Clinics* for the opportunity to guest edit this issue.

Ran Lee, MD, FACC
Sydell and Arnold Miller Family
Heart Vascular and Thoracic Institute
Department of Cardiovascular Medicine
Section of Critical Care Cardiology
Section of Advanced Heart Failure/
Transplant Cardiology
Cleveland Clinic Foundation Main Campus
9500 Euclid Avenue
J3-4
Cleveland, OH 44195, USA

E-mail address:
Leer2@CCF.org

Cardiac Tamponade and Pericardiocentesis
Recognition, Standard Techniques, and Modern Advancements

Zachary J. Il'Giovine, MD[a], Ann Gage, MD[b], Andrew Higgins, MD[a],*

KEYWORDS

- Pericardiocentesis • Cardiac critical care • Tamponade

KEY POINTS

- Pericardiocentesis rapidly improves hemodynamics in cardiac tamponade, serving as a crucial diagnostic and therapeutic intervention.
- Ultrasonography, particularly echocardiographic guidance, has become the standard of care, enhancing the precision of pericardiocentesis in contemporary medical practice.
- The evolving use of advanced tools like micropuncture techniques, live ultrasonographic guidance, and fluoroscopy further refines pericardiocentesis, enhancing procedural efficiency and safety.
- Fluid analysis during pericardiocentesis aids in diagnosing cases with uncertainty, contributing to a comprehensive understanding of the patient's condition.
- With experienced operators, pericardiocentesis stands as a safe, effective, and potentially life-saving procedure in the hands of skilled medical professionals.

INTRODUCTION

The pericardium is a thin fibroelastic sac surrounding the heart that typically contains a small fluid layer. Although it contains only 10 to 50 mL of fluid under normal conditions, it can accommodate significantly larger volumes without significant hemodynamic consequences provided the accumulation is gradual.[1] When its maximal constraints are exceeded by volume, rapid accumulation of fluid, or a loss of pericardial elasticity (as may be seen in constrictive/effusive constrictive pericarditis), hemodynamic consequences may result. Specifically, due to the fixed intrapericardial volume, external pressure is placed on the cardiac chambers resulting in chamber compression and augmented ventricular interdependence as the right and left heart compete for the fixed space. This clinical syndrome is referred to as cardiac tamponade and can lead to impaired venous return, impaired cardiac output (with respiratory variation), and if allowed to progress, eventual hemodynamic collapse. Importantly, cardiac tamponade is a clinical diagnosis supported by physical examination and imaging findings that must be recognized early and addressed urgently.

Pericardiocentesis is a procedure that is performed to percutaneously remove pericardial fluid and can be done urgently or emergently when necessary to acutely relieve the hemodynamic effects of cardiac tamponade.[2] It can also aid in distinguishing the cause of pericardial effusions. It is an important therapeutic and diagnostic tool that, when performed by experienced operators, is a safe and effective procedure. The following will detail the clinical recognition and adjunct testing to support the diagnosis of cardiac tamponade

a Department of Cardiovascular Medicine, Heart, Vascular, and Thoracic Institute, Cleveland Clinic Foundation, 9500 Euclid Avenue, Cleveland, OH 44106; b Centennial Heart, Tristar Centennial Medical Center, 2300 Patterson Street, Nashville, TN 37203
* Corresponding author.
E-mail address: higgina@ccf.org

Cardiol Clin 42 (2024) 159–164
https://doi.org/10.1016/j.ccl.2024.02.004
0733-8651/24/© 2024 Elsevier Inc. All rights reserved.

and describe contemporary techniques and best practices for performing pericardiocentesis.

DIAGNOSIS OF CARDIAC TAMPONADE

As previously noted, cardiac tamponade is a clinical diagnosis. Although classically taught as Beck's triad with hypotension, jugular venous distension, and diminished cardiac sounds on auscultation, this constellation is a late finding and relatively insensitive in the modern echocardiographic era, with one series reporting it as 0% sensitive.[3] In its earliest phases, there is a progressive increase in ventricular filling pressures that may initially be subclinical.

As venous return becomes impaired, pulsus paradoxus may be apparent. Although a small respirophasic variation in blood pressure is physiologic, changes in systolic blood pressure of greater than 10 mm Hg with respiration may be abnormal and is known as pulsus paradoxus. Either detected via auscultation with the deflation of a blood pressure cuff or visualized on an arterial line tracing, pulsus paradoxus is driven in tamponade by augmented ventricular interdependence in a fixed pericardial space. During inspiration, there is an increase in venous blood return to the right heart. In order for the right ventricle to accommodate this, the intraventricular septum must bow into the left ventricle, thereby decreasing left ventricular filling, stroke volume, and cardiac output. This decreased cardiac output results in the drop in systolic blood pressure typical of pulsus paradoxus. It should be noted that pulsus paradoxus is not unique to cardiac tamponade and may be present in other conditions that augment intrathoracic respirophasic pressure variation or confer partial cardiac compression, including compensatory hyperpnea in acidosis or sepsis, asthma, chronic obstructive pulmonary disease, pneumothorax, pleural effusions, pectus excavatum, or constrictive pericarditis. Notably, pulsus paradoxus may be absent in the presence of tamponade in certain disease states (such as tamponade while on temporary or durable mechanical circulatory support or in conditions which will protect the left ventricle from diastolic underfilling such as severe aortic regurgitation).

As tamponade progresses, a compensatory tachycardia will typically emerge if not blunted by conduction system disease or nodal blockade. Gradually, pericardial pressures will begin to exceed right ventricular and ultimately left ventricular pressure, resulting in rapid deterioration and hemodynamic collapse.

In addition to clinical findings and a high index of suspicion based on history, there are several diagnostic adjuncts including electrocardiogram (ECG), invasive hemodynamics (like a pulmonary artery catheter), or echocardiography that can aid in the diagnosis of tamponade. On routine ECG, variation in QRS amplitude as the heart swings toward and away from the electrodes, known as electrical alternans may be present and may suggest a pericardial effusion. A pulmonary artery catheter, if present, will show progressive equalization of diastolic pressures across all chambers.

Echocardiography is fundamental to the evaluation of a pericardial effusion. Although tamponade is more likely to occur as pericardial effusion size increases, a focal or rapidly developing effusion, even if small, may impair filling and precipitate tamponade if occurring in certain locations. Other echocardiographic stigmata of pericardial tamponade include right atrial collapse during ventricular systole (often the earliest sign), a plethoric inferior vena cava with minimal respiratory variation (which, though sensitive, may be confounded by positive pressure ventilation), diastolic collapse of the right ventricle, and augmented respirophasic inflow variation across the mitral or tricuspid valves (defined as an inspiratory decline in E wave velocity of greater than 25% for the mitral or inspiratory increase greater than 40% for the tricuspid).[4,5]

TECHNIQUES FOR PERICARDIOCENTESIS
Echocardiographic Guidance

Pericardiocentesis with echocardiographic guidance is the most common contemporary approach, especially given the wide availability of ultrasound. Patients are placed either in supine or in a slightly left lateral decubitus position and echocardiographic assessment is performed for the identification of the most appropriate window to access the effusion, the size of the effusion, and the depth at which the needle will reach the fluid. Selection of the most appropriate window is made on an individual basis while considering the location of the effusion and proximity to adjacent vital structures.

The 3 most common windows of approach are the subcostal, apical, and parasternal windows. The subcostal approach is regarded as having the lowest risk of causing pneumothorax, but the greatest risk of injuring the liver or gastrointestinal structures. This approach may be particularly challenging based on patient body habitus, as the subcostal approach may require the operator to traverse the furthest distance from skin to effusion. The apical approach has a lower risk of pneumothorax or injury to major vascular structures (coronary arteries or internal thoracic artery) but has a higher risk of left ventricular injury. When planning an apical approach, it is useful to obtain extreme apical views posteriorly, laterally, and/or inferiorly until the largest pocket of pericardial fluid with the best separation from adjacent structures. Finally, the parasternal approach has the advantage of small distance between the thoracic wall and the pericardium but due to positioning has a higher risk of pneumothorax or damage to an internal thoracic artery. A computed tomographic (CT) scan, if available, may be helpful in identifying the ideal target to approach.

Even when a high-quality echocardiogram is available, it is also critical for the proceduralist to reimage the patient immediately prior to sampling, as subtle shifts in patient positioning may have an outsized effect on approachability; moreover, standard echocardiographic views are obtained by sonographers with a goal of completing a standardized examination and not necessarily for procedural planning. In all of these approaches, the goal of imaging with echocardiography is to (1) identify the distance to the pericardial fluid and (2) utilize the position and angle of the probe as a surrogate for the trajectory of the needle. Variation in needle trajectory from the acoustic window obtained by the echo probe can cause difficulty in accessing the pericardial fluid and increases the risk of damaging surrounding structures. Live guidance of the needle tip is not always possible, so taking note of and maintaining the same trajectory with the needle that was obtained during echocardiographic assessment is of utmost importance.

Procedural Preparation and Technique

Once the most appropriate window is selected, the probe's location is marked with a permanent marker and scrubbed with sterile chlorhexidine—alcohol or povidone—iodine solution. Again the operator should take careful note of the probe's trajectory to recapitulate it with the needle during the procedure. The patient should not move between the echocardiographic examination and the procedure. To facilitate repeat or tandem ultrasound use during the procedure, once the patient is prepped and draped in a sterile manner, a sterile sleeve may be placed over the probe so that it is available as needed throughout pericardiocentesis.

For needle selection, historically an 18 gauge Cook needle or sheathed catheter was used. Our institution now routinely utilizes a small 21 gauge finder needle coupled with a 4 Fr micropuncture catheter that can be upsized after appropriate needle placement is confirmed. If this technique is employed, it is important that an appropriately stiff catheter and dilator are employed to avoid

bending within the subcutaneous tissue. Local anesthetic should be applied to the skin and subcutaneous tissue at the site of needle entry. If a chest wall approach is used, deeper anesthetic is also given over the superior aspect of the rib. Care must be taken when using an apical or intercostal approach to avoid damaging the neurovascular bundle at the lower edge of the rib at the superior aspect of the rib space.

To enter the pericardium and confirm appropriate needle positioning, our current technique is as follows. Outside of emergent situations (and even sometimes in emergencies), a micropuncture kit with a 21 gauge needle on a syringe is advanced through the anesthetized tract while maintaining negative pressure on the syringe. From apical or parasternal approaches, the needle should pass over the rib to avoid the neurovascular bundle, along the same trajectory established by ultrasound, until fluid is aspirated. Upon aspiration of fluid, the micropuncture wire (typically a 0.018 in guidewire) is threaded through the needle while monitoring for ventricular ectopy; the needle is then exchanged for the 4 Fr micropuncture catheter. It is important to note that the micropuncture wire may not be clearly visualized on ultrasound, though the subsequent 0.035 in wire is echogenic and may be visualized on either linear or phased array ultrasonography. If not using a micropuncture technique, a standard J-tip wire can be passed through an 18 gauge needle in a similar manner. It must be noted that fluid aspiration is not adequate confirmation of access to the pericardial space, as pleural or peritoneal fluid collections may be traversed by the needle based on approach. Further confirmation can be done by injecting agitated saline contrast through the 4 Fr micropuncture catheter while performing simultaneous echocardiography. The appearance of bubbles in the pericardial space confirms an appropriate location. Bubbles appearing within a cardiac chamber suggest that the heart has been perforated and that the needle or catheter should be withdrawn. If agitated saline cannot be visualized, either the needle/catheter position must be reconsidered and adjusted or another echocardiographic window should be obtained (in case there is no communication between pericardial fluid pockets). It should also be noted that direct echocardiographic guidance during access to the pericardial space can be performed by experienced operators with an assistant to help with probe manipulation, but extreme care must be taken to understand that needle trajectory and ensure that the true tip of the needle is being visualized.

Occasionally, bloody fluid is aspirated during pericardiocentesis. When this occurs, it is imperative to ensure the fluid is indeed pericardial fluid and not blood being withdrawn after chamber perforation or vascular complication. It has historically been taught that a small amount of the bloody aspirate may be ejected onto a gauze pad and monitored for coagulation to be placed on a gauze pad, with ex vivo coagulation suggesting whole blood from a cardiac perforation and a lack of coagulation suggesting a pericardial origin. Unfortunately, this lacks specificity, as hemorrhagic effusions secondary to cardiac rupture, dissection, or ongoing bleeding into the pericardial space may clot upon aspiration. Definitive testing requires testing the hematocrit of the fluid.

After entry into the pericardial space is confirmed, a pericardial drain may be placed. If using a micropuncture kit, after the 4 Fr microcatheter is placed, a J-tipped, 0.035 in guidewire is inserted into the pericardial space. The 4 Fr catheter is removed and a scalpel blade is then used to nick the skin, a dilator is used to broaden the tract into the pericardium, and the pericardial drainage catheter is threaded over the wire well into the pericardial space. If using other forms of access needles, the needle may be wired using a 0.035 in wire and the needle withdrawn. The next step is to make a skin-nick with a scalpel, followed by use of a dilator to increase the diameter of the tract. The drain can then be placed and sutured to the skin after the wire is removed.

Fluoroscopic Guidance

Fluoroscopy is sometimes utilized based on operator experience and training, particularly from the subxiphoid approach. For this approach, a needle with an attached syringe is directed to the left shoulder and toward the anterior diaphragmatic border of the right ventricle, at a 30° angle to the skin. The purpose is to avoid the coronary, pericardial, and internal mammary arteries with this direction and angulation. As the needle is advanced, negative pressure should be applied to the syringe. Once there is fluid "flash" in the syringe, a small amount of radiopaque contrast can be injected to confirm position. When contrast is injected, the pericardial silhouette should be visualized on fluoroscopy, a so-called halo sign, making sure that no contrast appears to be entering any of the cardiac chambers. After confirmation of access to the pericardial space, a wire can be advanced through the needle. The wire's trajectory may then be visualized fluoroscopically (ideally it should track around the entire cardiac silhouette) and a pericardial drain can be placed using standard Seldinger technique.

Electrocardiographic Guidance

ECG-guided pericardiocentesis is another alternative approach, also typically performed from the subxiphoid window, in which electrical monitoring is used to confirm position as the needle is advanced while looking for an electrical current of injury that would suggest the myocardium has been reached. It may be used either if echocardiography or fluoroscopy is not available or in conjunction with these approaches. However, the benefit or additive safety of this technique in addition to modern ultrasonographic techniques is undefined.

To perform and ECG-guided pericardiocentesis, ECG limb leads are attached to the patient in the usual manner, and a sterile alligator clip is affixed to the metal hub of the needle and connected to the V lead of the ECG monitor. As the needle is advanced, the operator should monitor for ST elevations or premature ventricular contractions to indicate that the needle is encountering the right ventricle, or PR-segment elevation or frequent PACs that might indicate that the needle is penetrating the right atrium.

Linear Ultrasound Probe Guidance

An emerging technique to aid in pericardiocentesis, especially in the parasternal approach, is using linear (high frequency) ultrasound with live guidance[6] in addition to echocardiography. Once an appropriate fluid pocket is identified on echocardiography, a linear ultrasound probe in a sterile sleeve is placed on the field. The patient is anesthetized in a standard manner, and then the linear probe is placed parallel to the rib space so that the entirety of the needle trajectory can be completely visualized. When ready, a needle and syringe is advanced with negative pressure between the ribs while the needle tip entering the pericardium is visualized under live ultrasound guidance. Care is again taken to avoid the neurovascular bundle of the rib. Fluid is aspirated, and needle position can be additionally confirmed with agitated saline and echocardiography as described earlier. This technique may allow entry into small fluid collections with relatively narrow margins of safety, although maintaining a stable ultrasonographic plane on the chest wall during respiration represents a technical challenge.

Blind Approach

Pericardiocentesis with no form of guidance, a so-called blind pericardiocentesis, is an emergent technique and should not be performed in nonemergent situations. There may be times in emergent conditions, such as cardiopulmonary arrest, in which a blind pericardiocentesis attempt is necessary. Even during emergent situations, it is often possible to utilize ultrasound guidance. However, when a blind approach must be used, the subxiphoid approach is often favored, with needle angulation toward the left shoulder. A needle with syringe should be advanced with negative pressure until fluid is aspirated. If cardiac tamponade is the etiology of the arrest, removal of even small amounts (50–100 mL) of fluid has the potential to improve hemodynamic conditions and may aid in the return of spontaneous circulation (ROSC). Because of this, we favor fluid removal with the needle and syringe to facilitate ROSC, and then subsequent placement of a pericardial drain. It should be stressed that because of the significantly higher risk of complications with a blind approach, it should be reserved only when absolutely necessary and when ultrasound is not available.

Contraindications to Pericardiocentesis

As with all invasive procedures, thoughtful patient selection and consideration of the risks and benefits is necessary. In an emergent situation such as cardiac tamponade resulting in cardiopulmonary arrest or when circulatory collapse is imminent, there are no absolute contraindications and pericardiocentesis may be a life-saving intervention. Outside of these emergent instances, there are relative contraindications to pericardiocentesis that must be considered and weighed against the potential benefits of the procedure. These include active anticoagulation and/or thrombocytopenia. While the risk of major bleeding during pericardiocentesis is low, routine laboratory testing should include a complete blood count, prothrombin, and activated partial thromboplastin time (aPTT). Although not a formal guideline, when the international normalized ratio is greater than 1.8 or an aPTT is greater than twice the normal range, this writing group routinely aims to correct with fresh frozen plasma before intervention. Likewise, a platelet count of greater than 50,000 is preferred in nonemergent cases.

Other relative contraindications to pericardiocentesis are conditions in which surgical management should be strongly considered. This includes traumatic hemopericardium, hemopericardium in association with an acute type A aortic, and subacute ventricular free wall rupture. However, in situations where tamponade and circulatory collapse are imminent, pericardiocentesis as a temporizing measure can be considered to facilitate definitive surgical management. This may risk disrupting

nascent clot formation and precipitating more rapid bleeding into the pericardial space, and the operator should be prepared for this possibility. Autotransfusion of aspirated blood may be necessary.

In certain conditions associated with pericardial effusion, surgical management (eg, with a pericardial window) is preferred due to the high risk for recurrence. These include purulent, tuberculous, or recurrent malignant effusions, though percutaneous aspiration may be employed preoperatively to facilitate stability at the time of anesthesia induction.

Lastly, small, loculated, or very posterior pericardial effusions may be more appropriate for the evaluation by interventional radiology to utilize a CT-guided approach.

COMPLICATIONS AND SAFETY

The most feared complications of pericardiocentesis are ventricular perforation, pneumothorax, and injury to other vascular structures like the coronary or intercostal arteries. Other potential complications include infection, bleeding, or precipitation of ventricular or atrial arrythmias. It should be noted these risks vary based on the window of approach and what techniques (echocardiography, fluoroscopy, and so forth) are used. The following are several series that tracked complication rates from pericardiocentesis. It is also important to note that the following studies on safety largely do not routinely utilize micropuncture kit use, and thus, actual rates may be different with increasing adoption of the micropuncture technique.

In a large series from the Mayo Clinic,[7] the use of echocardiographic guidance was associated with a relatively low complication rate. Among the 1127 procedures recorded, major complications occurred in just 1.2% of cases, including one death from right ventricular perforation and 5 nonfatal perforations in which surgical intervention was required. There was also one intercostal artery injury and 5 cases of pneumothorax. In comparison, fluoroscopy-alone guidance was associated with a higher rate of complications.[8] Finally, as expected, blind pericardiocentesis is has been associated with the highest rates of complications. For these reasons, we continue to advocate for echocardiographic guidance, even in urgent or emergent situations, whenever possible.

SUMMARY

Pericardiocentesis is an important diagnostic and therapeutic procedure. In the setting of cardiac tamponade, pericardiocentesis can rapidly improve hemodynamics, and in cases of diagnostic uncertainty, pericardiocentesis allows for fluid analysis to aid in diagnosis. In contemporary practice, the widespread availability of ultrasonography has made echocardiographic guidance the standard of care. Additional tools such as micropuncture technique, live ultrasonographic guidance, and adjunctive tools including fluoroscopy continue to advance and enhance procedural efficiency and safety. When performed by experienced operators, pericardiocentesis is a safe, effective, and potentially life-saving procedure.

CLINICS CARE POINTS

- Thorough bedside echocardiography by the proceduralist, coupled with appropriate patient preparation and positioning, are critical for success. Off-axis or unusual views, outside of those typically obtained by cardiac sonographers, may identify an angle of approach missed on routine echocardiography.

- The balance of risk versus benefit in pericardiocentesis will shift with operator experience; while some effusions may be easily approached, more challenging effusions may be better managed by a more experienced proceduralist.

- If there is ambiguity about the need for drainage of a specific effusion, time and careful clinical monitoring may be a reasonable choice: effusions that fail to improve with conservative management may become more easily accessible with expansion.

REFERENCES

1. Ivens EL, Munt BI. Pericardial disease: what the general cardiologist needs to know. Heart 2007;93(8):993–1000.

2. Adler Y, Charron P, Imazio M, et al. 2015 ESC guidelines for the diagnosis and management of pericardial diseases: the Task Force for the diagnosis and management of pericardial diseases of the European Society of Cardiology (ESC)endorsed by: the European association for Cardio-thoracic Surgery (EACTS). Eur Heart J 2015;36(42):2921–64.

3. Stolz L, Valenzuela J, Situ-LaCasse E, et al. Clinical and historical features of emergency department patients with pericardial effusions. World J Emerg Med 2017;8(1):29–33.

4. Alerhand S, Carter JM. What echocardiographic findings suggest a pericardial effusion is causing tamponade? Am J Emerg Med 2019;37(2):321–6.

5. Klein AL, Abbara S, Agler DA, et al. American Society of echocardiography clinical recommendations for multimodality cardiovascular imaging of patients with pericardial disease: endorsed by the Society for Cardiovascular Magnetic Resonance and Society of Cardiovascular computed tomography. J Am Soc Echocardiogr Off Publ Am Soc Echocardiogr 2013;26(9):965–1012.e15.

6. Osman A, Wan Chuan T, Ab Rahman J, et al. Ultrasound-guided pericardiocentesis: a novel parasternal approach. Eur J Emerg Med 2018;25(5):322–7.

7. Tsang TSM, Enriquez-Sarano M, Freeman WK, et al. Consecutive 1127 therapeutic echocardiographically guided pericardiocenteses: clinical profile, practice patterns, and outcomes spanning 21 years. Mayo Clin Proc 2002;77(5):429–36.

8. Duvernoy O, Borowiec J, Helmius G, et al. Complications of percutaneous pericardiocentesis under fluoroscopic guidance. Acta Radiol Stockh Swed 1987 1992;33(4):309–13.

Acute Heart Failure
From The Emergency Department to the Intensive Care Unit

Megan Sheehan, MD, MS[a], Lara Sokoloff, MD[a], Nosheen Reza, MD[b],*

KEYWORDS

- Acute heart failure • Cardiogenic shock • Guideline-directed medical therapy
- Emergency department • Intensive care unit

KEY POINTS

- Acute heart failure (AHF) is a leading cause of hospitalization and generates a significant economic burden worldwide.
- Diagnostic tools and management vary by clinical acuity and phase of care.
- Hospitalization is an opportunity to initiate evidence-based care in de novo heart failure and optimize therapy for those with acute decompensations.
- More research is needed to guide risk stratification and optimize linkage to outpatient care post-hospitalization.

INTRODUCTION

Acute heart failure (AHF) is one of the most frequent reasons for hospitalization in the United States (U.S.) and across the world. In the U.S., there are over 1 million hospitalizations annually for AHF, costing on average almost $16,000 per admission.[1] Among those older than 65 years, AHF is the most common reason for emergency hospital admission and carries an estimated in-hospital mortality of 4% to 12% for those with acute on chronic heart failure (HF) and up to 60% for those presenting with cardiogenic shock.[2] Moreover, individuals who survive an AHF hospitalization remain at elevated risk for poor post-discharge outcomes including readmission and mortality. In recent years, many advances in the care of patients with AHF have occurred, and this subtype of HF remains an active area of investigation. In this article, we summarize contemporary data on the epidemiology, presentation, evaluation, and management of patients with AHF across phases of care, from the emergency room to the intensive care unit (ICU).

DEFINITIONS AND CLASSIFICATIONS OF ACUTE HEART FAILURE

Definitions used in registries of AHF often include both acute de novo HF and acute decompensated HF. Acute de novo HF represents the first episode of cardiac decompensation in patients without a previously known history of HF, while acute decompensation occurs in patients with known chronic HF.[3] Variation exists across registries and guidelines, but most AHF definitions include (1) now or worsening symptoms, (2) escalation of care to urgent or emergent medical centers, and (3) treatment with intravenous or invasive therapies.[4] Even among those who meet criteria for AHF, there is marked heterogeneity in presentation, etiology of AHF, and subsequent management, which is challenging to encapsulate in a single

a Division of Internal Medicine, Department of Medicine, Perelman School of Medicine at the University of Pennsylvania, Maloney Building 5th Floor, 3400 Spruce Street, Philadelphia, PA 19104, USA; b Division of Cardiovascular Medicine, Department of Medicine, Perelman School of Medicine at the University of Pennsylvania, 3400 Civic Center Boulevard, 11th Floor South Pavilion, Room 11-145, Philadelphia, PA 19104, USA
* Corresponding author.
E-mail address: nosheen.reza@pennmedicine.upenn.edu
Twitter: @noshreza (N.R.)

Cardiol Clin 42 (2024) 165–186
https://doi.org/10.1016/j.ccl.2024.02.005

definition. Recent revisions to the 2021 European Society of Cardiology guidelines stratify patients with AHF into 4 distinct subtypes: acute decompensated HF, acute pulmonary edema, isolated right ventricular failure, and cardiogenic shock, with different management algorithms for each.[5] There is also some disagreement about the distinct nature of AHF, particularly in patients who are hospitalized with gradual worsening of chronic symptoms rather than an acute precipitant.[6] For this article, both acute *de novo* and acute decompensated HF are addressed, and diagnostic tools and management are stratified by phase of care.

EPIDEMIOLOGY OF ACUTE HEART FAILURE

Large-scale registries like Acute Decompensated Heart Failure National Registry (ADHERE), Organized Program to initiate Life Saving Treatment in Hospitalized Patients with Heart Failure (OPTIMIZE-HF), and Acute Heart Failure Global Registry of Standard Treatment (ALARM-HF) provide epidemiologic insight into AHF, although the majority of these registries are based in the U.S. or Europe.[7,8] Male sex and advanced age are risk factors for development of AHF. Acute decompensation in those with known chronic HF, make up 70% of all AHF presentations, while *de novo* presentation is less common. The most common comorbidities include hypertension, coronary artery disease, and diabetes mellitus.[7] Patients presenting with *de novo* episodes of AHF are on average younger with less comorbidity and have higher inpatient mortality compared to those with chronic decompensated HF.[3] In-hospital mortality ranges from 4% to 14%, with highest in-hospital mortality for those requiring intensive care.[3,9] Mortality after discharge for AHF remains high despite advancements in therapy, and in some registries is up to 30% at 1 year post-discharge.[10] Almost 40% of all deaths and re-hospitalizations in the year following discharge are due to non-cardiac causes, reflecting the significant comorbidity burden of many patients hospitalized with AHF.[11]

Acute HF is commonly precipitated by acute coronary syndrome and ischemia, particularly for patients with *de novo* HF. Other precipitants include uncontrolled hypertension, arrhythmias, pulmonary emboli, valvular dysfunction, or systemic infection. For those with known HF, non-adherence to medications is a frequent cause of acute decompensation. Uncontrolled endocrine disorders (eg, hyperthyroidism, adrenal crisis), surgeries, anemia, and changes in medications that increase sodium retention are other possible acute precipitants.[12] For some patients, a cause may never be clearly identified. An expanded discussion on the precipitants of AHF is beyond the scope of this article and has been summarized elsewhere.[13–15]

PHASE OF CARE: EMERGENCY DEPARTMENT
Presentation

There are over 1 million emergency department (ED) visits for AHF in the U.S. each year.[16] Most patients present with congestive symptoms, with dyspnea being the most common reason for emergency evaluation.[7,8] The nonspecific nature of presenting symptoms can make the timely diagnosis of AHF challenging. In a meta-analysis of index tests to diagnose AHF in the ED, the presence of an S3 on physical examination had the highest positive likelihood ratio (4.0, 2.7 to 5.9) among all history and physical exam elements evaluated.[17] As there is no single clinical history or physical exam finding that can reliably rule in or rule out AHF, further diagnostic testing is essential.

Diagnostics

Initial imaging should include a chest x-ray, which may show pulmonary venous congestion, pleural effusions, interstitial edema, or cardiomegaly. However, up to 20% of patients with AHF have a normal chest x-ray, so lack of congestion on imaging is not sufficient to exclude an HF diagnosis.[18] Point-of-care ultrasonography is being increasingly used to evaluate cardiac function expediently at the bedside. Obtaining views and estimates of the left ventricular ejection fraction, the inferior vena cava collapsibility, and the pleural space for signs of interstitial edema by experienced users has a specificity of nearly 100% for the diagnosis of AHF.[19] If a patient has new onset HF with no known clinical history, a formal echocardiogram should be obtained as soon as possible. Laboratory testing should include a complete blood count, electrolytes, creatinine and blood urea nitrogen, glucose, and cardiac troponin. Blood levels of natriuretic peptides, either b-type natriuretic peptide (BNP) or N-terminal proBNP (NT-proBNP), are highly sensitive and helpful to rule out AHF as the cause of presenting symptoms. A BNP of less than 100 pg/mL or NT-proBNP less than 300 pg/mL effectively excludes HF.[20] These biomarkers increase in response to ventricular dilatation and increased pressure, and the magnitude of elevation is correlated with illness severity and risk for mortality.[20,21] Of note, natriuretic peptide abnormalities should be interpreted with caution in patients with obesity or renal dysfunction, as obesity may falsely lower the value and renal dysfunction may falsely elevate it.[22,23] Sepsis, pulmonary hypertension, arrhythmia, and age also affect baseline natriuretic peptide levels. In patients with chronic HF, change from individual baseline is more accurate for identifying acute decompensation than interpreting the absolute value, which may always be elevated above normal range.[20] It is also important to identify emergent causes of AHF for rapid intervention, for example, acute coronary syndromes, pulmonary embolism, and acute lung pathologies.

Management

Assessment of respiratory status and risk of respiratory failure or hemodynamic compromise is essential immediately upon arrival to the emergency room. In AHF-related respiratory distress, noninvasive ventilation has been shown to reduce mortality and the need for intubation.[24] Intravenous loop diuretics should also be administered without delay, as early treatment is associated with reduced in-hospital mortality.[25] Intravenous vasodilators like nitroglycerin may also provide symptomatic relief, although they are contraindicated in patients with hypotension and concern for impending shock.[26]

Disposition

Over 80% of patients presenting to the emergency room for AHF are admitted to the hospital, with the majority receiving care on inpatient units and 5% to 10% going directly to intensive care.[16] Patients with respiratory compromise or those who require noninvasive ventilation or endotracheal intubation in the ED should receive further care in the ICU. Hemodynamic instability measured by heart rate less than 40 or greater than 130 beats per minute or systolic blood pressure less than 90 or requiring intravenous inotropic or vasopressor support, is also an indication for transfer to a higher level of care.[27] The majority of patients without these signs can be safely managed on the inpatient floors.

Identifying lower risk patients with AHF who can be discharged home safely is challenging, and various risk stratification tools have been developed to guide disposition decisions in the ED. The Ottawa Heart Failure Risk Scale (OHFRS), Emergency Heart Failure Mortality Risk Group (EHMRG), Multiple Estimation of Risk Based on the Emergency Department Spanish Score in Patients with AHF (MEESSI-AHF), and St. Thomas Risk Assessment Tool in Falling elderly inpatients (STRATIFY) tools have been prospectively derived from patients in the ED with AHF to predict major adverse events at 30 days post-discharge (**Table 1**).[28] Most of these tools rely on readily available clinical variables obtained in the initial evaluation of AHF, but implementation and evaluation of subsequent patient-centered outcomes has been challenging.[29] Even

in symptomatically improved patients, direct discharge from the emergency room to home is difficult to coordinate. High comorbidity burden, complex post-discharge follow-up needs, and elevated risk for higher post-discharge event rates and readmissions with direct discharge from the ED are contributing factors.[30] Patients may be admitted to observation units from the emergency room; however, studies comparing patients in observation have shown higher rates of cardiac and all-cause readmissions compared to those with inpatient stays, suggesting that the current admissions system still does not appropriately risk-stratify patients appropriate for observation status.[31] Further studies on risk stratification from the ED and randomized trials of these scoring systems are needed to improve patient outcomes and health system efficiency and resource utilization.

PHASE OF CARE: INPATIENT FLOORS
Diagnostics

Evaluation for the etiology of AHF and possible exacerbating factors should continue on the inpatient floor. This includes telemetry and blood pressure monitoring and evaluation for underlying infection. Signs and symptoms of congestion should be assessed daily. Screening for sleep apnea through careful history should also be performed on admission. Nutritional status and frailty should be assessed and multidisciplinary teams, including dieticians, physical therapy, and occupational therapy should be involved in care.[32]

For patients with newly diagnosed AHF, transthoracic echocardiography should be performed during the admission. In those with known chronic HF, echocardiography is indicated if there is a suspected significant change in cardiac function based on presentation.[32] Based on the history obtained from the patient and results of initial evaluation, catheterization, advanced imaging, or other laboratory tests may be indicated as well.[33]

Management

Loop diuretics are the mainstay for decongestion, although direct evidence supporting their use in comparison to other diuretics and specific dosing regimens in AHF is lacking.[34] If decongestion remains challenging, the diuretic dose can be increased, or additional medications like thiazide diuretics, metolazone, or acetazolamide can be added for benefit. In the Acetazolamide in Decompensated Heart Failure with Volume Overload (ADVOR) trial, acetazolamide in combination with loop diuretics led to more successful decongestion and natriuresis in patients admitted to the hospital with AHF when compared with loop diuretic alone,

Table 1
Selected risk stratification tools in acute heart failure

Location	Risk Tool	Year	Predicted Outcome	Variables and Performance
Emergency Department	Multiple Estimation of Risk Based on the Emergency Department Spanish Score in Patients with AHF (MEESSI-AHF)[84]	2019	30-d mortality	Incorporates 13 variables, including Barthel Index at ED admission, vital signs and ED labs, NYHA class, low output symptoms, ACS symptoms, and hypertrophy on ECG c-statistic = 0.83
	Emergency Heart Failure Mortality Risk Group (EHMRG)[85]	2019, 2012	7- and 30-d mortality	Incorporates 10 variables to identify patients at low risk for mortality, including ED vitals and labs, history of active cancer, transport by emergency medical services, and metolazone at home c-statistic = 0.80
	Ottawa Heart Failure Risk Scale[86]	2017, 2013	30-d SAE (death, admission to monitored unit, intubation, ventilation, myocardial infarction, or relapse resulting in hospital admission within 14 d	Incorporates 10 variables including history of stroke/TIA, prior intubation, ED vital signs and labs, and ischemic ECG changes c-statistic = 0.78
	STRATIFY[87]	2015	5- and 30-d hierarchical SAE (acute coronary syndrome, coronary revascularization, emergent dialysis, intubation, mechanical cardiac support, cardiopulmonary resuscitation, and death)	Age, BMI, ED vital signs and laboratory values, dialysis, supplemental oxygen use, and QRS duration c-statistic = 0.68
	Kaiser Permanente Northern California (KPNC) ED AHF[88]	2020	30-d SAE (acute coronary syndrome, coronary revascularization, emergent dialysis, intubation, mechanical cardiac support, cardiopulmonary resuscitation, and death)	Using STRATIFY as its base, this risk tool added 58 additional variables, including medical comorbidities, medications, health care utilization and additional ED vital signs, among others c-statistic = 0.85

Setting	Model	Year	Outcome	Description
Inpatient	ADHERE[55]	2005	In-hospital mortality	Simple model incorporating BUN, creatinine, systolic blood pressure; c-statistic = 0.75
	OPTIMIZE-HF[9]	2008	In-hospital mortality	Age, race, admission labs, history of liver disease, stroke, peripheral vascular disease, or chronic obstructive lung disease, previous HF hospitalization, systolic blood pressure; c-statistic = 0.72
	ELAN-HF[56]	2014	180-d mortality post-discharge	NT-proBNP at discharge and reduction in admission, age, peripheral edema, serum sodium and urea, systolic blood pressure, NYHA class on admission; c-statistic = 0.75
	ADHF/NT-proBNP risk score[57]	2013	6-mo mortality post-discharge	NT-proBNP, history of chronic obstructive pulmonary disease, serum sodium, hemoglobin, and glomerular filtration rate, left ventricular ejection fraction and tricuspid regurgitation, systolic blood pressure; C-statistic = 0.77
Intensive care	Society for Cardiovascular Angiography and Interventions (SCAI) stages[63]	2019	In-hospital mortality from cardiogenic shock	Stages patients into 5 categories (Stage A through E) based on physical exam findings, creatinine, lactate, liver function tests, BNP, and hemodynamic data, as well as response to intensive treatment. Increasing stage is associated with higher in-hospital mortality

Abbreviations: ACS, acute coronary syndrome; BMI, body mass index; BUN, blood urea nitrogen; ECG, electrocardiogram; ED, emergency department; HF, heart failure; NYHA, New York Heart Association; SAE, serious adverse event; TIA, transient ischemic attack.

along with shorter hospitalizations and reduced signs of volume overload on discharge.[35] Decongestion should continue until euvolemia is reached.[36] Physical markers of euvolemia include jugular venous pressure (JVP) reduction to less than 8 cm, resolved dyspnea at rest, and resolution of any orthopnea or edema noted on admission. Incomplete resolution of signs and symptoms of volume overload at the time of discharge is associated with higher rates of re-hospitalization and death.[37] Monitoring of electrolytes and kidney function should continue at least daily during diuresis. Transient rise in serum creatinine during diuresis is expected and does not represent worsening renal function or renal injury.[38] For most patients with AHF, pulmonary artery catheterization for clinical assessment of volume status is not indicated.[12] The use of invasive hemodynamics has not been shown to affect overall mortality and hospitalization rates for patients not at risk for the development of cardiogenic shock.[39] For some patients, invasive hemodynamic monitoring may be useful for guide treatment; clinical trials (eg, NCT05485376) are currently ongoing for further investigation from which patients may benefit.[40]

Once euvolemia is reached, patients are typically transitioned to oral diuretic doses for maintenance and monitored for at least 24 hours on oral medications alone. However, recent evidence suggests that this practice does not benefit patients and may only increase length of hospital stay, as no association between in-hospital observation on oral diuretics and accurate outpatient diuretic dosing or reduction in readmissions was observed in a multicenter cohort.[41]

For patients with AHF with reduced ejection fraction, hospitalization is an opportunity to titrate and optimize medication regimens. Patients already on guideline-directed medical therapy (GDMT) prior to admission should continue their home medications unless there is a clear contraindication, as there is mortality benefit to continuing all forms of GDMT during hospitalization (**Tables 2** and **3**). Beta blockers should only be held or dose-reduced in patients with low cardiac output and features concerning for cardiogenic shock. In OPTIMIZE-HF, discontinuation of beta blockers in the inpatient setting was associated with higher risk of mortality.[42] Discontinuation of angiotensin-converting enzyme inhibitors (ACEi) or angiotensin II receptor blockers (ARB) among hospitalized patients in the Get With The Guidelines-Heart Failure (GWTG-HF) registry was also associated with higher mortality and readmission rates.[43] Mineralocorticoid receptor antagonists like spironolactone should also be continued, as continuation was shown to decrease rates of rehospitalization

and 30-day mortality in the Comparison of Outcomes and Access to Care (COACH) study.[44] These therapies should be continued despite mild fluctuations in creatinine with diuresis, which are expected and do not represent a true renal tubular injury but likely represent changes in filtration as a result of diuresis and medication adjustments.[45]

Patients with newly diagnosed HF with reduced ejection fraction should be initiated on GDMT during the index admission (see **Tables 2** and **3**). Several trials studying initiation of beta blockers, ACEi/ARB/angiotensin receptor/neprilysin inhibitor (ARNI), mineralocorticoid receptor antagonists, and sodium-glucose cotransporter 2 (SGLT2)-inhibitors have shown improvements in mortality and decreased readmission rates with in-hospital prescription and uptitration prior to discharge.[43,46,47]

Iron deficiency is common among patients with AHF and associated with worse outcomes.[48,49] In the AFFIRM-HF trial, patients hospitalized with AHF with reduced ejection fraction and transferrin saturation less than 20% were treated with intravenous repletion with ferric carboxymaltose. This led to reduced cardiovascular deaths and recurrent hospitalizations for HF.[50] Iron studies should be checked on all patients hospitalized with AHF and repleted if indicated, regardless of hemoglobin level.

For patients with AHF with preserved ejection fraction, evidence-based therapies are more limited. Diuresis should be similarly used to improve symptoms and reach euvolemia. As poorly controlled hypertension is often a precipitant of this type of HF, control of blood pressure and medication titration while inpatient may be beneficial.[51] SGLT2 inhibitors have also shown benefit in this population, demonstrating a significant reduction in HF hospitalizations and improvement in quality of life in the EMPEROR-Preserved Trial.[52] Safety and tolerability of in-hospital SGLT2 inhibitor initiation was shown in the EMPULSE trial, and patients accrued significant clinical benefit even up to 90 days after discharge.[53]

Disposition

Several prognostic models have been developed to predict in-hospital and post-hospitalization outcomes in patients with AHF, although clinical application of these models remains difficult (see **Table 1**). Most of these risk scores use various combinations of presenting vital signs, comorbidities, and objective data including measures of renal function and electrolytes as predictive variables, but applicability at an individual patient-level is difficult to ascertain, and there is marked variability

Table 2
Selected observational studies of contemporary guideline-directed medical therapy in acute heart failure

Medication Class	Trial/Study (Author, Year)	Source of Data	Number of Patients	Follow-up Duration	Endpoints of Interest	Results
Beta-blocker (BB)	OPTIMIZE-HF (Fonarow et al., 2008)[42]	91 hospitals participating in the OPTIMIZE-HF hospital registry	2373 patients eligible for BB at discharge 1350 (56.9%) on BB before admission and continued on 632 (26.6%) BB newly started 79 (3.3%) BB withdrawn 303 (12.8%) BB eligible but not treated	60- to 90-d post-discharge	Post-discharge death and death/ rehospitalization	BB continuation associated with lower post-discharge death (HR: 0.60; 95% CI: 0.37–0.99, P = .044) and death/ rehospitalization (OR 0.69; 95% CI: 0.52–0.92, P = .012) risk compared with no BB BB withdrawal associated with higher mortality compared with BB continuation (HR: 2.3; 95% CI: 1.2–4.6, P = .013)
Mineralocorticoid receptor antagonists (MRA)	ALARM-HF (Bistola V et al., 2018)[89]	Acute Heart Failure Global Registry of Standard Treatment study cohort	4953 patients in original study cohort 1439 MRA-treated and 3514 untreated Propensity score with 1:1 matching yielded N = 1003 in each group	Up to 30 d from discharge	All-cause death during hospitalization	4.2% vs 10.8% in MRA treated vs untreated patients Treatment with MRAs was associated with a reduction of in-hospital mortality [HR 0.372 (95% CI, 0.261–0.532, P < .001)
	Yaku et al.,[90] 2019	Kyoto Congestive Heart Failure registry	3717 patients hospitalized for ADHF 1678 (45.1%) received MRA at discharge, 2039 (54.9%) did not	Mean 470 d (357–649 d)	Composite of all-death or heart failure hospitalization after discharge	MRA use was associated with lower incidence of HF hospitalization (18.7% vs 24.8%, HR 0.70, 95% CI 0.60–0.86; P < .001)

(continued on next page)

Table 2
(continued)

Medication Class	Trial/Study (Author, Year)	Source of Data	Number of Patients	Follow-up Duration	Endpoints of Interest	Results
			Matched cohort N = 1034			No difference in mortality between the 2 groups (15.6% vs 15.8%; HR 0.98, 95% CI 0.82–1.18, P = .85) or in all-cause hospitalization (35.3% vs 38.2%; HR, 0.88; 95% CI, 0.77–1.01; P = 0.07)
Angiotensin neprilysin inhibitor (ARNI)	Carnicelli et al,[91] 2021	Get With the Guidelines-Heart Failure registry linked with Medicare claims	897 patients discharged on sacubitril/ valsartan 295 (32.9%) PDC > 80% 602 (67.1%) PDC < 80%	Adherence 90 d post-discharge Follow up at 1 y	Adherence, assessed using medication fills to calculate proportion of days covered (PDC) Risk of readmission and death within 1 y	Adherence to sacubitril-valsartan was associated with lower risk of all cause rehospitalization (HR: 0.66 [95% CI: 0.48–0.89] and death (HR: 0.42 [95% CI: 0.22–0.79]) at 90 d and at 1 y (HR: 0.69 [95% CI: 0.56–0.86] and HR: 0.53 [95% CI: 0.38–0.74], respectively)

SGLT2 inhibitor	Martin et al,[92] 2021		102 patients discharged for acute HF 45 (44.1%) prescribed canagliflozin 57 (55.9%) not prescribed any SGLT-2 inhibitor	22 mo	Adverse clinical events (HF rehospitalization and cardiovascular death) NT-proBNP changes	Canagliflozin use was associated with a lower risk of HF readmission at first year (22.2% vs 49.1%, HR: 0.45; 95% CI: 0.21–0.96; $P < .039$) Composite outcome (hospitalization for HF, death from cardiovascular cause) was lower in the canagliflozin group vs control (37.8% vs 70.2%, HR: 0.51; 95% CI: 0.27–0.95; $P < .035$)
	Perez-Belmonte et al,[93] 2022	Four hospitals in Malaga, Spain	208 of 518 patients hospitalized with T2DM for AHF were > 80 year old 99 (47.6%) continued empagliflozin, 109 (52.4%) on basal bolus 79 propensity matched patients in each group	Discontinued due to loss of funding	Clinical efficacy (measured by visual analogue dyspnea score, NT-proBNP level, diuretic response, cumulative urine output) Safety endpoints: adverse events, worsening HF, discontinuation of empagliflozin, length of stay, in-hospital deaths	Empagliflozin was associated with lower NT-proBNP levels (1699 ± 522 vs 2303 ± 598 pg/mL, $P = .021$) Empagliflozin led to a greater diuretic response (weight loss/40 mg furosemide) and cumulative urine output (−0.14 ± −0.06 vs −0.24 ± −0.10, $P = .044$; and 16,100 ± 1510 vs 13,900 ± 1220 mL, $P = .037$, respectively)

Abbreviations: ADHF, acute decompensated heart failure; CI, confidence interval; HF, heart failure; HR, hazard ratio; OR, odds ratio; T2DM, type 2 diabetes mellitus.

Table 3
Selected ongoing and completed randomized trials of contemporary guideline-directed medical therapy in acute heart failure

Medication Class	Trial/Study (Author, Year)	Source of Data	Patient Population	Number of Patients & Trial Arms	Primary Endpoint	Results
Beta-blocker (BB)	IMPACT-HF (Gattis et al,[94] 2004)	Multicenter (45) across U.S.	LVEF < 40% + hospitalized for HF	N = 185 pre-discharge carvedilol initiation N = 178 physician discretion post-discharge initiation	Number of patients treated with any BB at 60 d after randomization	Patients randomized to carvedilol initiation predischarge arm were more likely to be treated with any BB at 60 d vs those randomized to the physician-discretion post-discharge BB initiation arm (91.2% vs 73.4%, $P < .0001$)
Mineralocorticoid receptor antagonists (MRA)	Ferreira et al,[95] 2013	Prospective, experimental single-center, single-blinded	Hospitalization due to decompensated chronic heart failure	N = 100 patients enrolled N = 50 patients in treatment group, 50 patients in placebo	Proportion of patients free of congestion at day 3 (defined as JVP < 8 cm, no orthopnea, no lower extremity edema)	Patients treated with spironolactone were more likely to be free of congestion at day 3: lack of edema (32% vs 66%, $P = .001$), no rales (24% vs 66%; $P < .001$), JVP < 8 cm (90% vs 100%; $P = .02$), and no orthopnea (76% vs 96%; $P = .004$)

ATHENA-HF (Butler et al,[96] 2017)	Double-blind randomized clinical trial in 22 US acute care hospitals	Hospitalized patients with AHF who previously receiving no or low dose spironolactone, NT-proBNP > 1000 pg/mL, BNP > 250 pg/mL	N = 360 patients enrolled. N = 182 (50.6%) patients randomized to receive spironolactone. N = 178 (49.4%) to usual care alone. N = 132 placebo, 46 low-dose spironolactone	Change in NT-proBNP levels from baseline to 96 h	There was no significant reduction in log NT-proBNP level between two groups: −0.55 [95% CI, −0.92 to −0.18] with high-dose spironolactone and −0.49 [95% CI, −0.98 to −0.14] with usual care, P = .57. No significant difference in 30-d all-cause mortality or heart failure hospitalization rate
EARLIER (Asakura et al,[97] 2022)	Multicenter, randomized, double-blind across 27 Japanese institutions	Age > 20 year old, LVEF < 40%	N = 300 patients. N = 149 (49.7%) in eplerenone. N = 151 (50.3%) in placebo group	Composite cardiac death or first re-hospitalization due to cardiovascular disease within 6 mo	The study was inadequately powered to detect a significant association between initiation of eplerenone and rates of cardiac death or hospitalization (19.5% vs 17.2%, HR 1.09, 95% CI 0.642–1.855)

(continued on next page)

Table 3
(continued)

Medication Class	Trial/Study (Author, Year)	Source of Data	Patient Population	Number of Patients & Trial Arms	Primary Endpoint	Results
Angiotensin neprilysin inhibitor (ARNI)	PIONEER-HF (Velazquez et al,[98] 2019)	Multicenter, randomized, double-blind trial across 129 sites in the United States	LVEF < 40%, or NT-proBNP > 1600 pg/mL, or BNP > 400 pg/mL, and received a diagnosis of ADHF	N = 881 patients randomized N = 440 sacubitril-valsartan N = 441 to receive enalapril	Time-averaged proportional change in NT-proBNP concentration through weeks 4 and 8	Initiation of sacubitril-valsartan led to a greater reduction in NT-proBNP level (0.53 vs 0.75, percent change, −46.7% vs −25.3%; ratio of change with sacubitril-valsartan vs enalapril, 0.71; 95% CI, 0.63–0.81; $P < .001$)
	TRANSITION (Wachter et al,[99] 2019)	Multicenter, randomized, open-label study	Hospitalized for an episode of ADHF, blood pressure > 100 mm Hg, LVEF < 40%	N = 1002 randomized N = 500 patients randomized to pre-discharge initiation N = 502 patients randomized to post-discharge initiation	Proportion of patients attaining 97/103 twice daily target dose after 10 wk	Comparable proportions of patients in each arm attained target dose after 10 wk ([45.4% vs 50.7%; RR 0.90; 95% CI 0.79–1.02], suggesting either in-hospital or shortly after discharge initiation is feasible
	PARAGLIDE-HF (Mentz et al,[100] 2023)	Double-blind, randomized control trial	LVEF > 40%, elevated NT-proBNP or BNP level	N = 466 patients N = 233 sacubitril/valsartan N = 233 valsartan	Time-averaged proportional change in NT-proBNP from baseline through weeks 4 and 8	Sacubitril/valsartan was associated with significant NT-proBNP reduction (ratio of change: 0.85; 95% CI: 0.73–0.999; $P = .049$).
	PREMIER[101]	Multicenter, open-label, blinded randomized control study	NYHA class II-IV, hospitalized for ADHF, currently taking an ACE-inhibitor or ARB, NT-proBNP > 1200 pg/mL, BNP > 300 pg/mL	N = 400 patients	Change in NT-proBNP concentrations from baseline to 8 wk	Estimated study completion date: March 2025

SGLT2 inhibitor						
	EMPA RESPONSE-AHF (Damman et al,[102] 2020)	Randomized, double blind, multicenter pilot study	Patients with and without T2DM, admitted for ADHF	N = 80, randomized 1:1 to receive empagliflozin 10 mg vs placebo	Change in visual analogue scale dyspnea score, diuretic response, change in NT-proBNP, and length of stay	Empagliflozin was associated with recued combined endpoint of in-hospital worsening of HF, rehospitalization, or death at 60 d (4 vs 13; P = .014), although no difference was observed in visual analogue scale dyspnea score, diuretic response, length of stay, or change in NT-proBNP level
	SOLOIST-WHF (Bhatt et al,[47] 2021)	Multicenter, double-blind trial	Patients with T2DM recently hospitalized for worsening HF	N = 1222 randomized N = 608 to sotagliflozin N = 614 to placebo	Total number of deaths from cardiovascular events, hospitalizations, and urgent visits for HF	Sotagliflozin associated with significantly fewer primary endpoint events (245 vs 355, 51.0 vs 76.3; HR, 0.67; 95% CI, 0.52–0.85; P < .001)
	Tamaki et al,[103] 2021	Prospective, single-center, randomized, open label	Patients with T2DM admitted for ADHF	N = 59 consecutive patients N = 30 to empagliflozin N = 29 to conventional glucose lowering therapy	Decongestion based on NT-proBNP levels	Empagliflozin was associated with significantly lower NT-proBNP level at 7 d (P = .040)
	EMPULSE (Voors et al,[53] 2022)	Multicenter, randomized, double blind trial across 118 sites in 15 countries	Hospitalized for AHF with 2 of the following: congestion on chest x-ray, rales on auscultation, elevated JVP, lower extremity edema	N = 530 randomized N = 265 empagliflozin N = 265 placebo	Hierarchical composite of death from any cause, number of HF events and time to first HF event, or a 5 point or greater difference in change from baseline in the	Empagliflozin was associated with clinical benefit over placebo (stratified win ratio 1.36, 95% CI 1.09–1.68, P = .0054)

(continued on next page)

Table 3
(continued)

Medication Class	Trial/Study (Author, Year)	Source of Data	Patient Population	Number of Patients & Trial Arms	Primary Endpoint	Results
	DELIVER (Solomon et al,[104] 2022)	Multicenter, double-blind randomized control	LVEF < 40%, evidence of structural heart disease, elevated BNP	N = 6263 patients randomized N = 3131 dapagliflozin N = 3132 placebo	Composite of worsening heart failure or cardiovascular death Kansas City Cardiomyopathy Questionnaire Total Symptoms Score, assessed using a win ratio	The primary outcome occurred less frequently in the dapagliflozin group (512 (16.4%) vs 610 (19.5%), HR, 0.82; 95% CI, 0.73–0.92; $P < .001$)
	Charaya et al,[105] 2022	Single-center, controlled, randomized study	AHF hospitalization with planned administration of loop diuretics, LVEF < 50%	N = 102 randomized N = 50 dapagliflozin N = 52 standard therapy	Renal function deterioration	Although GFR decreased in 48 h in the dapagliflozin (−4.2 (−11.03; 2.28) mL/min vs 0.3 (−6; 6) mL/min; $P = .04$), renal function did not differ on discharge (54.71 ± 19.18 mL/min and 58.92 ± 24.65 mL/min; $P = .36$)
	EMPAG-HF (Schulze et al,[106] 2022)	Single center, prospective, double-blind, placebo-controlled randomized study	BNP > 100 pg/mL, NT-proBNP > 300 pg/mL	N = 60 randomized	Cumulative urine output over 5 d	Use of empagliflozin increased urine output by 25% over 5 d (10.8 vs 8.7 L, 2.2 L difference, [95% CI, 8.4–3.6]; $P = .003$)

Study	Study design	Inclusion criteria	Participants	Primary endpoint	Results
Thiele et al,[107] 2022	Prospective, placebo-controlled, double-blind exploratory study	NT-proBNP > 1000 pg/mL	N = 19 study participants, received 10 mg or placebo	Cardiac output as determined by ClearSight System	Empagliflozin did not affect cardiac index or systemic vascular resistance, although reduced parameters of AKI (placebo: 1.1 ± 1.1 (ng/mL)2/1000; empagliflozin: 0.3 ± 0.2 (ng/mL)2/1000; $P = .02$)
DICTATE-AHF[108,109]	Prospective, multicenter, open-label randomized trial	Patients with T2DM hospitalized with AHF, GFR > 30	N = 240 patients planned for enrollment, randomized 1:1 to dapagliflozin 10 mg or usual care	Diuretic response, defined as cumulative change in weight per cumulative loop diuretic dose (40 mg IV furosemide equivalent)	Estimated study report date: August 2023
DAPA ACT HF-TIMI 68[110]	Multicenter, randomized, double-blind placebo controlled trial	For LVEF < 40%: NT-proBNP > 1600 pg/mL, BNP >400 pg/mL For LVEF ≥ 40%: NT-proBNP > 1200 pg/mL, BNP >300 pg/mL	N = 2400 participants	CV death or worsening heart failure	Estimated study completion date: March 2024
Ferric carboxymaltose — AFFIRM-AHF (Ponikowski et al,[50] 2020)	Multicenter, double-blind, randomized trial at 121 sites in Europe, South America, and Singapore	Hospitalized for acute heart failure with iron deficiency (ferritin < 100, or 100–299 with transferrin saturation < 20%), LVEF < 50%	N = 1132 randomly assigned N = 1108 with at least 1 post-randomization value (558 in ferric carboxymaltose vs 550 placebo)	Composite of total hospitalization for HF and CV death 52 wk after randomization	Treatment with ferric carboxymaltose was associated with lower rates of HF hospitalization (217 vs 294, RR 0.74; 95% CI 0.58–0.94, $P = .013$), although no effect on CV mortality (77 (14%) vs 78 (14%), HR 0.96, 95% CI 0.70–1.32, $P = .81$)

Abbreviations: ACE, angiotensin-converting enzyme; ADHF, acute decompensated heart failure; AHF, acute heart failure; AKI, acute kidney injury; ARB, angiotensin receptor blockers; CI, confidence interval; CV, cardiovascular; HF, heart failure; HR, hazard ratio; JVP, jugular venous pressure; LVEF, left ventricular ejection fraction; NYHA, new york heart association; RR, risk ratio.

among prognostic models depending on the variables selected.[54] Tools like the ADHERE score and OPTIMIZE-AF registry score have good performance predicting in-hospital mortality for admitted patients.[9,55] For outcomes post-discharge, the ELAN-HF score and ADHF/NT-proBNP risk score are effective for predicting 180 day and 1-year mortality post-discharge, respectively.[56,57]

Patients who achieve decongestion and have undergone therapeutic optimization can be discharged with clear plans for rescue dosing of diuretics in case of weight gain at home, as well as with instructions for fluid restriction and standing electrolyte supplementation if needed.[32] If medication or dietary nonadherence were suspected as triggers of decompensation, patient concerns and barriers to adherence should be fully addressed at the time of discharge.

Up to 25% of patients will be readmitted after 30 days after a hospitalization for AHF.[58] The transition between inpatient and outpatient care is a particularly vulnerable time, and efforts should be made during hospitalization to coordinate care and ensure close follow-up with a specialized team. A post-discharge clinic visit should occur within 1 week of hospitalization and should focus on review of symptom trajectory, medication reconciliation, management of comorbidities, safety, laboratory testing, patient education, and advance care planning. Titration of GDMT, assessment of volume status, and adjustments in diuretic dosing to maintain euvolemia should be focuses of initial outpatient follow-up.[59] For patients with *de novo* AHF, a repeat assessment of left ventricular systolic function should occur within 3 months of hospital discharge for evaluation of primary pretention defibrillator implantation.[12] A multidisciplinary approach, with case management involvement for high-risk patients, visits to the home, and outreach via phone or other mechanisms when possible is helpful to prevent readmissions and reduce mortality.[60] Cardiac rehabilitation referrals should be in place for all patients discharged from the hospital, as supported by the REHAB-HF trial which showed that cardiac rehabilitation participation led to improvements in physical functioning without causing harm, even in the elderly or frail.[61]

Inability to achieve decongestion despite escalating diuretic doses is 1 indication for transfer to a higher level of care. These patients may require transfer to the ICU for invasive monitoring and consideration of mechanical support in case of worsening cardiogenic shock. Invasive hemodynamic monitoring with pulmonary artery catheterization may provide helpful guidance for effective diuresis and augmentation from intravenous vasodilators or inotropic therapy.

INTENSIVE CARE UNIT
Presentation

An estimated 20% of patients hospitalized with HF require admission to the ICU at some point during their stay.[62] Patients with AHF requiring ICU support often present in cardiogenic shock, characterized by hypotension (systolic blood pressure < 90 mm Hg or mean arterial blood pressure <60 mm Hg) with other signs of hypoperfusion, including cold extremities, low urine output, altered mental status, or elevated lactate.[63] Mortality rates are high for this population, with some studies estimating short-term mortality of almost 40%.[64] Physical examination is the first important step in diagnosing AHF and cardiogenic shock. Many patients present with a "cold and wet" hemodynamic profile, although some with decompensated chronic HF may present without signs of overt congestion.[62]

Diagnostics

In addition to the previously discussed diagnostic tools, pulmonary artery catheterization for hemodynamic monitoring is associated with lower mortality in patients with cardiogenic shock.[65] The 2022 American Heart Association/American College of Cardiology/Heart Failure Society of America HF guidelines recommend obtaining invasive hemodynamic data when escalation to mechanical support is being considered or when there is diagnostic uncertainty regarding the etiology of shock in patients with AHF.[12]

Management

Careful monitoring of respiratory status is essential, as elevated ventricular filling pressures and subsequent cardiogenic pulmonary edema can cause significant hypoxemia and hypercarbia. Noninvasive positive pressure ventilation (NIPPV) helps to reduce work of breathing, increase lung compliance, and recruit alveoli.[66] Studies have shown reduction in both intubation rates and in-hospital mortality with use of NIPPV.[67] If hypoxemia and hypercarbia persists with NIPPV, endotracheal intubation can decrease left ventricular afterload and improve both oxygenation and cardiac index.[66] Caution is warranted, as anesthesia induction and continued sedation may cause more harm in those with significant right ventricular dysfunction.

In patients with cardiogenic shock, vasopressors and inotropes should be considered to address hemodynamic instability and rapidly improve organ perfusion. Dobutamine and milrinone are common first choice agents in cardiogenic shock because of both inotropic and vasodilatory properties.[62] Studies have shown no difference in in-hospital mortality or adverse effects between the 2 agents.[68] Norepinephrine is the first-line vasopressor of choice in HF and increases both systemic vascular resistance and cardiac output. Epinephrine is associated with increased incidence of arrhythmia and refractory shock compared to norepinephrine and is less frequently used.[69,70] Dopamine is similarly associated with increased risk of death in patients with cardiogenic shock.[71] Vasopressin is often used in addition to norepinephrine and is particularly beneficial in right ventricular failure due to increase in pulmonary vasodilation.[62] While vasopressors can help sustain mean arterial pressure, their use increases left ventricular afterload and can cause myocardial ischemia.[62]

Mechanical circulatory support (MCS) provides increased circulatory support beyond what can be achieved through inotropic infusions. Temporary forms of MCS help to stabilize patients in the acute setting and allow time for either recovery or multidisciplinary discussions about transitions to durable MCS or cardiac transplantation. While there is a paucity of data directly comparing MCS options, and most studies have been performed in patients with acute myocardial infarction and subsequent shock, MCS use has increased exponentially over the last few decades even in patients with AHF unrelated to myocardial infarction.[72]

Current U.S. society guidelines list temporary MCS as a class 2a recommendation for the management of patients with cardiogenic shock.[12] The intra-aortic balloon counter-pulsation pump is the most frequently used device as first-line temporary circulatory support for patients in AHF.[73] The Intra-aortic Balloon Counterpulsation in Cardiogenic Shock II trial showed that use of intra-aortic balloon pump (IABP) did not significantly reduce 30- or 1-year mortality for patients with cardiogenic shock from acute myocardial infarction (AMI-CS).[74] However, in patients with cardiogenic shock from HF (HF-CS), IABP use is associated with improved outcomes when used as a bridge to durable MCS or cardiac transplantation.[75] This patient population is currently being enrolled in the Altshock-2 trial, a prospective, randomized, multicenter, open-label study in which patients with acute HF-CS will be randomized to early IABP implantation or to vasoactive treatments with a primary end point of 60 days patients' survival or successful bridge to heart replacement therapy.[76] The Impella is a continuous-flow axial pump placed across the aortic valve into the left ventricle, which produces flow from the left ventricle to the ascending aorta at set rates, reducing myocardial oxygen demand

and ventricular wall stress. Retrospective studies have not shown a mortality benefit of the Impella compared to the IABP in patients with AMI-CS,[77] and there are a number of ongoing studies and registries of Impella use in CS. Venoarterial extracorporeal membrane oxygenation is an additional temporary MCS strategy and has been associated with worse survival compared with IABP and other temporary MCS platforms in patients being bridged to durable MCS.[78]

A high proportion of patients who are bridged to durable left ventricular assist device reach discharge, and this may serve as destination therapy for some.[79] Patients with refractory HF may also be considered for heart transplantation. Those who do not experience recovery and are not deemed to benefit from advanced therapies should be palliated.

Outcomes and Disposition

Patients who require intensive care at any point during their hospitalization have higher mortality at 30-days and 1 year after hospitalization, as well as higher rates of readmission.[80] Elevated biventricular filling pressures, low systemic blood pressure, and elevated markers of end-organ perfusion on admission to intensive care are associated with higher mortality.[73] The Society for Cardiovascular Angiography and Interventions (SCAI) staging system use some of these biochemical and hemodynamic findings to risk stratify patients with cardiogenic shock and increasing shock severity stage is associated with increased in-hospital mortality for patients in AHF.[81]

Those who improve in intensive care will transition to inpatient floors, where their medications can be adjusted and optimized in preparation for discharge. However, there are a significant proportion of patients who do not survive to discharge from the ICU. For these patients, palliative care is an integral part of their care. Early integration of palliative care can ensure patients' wishes are respected in the setting of critical illness and are an essential part of compassionate, patient-centered care at the end of life.[82] Patients who participate in interdisciplinary palliative care intervention have improvements in quality of life, anxiety, depression, and spiritual well-being.[83]

SUMMARY

AHF remains a significant public health challenge, and as the prevalence of HF continues to rise, an increasing number of individuals will be at elevated risk for hospital readmission and mortality. There is a paucity of high-quality evidence to guide the care of patients with AHF, and further studies focused on optimal timing of deployment of stabilizing therapies are urgently needed. Nevertheless, the AHF period is an opportune time to optimize evidence-based medical therapy for HF, and linkage to outpatient care is essential to improve outcomes.

CLINICS CARE POINTS

- Among those older than 65 years, AHF is the most common reason for emergency hospital admission.
- Acute decompensated HF in those with known chronic HF make up 70% of all AHF presentations.
- For patients with AHF with reduced ejection fraction, hospitalization is a golden opportunity to optimize guideline directed medical therapy.
- Discontinuation of guideline directed medical therapy for HFwith reduced ejection fraction during hospitalization for AHF has been associated with higher risk of mortality and higher readmission rates.

DISCLOSURE

N. Reza is supported by the National Heart, Lung, And Blood Institute of the National Institutes of Health under Award Number K23HL166961. The content is solely the responsibility of the author and does not necessarily represent the official views of the National Institutes of Health. N.R. reports speaking honoraria from Zoll, Inc. and consulting for Roche Diagnostics.

REFERENCES

1. Urbich M, Globe G, Pantiri K, et al. A systematic review of medical Costs associated with heart failure in the USA (2014–2020). Pharmacoeconomics 2020;38(11):1219–36.
2. Bazmpani MA, Papanastasiou CA, Kamperidis V, et al. Contemporary data on the status and medical management of acute heart failure. Curr Cardiol Rep 2022;24(12):2009–22.
3. Follath F, Yilmaz MB, Delgado JF, et al. Clinical presentation, management and outcomes in the acute heart failure Global Survey of standard treatment (ALARM-HF). Intensive Care Med 2011;37(4):619–26.
4. Bozkurt B. Proposed new Conceptualization for definition of decompensated HF: Taking the acute out of decompensation. JACC Heart Fail 2023; 11(3):368–71.
5. McDonagh TA, Metra M, Adamo M, et al. 2021 ESC Guidelines for the diagnosis and treatment of acute and chronic heart failure: developed by the Task Force for the diagnosis and treatment of acute and chronic heart failure of the European Society of Cardiology (ESC) with the special contribution of the Heart Failure Association (HFA) of the ESC. Eur Heart J 2021;42(36):3599–726.
6. Straw S, Napp A, Witte KK. 'Acute heart failure': should We Abandon the term Altogether? Curr Heart Fail Rep 2022;19(6):425–34.
7. Adams KF, Fonarow GC, Emerman CL, et al. Characteristics and outcomes of patients hospitalized for heart failure in the United States: rationale, design, and preliminary observations from the first 100,000 cases in the Acute Decompensated Heart Failure National Registry (ADHERE). Am Heart J 2005;149(2):209–16.
8. Fonarow GC, Stough WG, Abraham WT, et al. Characteristics, treatments, and outcomes of patients with preserved systolic function hospitalized for heart failure: a report from the OPTIMIZE-HF registry. J Am Coll Cardiol 2007;50(8):768–77.
9. Abraham WT, Fonarow GC, Albert NM, et al. Predictors of in-hospital mortality in patients hospitalized for heart failure: insights from the Organized program to initiate Lifesaving treatment in hospitalized patients with heart failure (OPTIMIZE-HF). J Am Coll Cardiol 2008;52(5):347–56.
10. Chioncel O, Collins SP, Ambrosy AP, et al. Improving post-discharge outcomes in acute heart failure. Am J Ther 2018;25(4):e475–86.
11. Maggioni AP, Orso F, Calabria S, et al. The real-world evidence of heart failure: findings from 41 413 patients of the ARNO database. Eur J Heart Fail 2016;18(4):402–10.
12. Heidenreich PA, Bozkurt B, Aguilar D, et al. 2022 AHA/ACC/HFSA guideline for the management of heart failure: a report of the American College of Cardiology/American heart association Joint Committee on clinical practice guidelines. Circulation 2022;145(18):e895–1032.
13. Arrigo M, Gayat E, Parenica J, et al. Precipitating factors and 90-day outcome of acute heart failure: a report from the intercontinental GREAT registry. Eur J Heart Fail 2017;19(2):201–8.
14. Tsuyuki RT, McKelvie RS, Arnold JMO, et al. Acute precipitants of congestive heart failure Exacerbations. Arch Intern Med 2001;161(19):2337–42.
15. Fonarow GC, Abraham WT, Albert NM, et al. Factors identified as precipitating hospital admissions for heart failure and clinical outcomes: findings from OPTIMIZE-HF. Arch Intern Med 2008;168(8): 847–54.
16. Storrow AB, Jenkins CA, Self WH, et al. The burden of acute heart failure on U.S. emergency departments. JACC Heart Fail 2014;2(3):269–77.

17. Martindale JL, Wakai A, Collins SP, et al. Diagnosing acute heart failure in the emergency department: a systematic review and meta-analysis. Acad Emerg Med 2016;23(3):223–42.

18. Collins SP, Lindsell CJ, Storrow AB, et al. Prevalence of Negative chest Radiography results in the emergency department patient with decompensated heart failure. Ann Emerg Med 2006;47(1):13–8.

19. Anderson KL, Jenq KY, Fields JM, et al. Diagnosing heart failure among acutely dyspneic patients with cardiac, inferior vena cava, and lung ultrasonography. Am J Emerg Med 2013;31(8):1208–14.

20. Weintraub NL, Collins SP, Pang PS, et al. Acute heart failure syndromes: emergency department presentation, treatment, and disposition: current approaches and future aims: a scientific statement from the American Heart Association. Circulation 2010;122(19):1975–96.

21. Lassus J, Gayat E, Mueller C, et al. Incremental value of biomarkers to clinical variables for mortality prediction in acutely decompensated heart failure: the Multinational Observational Cohort on Acute Heart Failure (MOCA) study. Int J Cardiol 2013;168(3):2186–94.

22. Krauser DG, Lloyd-Jones DM, Chae CU, et al. Effect of body mass index on natriuretic peptide levels in patients with acute congestive heart failure: a ProBNP Investigation of Dyspnea in the Emergency Department (PRIDE) substudy. Am Heart J 2005;149(4):744–50.

23. Anwaruddin S, Lloyd-Jones DM, Baggish A, et al. Renal function, congestive heart failure, and amino-terminal pro-brain natriuretic peptide measurement: results from the ProBNP Investigation of Dyspnea in the Emergency Department (PRIDE) Study. J Am Coll Cardiol 2006;47(1):91–7.

24. Masip J, Roque M, Sánchez B, et al. Noninvasive ventilation in acute cardiogenic pulmonary edema: systematic review and meta-analysis. JAMA 2005;294(24):3124–30.

25. Matsue Y, Damman K, Voors AA, et al. Time-to-Furosemide treatment and mortality in patients hospitalized with acute heart failure. J Am Coll Cardiol 2017;69(25):3042–51.

26. Peacock WF, Emerman C, Costanzo MR, et al. Early vasoactive drugs improve heart failure outcomes. Congest Heart Fail Greenwich Conn 2009;15(6):256–64.

27. 2016 ESC Guidelines for the diagnosis and treatment of acute and chronic heart failure | European Heart Journal | Oxford Academic. Available at: https://academic.oup.com/eurheartj/article/37/27/2129/1748921. [Accessed 13 April 2023].

28. Sax DR, Mark DG, Rana JS, et al. Current emergency department disposition of patients with acute heart failure: an opportunity for improvement. J Card Fail 2022;28(10):1545–59.

29. Miró Ò, Rossello X, Platz E, et al. Risk stratification scores for patients with acute heart failure in the Emergency Department: a systematic review. Eur Heart J Acute Cardiovasc Care 2020;9(5):375–98.

30. Rame JE, Sheffield MA, Dries DL, et al. Outcomes after emergency department discharge with a primary diagnosis of heart failure. Am Heart J 2001;142(4):714–9.

31. Masri A, Althouse AD, McKibben J, et al. Outcomes of heart failure admissions under observation versus short inpatient stay. J Am Heart Assoc 2018;7(3):e007944.

32. Hollenberg SM, Warner Stevenson L, Ahmad T, et al. 2019 ACC expert consensus decision Pathway on risk assessment, management, and clinical trajectory of patients hospitalized with heart failure: a report of the American College of Cardiology Solution set Oversight Committee. J Am Coll Cardiol 2019;74(15):1966–2011.

33. Arrigo M, Jessup M, Mullens W, et al. Acute heart failure. Nat Rev Dis Primer 2020;6(1):1–15.

34. Felker GM, Ellison DH, Mullens W, et al. Diuretic therapy for patients with heart failure: JACC State-of-the-Art review. J Am Coll Cardiol 2020;75(10):1178–95.

35. Mullens W, Dauw J, Martens P, et al. Acetazolamide in acute decompensated heart failure with volume overload. N Engl J Med 2022;387(13):1185–95.

36. Felker GM, Lee KL, Bull DA, et al. Diuretic strategies in patients with acute decompensated heart failure. N Engl J Med 2011;364(9):797–805.

37. Rubio-Gracia J, Demissei BG, Ter Maaten JM, et al. Prevalence, predictors and clinical outcome of residual congestion in acute decompensated heart failure. Int J Cardiol 2018;258:185–91.

38. Greene SJ, Gheorghiade M, Vaduganathan M, et al. Haemoconcentration, renal function, and post-discharge outcomes among patients hospitalized for heart failure with reduced ejection fraction: insights from the EVEREST trial. Eur J Heart Fail 2013;15(12):1401–11.

39. Binanay C, Califf RM, Hasselblad V, et al. Evaluation study of congestive heart failure and pulmonary artery catheterization effectiveness: the ESCAPE trial. JAMA 2005;294(13):1625–33.

40. Tufts medical center. The pulmonary artery catheter in cardiogenic shock trial. clinicaltrials.gov. 2022. Available at: https://clinicaltrials.gov/ct2/show/NCT05485376. [Accessed 17 June 2023].

41. Ivey-Miranda JB, Rao VS, Cox ZL, et al. In-hospital observation on oral diuretics after treatment for acute decompensated heart failure: Evaluating the utility. Circ Heart Fail 2023;16(4):e010206.

42. Fonarow GC, Abraham WT, Albert NM, et al. Influence of beta-blocker continuation or withdrawal on outcomes in patients hospitalized with heart failure: findings from the OPTIMIZE-HF program. J Am Coll Cardiol 2008;52(3).190–9.

43. Gilstrap LG, Fonarow GC, Desai AS, et al. Initiation, continuation, or withdrawal of angiotensin-converting enzyme inhibitors/angiotensin receptor blockers and outcomes in patients hospitalized with heart failure with reduced ejection fraction. J Am Heart Assoc 2017;6(2):e004675.

44. Maisel A, Xue Y, van Veldhuisen DJ, et al. Effect of spironolactone on 30-day death and heart failure rehospitalization (from the COACH study). Am J Cardiol 2014;114(5):737–42.

45. Ahmad T, Jackson K, Rao VS, et al. Worsening renal function in patients with acute heart failure undergoing Aggressive diuresis is not associated with tubular injury. Circulation 2018;137(19):2016–28.

46. Bhatia V, Bajaj NS, Sanam K, et al. Beta-Blocker Use and 30-day all-cause readmission in Medicare Beneficiaries with systolic heart failure. Am J Med 2015;128(7):715–21.

47. Bhatt DL, Szarek M, Steg PG, et al. Sotagliflozin in patients with diabetes and recent worsening heart failure. N Engl J Med 2021;384(2):117–28.

48. Beavers CJ, Ambrosy AP, Butler J, et al. Iron deficiency in heart failure: a scientific statement from the heart failure society of America. J Card Fail 2023. https://doi.org/10.1016/j.cardfail.2023.03.025. S1071-9164(23)00121-5.

49. Klip IT, Comin-Colet J, Voors AA, et al. Iron deficiency in chronic heart failure: an international pooled analysis. Am Heart J 2013;165(4):575–82.e3.

50. Ponikowski P, Kirwan BA, Anker SD, et al. Ferric carboxymaltose for iron deficiency at discharge after acute heart failure: a multicentre, double-blind, randomised, controlled trial. Lancet Lond Engl 2020;396(10266):1895–904.

51. Jasinska-Piadlo A, Campbell P. Management of patients with heart failure and preserved ejection fraction. Heart 2023. https://doi.org/10.1136/heartjnl-2022-321097.

52. Anker SD, Butler J, Filippatos G, et al. Empagliflozin in heart failure with a preserved ejection fraction. N Engl J Med 2021;385(16):1451–61.

53. Voors AA, Angermann CE, Teerlink JR, et al. The SGLT2 inhibitor empagliflozin in patients hospitalized for acute heart failure: a multinational randomized trial. Nat Med 2022;28(3):568–74.

54. Passantino A, Monitillo F, Iacoviello M, et al. Predicting mortality in patients with acute heart failure: Role of risk scores. World J Cardiol 2015;7(12):902–11.

55. Fonarow GC, Adams KF, Abraham WT, et al. ADHERE Scientific Advisory Committee, Study Group, and Investigators. Risk stratification for in-hospital mortality in acutely decompensated heart failure: classification and regression tree analysis. JAMA 2005;293(5):572–80.

56. Salah K, Kok WE, Eurlings LW, et al. A novel discharge risk model for patients hospitalised for

acute decompensated heart failure incorporating N-terminal pro-B-type natriuretic peptide levels: a European coLlaboration on Acute decompeNsated Heart Failure: ELAN-HF Score. Heart Br Card Soc 2014;100(2):115–25.

57. Scrutinio D, Ammirati E, Guida P, et al. Clinical utility of N-terminal pro-B-type natriuretic peptide for risk stratification of patients with acute decompensated heart failure. Derivation and validation of the ADHF/NT-proBNP risk score. Int J Cardiol 2013;168(3):2120–6.

58. Chang PP, Wruck LM, Shahar E, et al. Trends in hospitalizations and survival of acute decompensated heart failure in four US Communities (2005-2014): ARIC study Community Surveillance. Circulation 2018;138(1):12–24.

59. Ostrominski JW, Vaduganathan M. Evolving therapeutic strategies for patients hospitalized with new or worsening heart failure across the spectrum of left ventricular ejection fraction. Clin Cardiol 2022;45(Suppl 1):S40–51.

60. Feltner C, Jones CD, Cené CW, et al. Transitional care interventions to prevent readmissions for persons with heart failure: a systematic review and meta-analysis. Ann Intern Med 2014;160(11):774–84.

61. Kitzman DW, Whellan DJ, Duncan P, et al. Physical rehabilitation for older patients hospitalized for heart failure. N Engl J Med 2021;385(3):203–16.

62. Cook DJ, Webb S, Proudfoot A. Assessment and management of cardiovascular disease in the intensive care unit. Heart 2022;108(5):397–405.

63. Baran DA, Grines CL, Bailey S, et al. SCAI clinical expert consensus statement on the classification of cardiogenic shock. Catheter Cardiovasc Interv 2019;94(1):29–37.

64. Harjola VP, Lassus J, Sionis A, et al. Clinical picture and risk prediction of short-term mortality in cardiogenic shock. Eur J Heart Fail 2015;17(5):501–9.

65. Hernandez GA, Lemor A, Blumer V, et al. Trends in utilization and outcomes of pulmonary artery catheterization in heart failure with and without cardiogenic shock. J Card Fail 2019;25(5):364–71.

66. Alviar CL, Miller PE, McAreavey D, et al. Positive pressure ventilation in the cardiac intensive care Unit. J Am Coll Cardiol 2018;72(13):1532–53.

67. Berbenetz N, Wang Y, Brown J, et al. Non-invasive positive pressure ventilation (CPAP or bilevel NPPV) for cardiogenic pulmonary oedema. Cochrane Database Syst Rev 2019;4(4):CD005351.

68. Mathew R, Di Santo P, Jung RG, et al. Milrinone as compared with dobutamine in the treatment of cardiogenic shock. N Engl J Med 2021;385(6):516–25.

69. Levy B, Clere-Jehl R, Legras A, et al. Epinephrine versus norepinephrine for cardiogenic shock after

acute myocardial infarction. J Am Coll Cardiol 2018;72(2):173–82.

70. Levy B, Perez P, Perny J, et al. Comparison of norepinephrine-dobutamine to epinephrine for hemodynamics, lactate metabolism, and organ function variables in cardiogenic shock. A prospective, randomized pilot study. Crit Care Med 2011;39(3):450–5.

71. De Backer D, Biston P, Devriendt J, et al. Comparison of dopamine and norepinephrine in the treatment of shock. N Engl J Med 2010;362(9):779–89.

72. Stretch R, Sauer CM, Yuh DD, et al. National trends in the utilization of short-term mechanical circulatory support: incidence, outcomes, and cost analysis. J Am Coll Cardiol 2014;64(14):1407–15.

73. Hernandez-Montfort J, Sinha SS, Thayer KL, et al. Clinical outcomes associated with acute mechanical circulatory support utilization in heart failure related cardiogenic shock. Circ Heart Fail 2021;14(5):e007924.

74. Thiele H, Zeymer U, Neumann FJ, et al. Intraaortic balloon support for myocardial infarction with cardiogenic shock. N Engl J Med 2012;367(14):1287–96.

75. Abraham J, Blumer V, Burkhoff D, et al. Heart failure-related cardiogenic shock: Pathophysiology, evaluation and management considerations: review of heart failure-related cardiogenic shock. J Card Fail 2021;27(10):1126–40.

76. Morici N, Marini C, Sacco A, et al. Early intra-aortic balloon pump in acute decompensated heart failure complicated by cardiogenic shock: rationale and design of the randomized Altshock-2 trial. Am Heart J 2021;233:39–47.

77. Schrage B, Ibrahim K, Loehn T, et al. Impella support for acute myocardial infarction complicated by cardiogenic shock. Circulation 2019;139(10):1249–58.

78. Hernandez-Montfort JA, Xie R, Ton VK, et al. Longitudinal impact of temporary mechanical circulatory support on durable ventricular assist device outcomes: an IMACS registry propensity matched analysis. J Heart Lung Transplant 2020;39(2):145–56.

79. den Uil CA, Akin S, Jewbali LS, et al. Short-term mechanical circulatory support as a bridge to durable left ventricular assist device implantation in refractory cardiogenic shock: a systematic review and meta-analysis. Eur J Cardio Thorac Surg 2017;52(1):14–25.

80. DeVore AD, Hammill BG, Sharma PP, et al. In-hospital worsening heart failure and associations with mortality, readmission, and healthcare utilization. J Am Heart Assoc 2014;3(4):e001088.

81. Thayer KL, Zweck E, Ayouty M, et al. Invasive hemodynamic assessment and classification of in-hospital mortality risk among patients with cardiogenic shock. Circ Heart Fail 2020;13(9):e007099.

82. Naib T, Lahewala S, Arora S, et al. Palliative care in the cardiac intensive care Unit. Am J Cardiol 2015;115(5):687–90.

83. Sidebottom AC, Jorgenson A, Richards H, et al. Inpatient palliative care for patients with acute heart failure: outcomes from a randomized trial. J Palliat Med 2015;18(2):134–42.

84. Wussler D, Kozhuharov N, Sabti Z, et al. External validation of the MEESSI acute heart failure risk score: a cohort study. Ann Intern Med 2019;170(4):248–56.

85. Lee DS, Stitt A, Austin PC, et al. Prediction of heart failure mortality in emergent care: a cohort study. Ann Intern Med 2012;156(11):767–75. W-261, W-262.

86. Stiell IG, Perry JJ, Clement CM, et al. Prospective and Explicit clinical validation of the Ottawa heart failure risk scale, with and without Use of Quantitative NT-proBNP. Acad Emerg Med 2017;24(3):316–27.

87. Collins SP, Jenkins CA, Harrell FE, et al. Identification of emergency department patients with acute heart failure at low risk for 30-day adverse events: the STRATIFY decision tool. JACC Heart Fail 2015;3(10):737–47.

88. Sax DR, Mark DG, Rana JS, et al. Risk adjusted 30-day mortality and serious adverse event rates among a large, multi-center cohort of emergency department patients with acute heart failure. J Am Coll Emerg Physicians Open 2022;3(3):e12742.

89. Bistola V, Simitsis P, Farmakis D, et al. Association of mineralocorticoid receptor antagonist use and in-hospital outcomes in patients with acute heart failure. Clin Res Cardiol Off J Ger Card Soc 2018;107(1):76–86.

90. Yaku H, Kato T, Morimoto T, et al. Association of mineralocorticoid receptor antagonist Use with all-cause mortality and hospital readmission in older Adults with acute decompensated heart failure. JAMA Netw Open 2019;2(6):e195892.

91. Carnicelli AP, Li Z, Greiner MA, et al. Sacubitril/Valsartan adherence and Postdischarge outcomes among patients hospitalized for heart failure with reduced ejection fraction. JACC Heart Fail 2021;9(12):876–86.

92. Martín E, López-Aguilera J, González-Manzanares R, et al. Impact of Canagliflozin in patients with type 2 diabetes after hospitalization for acute heart failure: a cohort study. J Clin Med 2021;10(3):505.

93. Pérez-Belmonte LM, Sanz-Cánovas J, Millán-Gómez M, et al. Clinical benefits of empagliflozin in very old patients with type 2 diabetes hospitalized for acute heart failure. J Am Geriatr Soc 2022;70(3):862–71.

94. Gattis WA, O'Connor CM, Gallup DS, et al. IMPACT-HF Investigators and Coordinators. Predischarge initiation of carvedilol in patients hospitalized for

decompensated heart failure: results of the initiation management Predischarge: Process for assessment of Carvedilol therapy in heart failure (IMPACT-HF) trial. J Am Coll Cardiol 2004;43(9): 1534–41.

95. Ferreira JP, Santos M, Almeida S, et al. Mineralocorticoid receptor antagonism in acutely decompensated chronic heart failure. Eur J Intern Med 2014;25(1):67–72.

96. Butler J, Anstrom KJ, Felker GM, et al. Efficacy and safety of spironolactone in acute heart failure: the ATHENA-HF randomized clinical trial. JAMA Cardiol 2017;2(9):950–8.

97. Asakura M, Ito S, Yamada T, et al. Efficacy and safety of early initiation of Eplerenone treatment in patients with acute heart failure (EARLIER trial): a multicentre, randomized, double-blind, placebo-controlled trial. Eur Heart J Cardiovasc Pharmacother 2022;8(2):108–17.

98. Velazquez EJ, Morrow DA, DeVore AD, et al. Angiotensin-neprilysin inhibition in acute decompensated heart failure. N Engl J Med 2019;380(6): 539–48.

99. Wachter R, Senni M, Belohlavek J, et al. Initiation of sacubitril/valsartan in haemodynamically stabilised heart failure patients in hospital or early after discharge: primary results of the randomised TRANSITION study. Eur J Heart Fail 2019;21(8): 998–1007.

100. Mentz RJ, Ward JH, Hernandez AF, et al. Angiotensin-neprilysin inhibition in patients with mildly reduced or preserved ejection fraction and worsening heart failure. J Am Coll Cardiol 2023. https://doi.org/10.1016/j.jacc.2023.04.019. S0735-1097(23)05429-3.

101. Program of angiotensin-neprilysin inhibition in admitted patients with worsening heart failure (PREMIER) - Full Text view - ClinicalTrials.gov. Available at: https://clinicaltrials.gov/ct2/show/NCT05164653. [Accessed 22 June 2023].

102. Damman K, Beusekamp JC, Boorsma EM, et al. Randomized, double-blind, placebo-controlled, multicentre pilot study on the effects of empagliflozin on clinical outcomes in patients with acute decompensated heart failure (EMPA-RESPONSE-AHF). Eur J Heart Fail 2020;22(4):713–22.

103. Tamaki S, Yamada T, Watanabe T, et al. Effect of empagliflozin as an Add-on therapy on decongestion and renal function in patients with diabetes hospitalized for acute decompensated heart failure: a prospective randomized controlled study. Circ Heart Fail 2021;14(3):e007048.

104. Solomon SD, McMurray JJV, Claggett B, et al. Dapagliflozin in heart failure with mildly reduced or preserved ejection fraction. N Engl J Med 2022; 387(12):1089–98.

105. Charaya K, Shchekochikhin D, Andreev D, et al. Impact of dapagliflozin treatment on renal function and diuretics use in acute heart failure: a pilot study. Open Heart 2022;9(1):e001936.

106. Schulze PC, Bogoviku J, Westphal J, et al. Effects of early empagliflozin initiation on diuresis and kidney function in patients with acute decompensated heart failure (EMPAG-HF). Circulation 2022;146(4): 289–98.

107. Thiele K, Rau M, Hartmann NUK, et al. Empagliflozin reduces markers of acute kidney injury in patients with acute decompensated heart failure. ESC Heart Fail 2022;9(4):2233–8.

108. Cox ZL, Collins SP, Aaron M, et al. Efficacy and safety of dapagliflozin in acute heart failure: rationale and design of the DICTATE-AHF trial. Am Heart J 2021;232:116–24.

109. Efficacy and safety of dapagliflozin in acute heart failure - Full Text view - ClinicalTrials.gov. Available at: https://clinicaltrials.gov/ct2/show/NCT04298229. [Accessed 22 June 2023].

110. Dapagliflozin and effect on cardiovascular events in acute heart failure -Thrombolysis in myocardial infarction 68 (DAPA ACT HF-TIMI 68) - Full Text view - ClinicalTrials.gov. Available at: https://clinicaltrials.gov/ct2/show/NCT04363697. [Accessed 22 June 2023].

Mechanical Circulatory Support in Cardiogenic Shock: Uses in the Emergency Setting

Ian Persits, DO[a], Ran Lee, MD, FACC[b],*

KEYWORDS

• Cardiogenic shock • Mechanical circulatory support • ECMO • IABP • Impella

KEY POINTS

- Cardiogenic shock is a state of systemic hypoperfusion as a result of myocardial dysfunction leading to low cardiac output. It is associated with a high rate of morbidity and mortality.
- The 2019 Society for Cardiovascular Angiography and Interventions shock classification is now recommended to classify, define, and guide shock recognition and management.
- Many temporary mechanical circulatory support devices exist which can help support individuals through cardiogenic shock. These can be separated by ventricular support, need for oxygenation, percutaneous, or surgical.
- Left ventricular specific support devices include the intra-aortic balloon pump, Impella, and TandemHeart left ventricular assist device. Right ventricular specific support devices include the TandemHeart Protek Duo and Impella RP.
- Biventricular support devices include veno-arterial extracorporeal membrane oxygenation, which can also provide pulmonary assistance in addition to cardiac support.

INTRODUCTION

Cardiogenic shock (CS) is often thought of as a condition characterized by hemodynamic instability, low cardiac output, and multiorgan hypoperfusion. However, CS exists on a spectrum, is often multifactorial, and carries high rates of morbidity/mortality.[1] Patients with CS can deteriorate rapidly, and thus early detection and swift intervention are crucial. The present review will focus on temporary mechanical circulatory support (tMCS) devices that may be used in the emergency setting for patients who develop more severe forms of CS.

Defining Cardiogenic Shock

The definition of CS has evolved over the years from early cases reporting signs of elevated central venous pressure in heart failure (HF) patients[2] to more recent descriptions that incorporate hemodynamic parameters, signs of end-organ hypoperfusion, and clinical gestalt. However, a universal definition has yet to be established. The original SHOCK (Should We Emergently Revascularize Occluded Coronaries for Cardiogenic Shock) trial (1999) was one of the first randomized trials to establish a concrete definition of CS: (i) systolic blood pressure (SBP) less than 90 mm Hg for $\geq$ 30 min; (ii) need for support measures such as vasopressors to maintain SBP greater than 90 mm Hg and signs of end-organ hypoperfusion (cool extremities or a urine output of < 30 mL/hr and a heart rate $\geq$ 60 beats per minute); or (iii) cardiac index (CI) $\leq$ 2.2 L • minute^{-1} • meter^{-2} and pulmonary-capillary wedge pressure (PCWP) $\geq$ 15 mm Hg.[3]

Sources of Funding: None.
[a] Department of Internal Medicine, Cleveland Clinic, Cleveland, OH, USA; [b] Department of Cardiovascular Medicine, Heart, Vascular, and Thoracic Institute, Cleveland Clinic, Mail Code J3-4, 9500 Euclid Avenue, Cleveland, OH 44195, USA
* Corresponding author.
E-mail address: leer2@ccf.org
Twitter: @RanLeeMD (R.L.)

Cardiol Clin 42 (2024) 187–193
https://doi.org/10.1016/j.ccl.2024.02.006
0733-8651/24/© 2024 Elsevier Inc. All rights reserved.

	IABP	Impella 2.5, CP, 5.0, 5.5	Impella RP	TandemHeart LVAD	TandemHeart RVAD/Protek Duo	VA-ECMO
Diagram						
Mechanism	Pneumatic Counterpulsation	Axial Flow Continuous Pump	Axial Flow Continuous Pump	Centrifugal Flow Continuous Pump	Centrifugal Flow Continuous Pump	Centrifugal Flow Continuous Pump
Inflow	N/A	LV	RA	LA	RA	RA
Outflow	N/A	Ao	PA	FA	PA	RA
Maximum Output Provided	0.5–1.5 L/min	2.5–5.5 L/min	4 L/min	5 L/min	5 L/min	7 L/min
Benefits/Uses						
Major Contraindications						
Relative Contraindications						
Complications						

Fig. 1. Device overview.

Most landmark randomized trials since that time have adopted similar definitions of CS.[4–7]

On the other hand, there are several societal guidelines that describe CS as a continuous spectrum, rather than a binary condition, manifesting with a variety of clinical profiles depending on etiology. Rapid hemodynamic deterioration that leads to CS often occurs because of an acute myocardial infarction resulting in a suppressed CI with simultaneous normal/elevated PCWP. This combination of hypoperfusion and volume overload, often referred to as "cold & wet," is the classically described flavor of CS but does not encompass the full picture. HF patients who develop CS tend to present more indolently with New York Heart Association class III/IV or American College of Cardiology (ACC)/

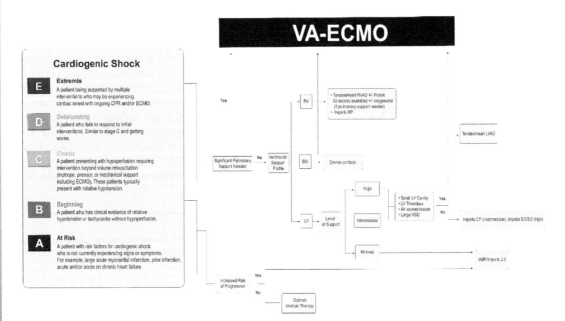

Fig. 2. Algorithm for device selection.

American Heart Association (AHA) stage C/D symptoms. Similarly, the Interagency Registry for Mechanically Assisted Circulatory Support (INTERMACS) incorporates a culmination of subjective markers such as the need for increasing inotropic, vasopressor, or intra-aortic balloon pump (IABP) support or evidence of end-organ hypoperfusion to classify patients on a scale of 1 (critical CS) to 7 (less severe CS). These categorizations allow for a more expansive definition of CS that accounts for the most common culprits. As such the Society for Cardiovascular Angiography and Interventions (SCAI) put forth a novel classification system in 2019 that incorporated the concepts of the prior ACC/AHA and INTERMACS definitions.[8] This unifying proposal described CS as a continuum of 5 stages (A–E) spanning those at risk to those in the most critical stages of shock.[9] Utilizing these systems, clinicians are more easily able to identify those at risk of requiring an initial tMCS device or even those who require device escalation to provide more robust support.

TEMPORARY MECHANICAL CIRCULATORY SUPPORT OVERVIEW
Intra-Aortic Balloon Pump

First reportedly used in human subjects in 1967, the IABP was the earliest tMCS device developed, and though rates of its use have declined over the past decade, it remains the most widely used form of mechanical circulatory support to date.[10] The IABP is a counterpulsation apparatus that is transcutaneously placed in the descending aorta, via a femoral or axillary approach, with its proximal end several centimeters distal to the origin of the left subclavian artery and distal end sitting above the renal arteries.[11] The balloon is set to rapidly deflate in systole, thereby creating a vacuum effect that modestly augments cardiac output (0.5–1.5 L/min). In diastole, the balloon inflates and increases coronary perfusion.

Given the length of time the device has been in clinical use and its wide availability, the IABP is the most popular device used in pre-shock or early stages of CS. Moreover, it can be placed via an axillary approach, as a substitute to the more commonly used femoral access, thereby preserving patient mobility while allowing providers an alternative in the event of difficult femoral access or significant peripheral arterial disease (PAD).[12] Once placed, the IABP is also relatively easy to manage and troubleshoot.

The major downside is the modest support it provides from a cardiac output standpoint in comparison to other tMCS devices. Aortic dissections are a major contraindication to its use given the location of the IABP in the descending aorta and its mechanism of action which increases aortic wall stress during balloon inflation. Additionally, balloon inflation during diastole can further exacerbate severe aortic insufficiency (AI) and thus is a contraindication as well. Though complications such as limb ischemia, venous thromboembolism, or air embolism from balloon rupture are rare, arrhythmias or significant ectopy are some of the more common complications that can lead to device desynchronization and mistiming within the cardiac cycle.

Impella (2.5, CP, 5.0, 5.5)

The Impella device is an axial flow device that is placed percutaneously or via surgical cutdown (in the case of the larger Impella 5.5 device) across the aortic valve in a retrograde fashion under fluoroscopic or echocardiographic guidance so that the inlet is seated in the left ventricle (LV) and outlet in the ascending aorta. This family of devices is the most used out of the LV-to-aorta (LV-Ao) devices available and comes in a variety of sizes that provide 2.5 to 5.5 L/min of continuous cardiac output depending on the model placed. The main mechanism of action of an Impella revolves around LV offloading which in turn decreases myocardial oxygen consumption.[13]

In comparison to an IABP, an Impella generates more cardiac power output, provides a greater level of cardiac output support, and can be used independently of tachyarrhythmias.[14] It does require larger catheters for its placement and a heparin-based purge fluid runs through the system itself to mitigate the risk of pump thrombosis which both contribute to increased bleeding risk.[15] Moreover, more complex insertion, device migration, and system maintenance require more attention and expertise from providers than an IABP does. There are several contraindications to its use such as a LV thrombus, large ventricular septal defect (VSD), severe AI, and aortic valve access issues that relate to the inlet's placement in the LV. Other complications include hemolysis, limb ischemia, mitral valve damage, and ventricular arrhythmias.

Impella RP

Like other versions of the Impella family, the Impella RP device is a continuous axial flow pump that is typically used for isolated right ventricular (RV) support as blood is aspirated from the RV and ejected into the pulmonary artery (PA). It can provide up to 4 L/min of cardiac output.[16]

Major contraindications to its placement include severe pulmonary or tricuspid valvulopathies, inferior vena cava (IVC) filters, and mural thrombus of the right atrium (RA) given the device is advanced via the IVC into the RA and through the tricuspid valve. The Impella RP has many of the same complications as other Impella devices with the addition of more frequent atrial arrhythmias.

TandemHeart (Heart Mate Left Ventricular Assist Device)

The TandemHeart left ventricular assist device (LVAD) is a relatively newer addition to tMCS options. The device is a continuous centrifugal flow pump placed via transfemoral venous access and transseptal atrial puncture to allow advancement of the inlet into the left atrium (LA). Blood is aspirated from the LA and after passing through the device is recirculated back into the outlet placed in the femoral artery (FA). This LA-FA device allows direct bypass and unloading of a failing LV while providing up to 5 L/min of cardiac output.[17,18]

This device generates a similar amount of cardiac output to the larger versions of the Impella device but has several notable benefits. The transseptal puncture into the LA eliminates any of the complications/contraindications that may occur with Impella placement into the LV such as a large VSD, LV thrombus, and arteriovenous access issues. However, the appropriate placement of the device does require more intraprocedural complexity and expertise.

TandemHeart Protek Right Ventricular Assist Device

The TandemHeart Protek right ventricular assist device (RVAD), also known as the Protek Duo, is similar to its LVAD counterpart but configured in a way to directly bypass the RV so that the inlet is in the RA and outlet is in the PA.[19] The are several benefits of this device which include a significant amount of cardiac output supplementation, as well as options for internal jugular access, specifically with the Protek cannula, that allows device placement in the event of IVC filters or lower extremity peripheral venous access issues. Absolute contraindications are related to device positioning and are similar to those of Impella RP placement.

Venoarterial Extracorporeal Membrane Oxygenation

Venoarterial extracorporeal membrane oxygenation (VA-ECMO) is a centrifugal flow continuous pump that aspirates blood from the RA, oxygenates it, and then ejects it into the descending aorta via FA access. This is considered the most advanced form of tMCS devices given that it can be used for biventricular failure to provide full cardiopulmonary support and provides the most amount of cardiac support in comparison to its counterparts.[20]

The major contraindication to the device is severe AI given the fact that the ejected blood into the aorta increases afterload and can thereby worsen the aortic valvular regurgitation. There is also a relative contraindication to placement in patients who have severe PAD. But aside from this, VA-ECMO also comes with a host of complications including but not limited to severe bleeding, thrombosis, limb ischemia, and north-south syndrome that limit long-term use.

DEVICE SELECTION

Selecting the appropriate tMCS device for patients with CS is a nuanced process that relies on numerous factors including hemodynamics, cardiac anatomy, device access, underlying shock culprit, and patient comorbidities (**Fig. 1**).

Shock Stage

Identifying the amount of support needed in relation to the stage of shock should be part of the initial survey when considering tMCS devices (**Fig. 2**). Several studies have evaluated the role of early tMCS initiation in the pre-shock stage (SCAI stage A & B) who are at higher risk of deteriorating clinically or require additional support despite optimal medical therapy. In these earlier stages, an IABP would be a viable choice.[21] However, once "classic shock" begins to develop (SCAI stage C), more advanced therapies can be considered based on the ventricular shock profile.

Ventricular Shock Profile

Assessing the ventricular shock profile is crucial to determining whether LV, RV, or biventricular support is needed. Echocardiography is helpful in terms of direct visualization and noninvasive hemodynamic measures that help guide the type of support needed. Moreover, PA catheterization calculations can provide invasive hemodynamic measures to better assess this.

LV support is most often needed based on the traditional culprits of CS. In pure LV failure, the device choice is heavily dependent on the level of support anticipated. If minimal/intermediate cardiac support is needed, an IABP or smaller versions of the Impella device, such as the 2.5 or CP, can be used. But with higher support needs, a TandemHeart LVAD or Impella 5.5 should be considered.

Pure RV failure is rarer, but when it occurs options are limited in terms of tMCS devices. Typically, the 2 main devices to consider would be an Impella RP device or a TandemHeart RVAD.

Biventricular failure has typically been managed with VA-ECMO. However, there have been recent advancements in using device combinations such as a TandemHeart RVAD/Protek with an Impella device to provide both left-sided and right-sided support. This choice is made individually depending on the underlying etiology, expected length of recovery, procedural complexity, provider comfortability, and numerous additional factors.

Is Pulmonary Support Needed?

Early in the decision-making tree, assessing the need for pulmonary support is required. In patients that require a significant amount of both pulmonary and cardiac support, VA-ECMO is the best option. However, in those that have isolated RV failure that may be contributing to the need for pulmonary support, a TandemHeart RVAD with an oxygenator can be used as well. The decision to pursue the TandemHeart versus VA-ECMO is often institution/practitioner dependent and can be based on the type of provider that inserts these devices (interventional cardiologists vs cardiothoracic surgeons). Other factors to consider such as access/anatomic issues and estimated length of time that a tMCS device may be required also factor into the decision-making with the TandemHeart RVAD being a more durable option in the short-term in comparison to VA-ECMO.

Anatomic/Access Considerations

Anatomic issues often provide challenges to choosing an appropriate tMCS device. Significant left-sided valvulopathies or pathologies within/ involving the LV often preclude the use of the Impella family of devices. In such cases where LV support is needed and there is either a mechanical aortic valve, severe AI, large VSD, or large LV thrombus, a TandemHeart LVAD can be considered instead. Moreover, many tMCS devices require peripheral arterial or venous cannulation and thus device placement may be precluded by those patients with significant PAD or venous access issues. As such, certain alternative device placement considerations can be made as in the TandemHeart Protek which can be placed via internal jugular cannulation or even an IABP and Impella 5.5 which can both be placed via an axillary approach.

COMPLICATIONS/TROUBLESHOOTING

With any tMCS, there are inherent risks and device misfunctions that require adjustments. With each device, there are common issues that can be encountered based on their positioning, method of insertion, and mechanism of action.

Intra-Aortic Balloon Pump

Ideally, the balloon portion of the IABP should be seated between the left subclavian artery and the renal artery. If the balloon travels too proximally or distally, this could ultimately lead to arterial occlusion. As such, positioning should be evaluated routinely with imaging such as a daily chest X ray and adjusted accordingly.

Inflation mistiming, either too early or too late, can lead to device malfunction. Ideally inflation occurs during diastole and deflation in systole. Monitoring the tracing on the IABP display is useful in determining the correct timing. When the device is being inflated too early the augmented peak diastolic pressure wave begins to merge with the unassisted peak systolic pressure. On the other hand, delayed augmentation can be seen when these peaks are too far apart from one another. In both cases, the timing of the balloon inflation can be reprogrammed.

Limb ischemia is a possibility and requires careful examination of the extremities. If this develops, consideration should be made to move from either a femoral to axillary pump or vice versa or even remove the device all together. Balloon and/or aortic rupture are rarer complications that often require device removal and/or prompt surgical evaluation.

Impella

For the traditional left-sided Impella Devices, the inlet cannula should be well seated within the LV, anywhere from 2.5 to 5.0 cm beyond the aortic valve depending on the device and model used. This is normally monitored with routine echocardiography and via the Impella device console. On the device display, there are different alarm settings that can alert to positioning being either too deep or shallow, but it is also important to pay attention to the motor current and placement signals that can provide more data. Deep positioning can lead to mitral valvular damage or obstruction, endocardial damage, or significant device suctioning. A shallow position would primarily result in inadequate cardiac output generation. Repositioning is performed under echocardiographic or fluoroscopic guidance. Aside from device positioning causing suctioning, this can occur if higher performance levels of the Impella are being utilized or if the LV cavity is underfilled. In such cases, downgrading the performance level should be attempted and volume status should be optimized.

Common complications shared by all Impella devices include hemolysis, bleeding, and limb ischemia which are inherent to the large cannulas used for placement and the centrifugal flow of the motor. Adjustments can be made to the purge fluid running through the device in the setting of bleeding, but significant bleeding and/or hemolysis would require device removal.

Venoarterial Extracorporeal Membrane Oxygenation

The primary complications with VA-ECMO involve coagulopathies. Bleeding is more common than thrombosis, but both can occur regularly. If patients are more prone to bleeding, lower anticoagulation goals should be targeted but with the simultaneous goal of targeting higher flow rates through the ECMO circuit. Similarly, limb ischemia is a possibility given the large cannulas used and thus reperfusion cannulas to provide blood flow distal to the ECMO entry site are often employed.

Given the significant amount of blood flow returned through the FA directed proximally into the aorta, there is a significant increase in afterload generated by the VA-ECMO circuit. To combat this, an LV venting strategy to offload the failed LV can be used by adding either an IABP or Impella device.

Harlequin syndrome (also known as north-south syndrome) occurs as the oxygenated blood removed from the IVC goes through the membrane oxygenator of the VA-ECMO circuit and is returned through the FA into the aorta. While the blood returning into the aorta is well oxygenated, the blood flowing from the super vena cava, into the intrinsic pulmonary circulation, and out of the LV is relatively oxygen deficient. This mixing of blood causes an overlap zone that can lead to upper limb or cerebral hypoperfusion. This risk can be managed by the placement of a reperfusion cannula in the right internal jugular vein and splitting arterial outflow with a Y connector which creates a veno-arterial-venous extracorporeal membrane oxygenation circuit, thereby delivering well-oxygenated blood through the intrinsic circulatory system. Alternatively, increasing flow rates on the VA-ECMO pump would push the watershed area more superiorly and could help lower the risk of north-south syndrome, but doing so also increases afterload on an already weakened LV and is thus not routinely advised.

UPGRADING DEVICE

While tMCS devices are initially placed to help provide additional cardiac support, there are often instances in which the amount of support provided is inadequate; in these cases, device upgrade should be considered. Typical signs of inadequate cardiac support include advancing SCAI shock stage, signs of worsening end-organ hypoperfusion, increasing chronotropic/inotropic dependence, or additional cardiac dysfunction (as in new LV or RV failure) despite maximal settings of the current device. The decision to upgrade is often undertaken by a multidisciplinary team that considers the underlying etiology, patient anatomy/physiology, echocardiographic/PA catheter data, and bridge to recovery, advanced therapies, or palliation.

With persistence or worsening of LV dysfunction, a device upgrade may be placing an Impella in someone who currently has an IABP or upgrading to a larger Impella or VA-ECMO in someone with a smaller Impella in place who are not being adequately supported by their current devices. In patients who develop a need for pulmonary support, the devices can be upgraded to include oxygenators in some cases or may even require transition to VA-ECMO. In some instances, patients develop RV dysfunction concomitantly with their LV dysfunction or vice versa and thus upgrades to biventricular support with device combinations for both left-sided and right-sided support or VA-ECMO should be considered. As such, daily evaluation and close monitoring are crucial to determining the trajectory patients take while on tMCS devices.

SUMMARY

The decision to pursue tMCS devices in the emergency setting for patients with CS is a nuanced decision that requires a multidisciplinary team to consider numerous patient-centered and institutional-centered factors. In-depth knowledge of specific device characteristics, indications for use, daily maintenance, and troubleshooting are imperative to success with this approach. With the ever-expanding evolution of device technology and practitioner comfortability, tMCS devices are becoming more readily used and may ultimately lead to improved patient outcomes.

CLINICS CARE POINTS

- Utility of a cardiogenic shock team to rapidly deploy these temporary mechanical circulatory support devices is crucial to best practice and standard of care for cardiogenic shock.
- Etiology, type of ventricular support, and oxygenation need can guide you at the bedside to rapidly deploy these devices.

ACKNOWLEDGMENTS

None.

DISCLOSURE

None.

REFERENCES

1. Shaefi S, O'Gara B, Kociol RD, et al. Effect of cardiogenic shock hospital volume on mortality in patients with cardiogenic shock. J Am Heart Assoc 2015; 4(1):e001462.
2. Boyer BH. Cardiogenic shock. N Engl J Med 1944; 230:226–9.
3. Hochman JS, Sleeper LA, Webb JG, et al. Early revascularization in acute myocardial infarction complicated by cardiogenic shock. SHOCK Investigators. Should we emergently revascularize occluded coronaries for cardiogenic shock. N Engl J Med 1999; 341(9):625–34.
4. Thiele H, Zeymer U, Neumann FJ, et al. Intraaortic balloon support for myocardial infarction with cardiogenic shock. N Engl J Med 2012;367(14): 1287–96.
5. Bauer T, Zeymer U, Hochadel M, et al. Use and outcomes of multivessel percutaneous coronary intervention in patients with acute myocardial infarction complicated by cardiogenic shock (from the EHS-PCI Registry). Am J Cardiol 2012;109(7):941–6.
6. Ponikowski P, Voors AA, Anker SD, et al. 2016 ESC Guidelines for the diagnosis and treatment of acute and chronic heart failure: the Task Force for the diagnosis and treatment of acute and chronic heart failure of the European Society of Cardiology (ESC) Developed with the special contribution of the Heart Failure Association (HFA) of the ESC [published correction appears in Eur Heart J. 2016 Dec 30. Eur Heart J 2016;37(27):2129–200.
7. Lee JM, Rhee TM, Hahn JY, et al. Multivessel percutaneous coronary intervention in patients with ST-segment elevation myocardial infarction with cardiogenic shock. J Am Coll Cardiol 2018; 71(8):844–56.
8. Abraham J, Blumer V, Burkhoff D, et al. Heart failure-related cardiogenic shock: pathophysiology, evaluation and management considerations: review of heart failure-related cardiogenic shock. J Card Fail 2021;27(10):1126–40.
9. Baran DA, Grines CL, Bailey S, et al. SCAI clinical expert consensus statement on the classification of cardiogenic shock: this document was endorsed by the American College of Cardiology (ACC), the American heart association (AHA), the society of critical care medicine (SCCM), and the society of thoracic Surgeons (STS) in April 2019. Catheter Cardiovasc Interv 2019;94(1):29–37.
10. Shah M, Patnaik S, Patel B, et al. Trends in mechanical circulatory support use and hospital mortality among patients with acute myocardial infarction and non-infarction related cardiogenic shock in the United States. Clin Res Cardiol 2018;107(4):287–303.
11. Papaioannou TG, Stefanadis C. Basic principles of the intraaortic balloon pump and mechanisms affecting its performance. ASAIO J 2005;51(3): 296–300.
12. Bhimaraj A, Agrawal T, Duran A, et al. Percutaneous left axillary artery placement of intra-aortic balloon pump in advanced heart failure patients. JACC Heart Fail 2020;8(4):313–23.
13. Glazier JJ, Kaki A. The Impella device: historical background, clinical applications and future directions. Int J Angiol 2019;28(2):118–23.
14. O'Neill WW, Kleiman NS, Moses J, et al. A prospective, randomized clinical trial of hemodynamic support with Impella 2.5 versus intra-aortic balloon pump in patients undergoing high-risk percutaneous coronary intervention: the PROTECT II study. Circulation 2012;126(14):1717–27.
15. Beavers CJ, DiDomenico RJ, Dunn SP, et al. Optimizing anticoagulation for patients receiving Impella support. Pharmacotherapy 2021 Nov;41(11):932–42.
16. Kanwar MK, Everett KD, Gulati G, et al. Epidemiology and management of right ventricular-predominant heart failure and shock in the cardiac intensive care unit. Eur Heart J Acute Cardiovasc Care 2022;11(7):584–94.
17. Kar B, Adkins LE, Civitello AB, et al. Clinical experience with the TandemHeart percutaneous ventricular assist device. Tex Heart Inst J 2006;33(2):111–5.
18. Megaly M, Gandolfo C, Zakhour S, et al. Utilization of TandemHeart in cardiogenic shock: insights from the THEME registry. Catheter Cardiovasc Interv 2020;101(4):750–63.
19. Kapur NK, Paruchuri V, Jagannathan A, et al. Mechanical circulatory support for right ventricular failure. JACC Heart Fail 2013;1(2):127–34.
20. Rajsic S, Treml B, Jadzic D, et al. Extracorporeal membrane oxygenation for cardiogenic shock: a meta-analysis of mortality and complications. Ann Intensive Care 2022;12(1):93.
21. Kimman JR, Van Mieghem NM, Endeman H, et al. Mechanical support in early cardiogenic shock: what is the role of intra-aortic balloon counterpulsation? Curr Heart Fail Rep 2020;17(5):247–60.

Initial Triage and Management of Patients with Acute Aortic Syndromes

Willard N. Applefeld, MD[a], Jacob C. Jentzer, MD[b],*

KEYWORDS

- Acute aortic syndrome • Aortic dissection • Intramural hematoma • Penetrating aortic ulcer
- Blunt traumatic thoracic aortic injury • Vascular emergency

KEY POINTS

- Acute aortic syndromes (AAS) encompass life-threatening conditions like aortic dissection, intramural hematoma, penetrating aortic ulcer, and traumatic thoracic aortic injury.
- AAS often manifests with classic ripping or tearing chest pain; however, diverse symptoms such as syncope, shock, or organ dysfunction may also occur. Therefore clinicians should maintaine a high index of suspicion.
- Timely diagnosis of AAS is crucial for initiating life-saving treatment; clinicians must remain vigilent and integrate patient presentation, comorbidities, and pre-test probability to guide diagnostic and therapeutic descision making.
- High-risk patients require immediate treatment, even before diagnostic imaging is completed. Acute treatment typically includes intravenous beta-blockers, vasodilators, and pain control to reduce heart rate and blood pressure.
- Surgical intervention for AAS is often necessary and should be tailored to patient anatomy and the extent of vascular compromise. A comprehensive approach to management is required.

INTRODUCTION

Acute aortic syndromes (AAS) are highly lethal vascular emergencies involving disruption of the aortic wall. First described by Morgagni in 1761 as a cause of death in a patient who suffered fatal pericardial tamponade after an aortic dissection (AD), AAS continued to remain a lethal disease without treatment until DeBakey, Cooley, and Creech described successful surgical repair techniques in 1955.[1] AAS represent a syndromically related series of diseases which include AD, intramural hematoma (IMH), and penetrating aortic ulcer (PAU); blunt traumatic thoracic aortic injury (BTTAI) results from a different mechanism but carries important similarities.[2] These conditions require urgent evaluation, prompt diagnosis, and emergent treatment which often includes surgical repair.

PATHOPHYSIOLOGY AND RISK FACTORS

The common pathophysiologic factor uniting all AAS is damage to the integrity of the aortic wall. ADs comprise the vast majority of AAS (85%–95% of all cases).[3] In acute AD, intramural hemorrhage with infiltration of blood products into the medial layers of the aortic wall results in the creation of a dissection plane with propagation of blood into a false lumen (**Fig. 1**).[4] Often, the inciting event is a tear in the intimal layer of the vessel wall which results in blood tracking along a dissection plane in the media. Aortic rupture can occur if the adventitial layer is disrupted. A second intimal

[a] Division of Cardiology, Department of Internal Medicine, Duke University School of Medicine, 2301 Erwin Road, Durham, NC 27710, USA; [b] Department of Cardiovascular Medicine, Mayo Clinic, 200 First Street Southwest, Rochester, MN 55905, USA
* Corresponding author.
E-mail address: Jentzer.Jacob@mayo.edu

Cardiol Clin 42 (2024) 195–213
https://doi.org/10.1016/j.ccl.2024.02.007
0733-8651/24/© 2024 Elsevier Inc. All rights reserved.

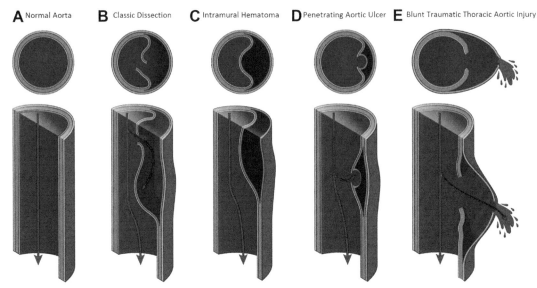

A Normal Aorta   **B** Classic Dissection   **C** Intramural Hematoma   **D** Penetrating Aortic Ulcer   **E** Blunt Traumatic Thoracic Aortic Injury

Fig. 1. Types of acute aortic syndromes. (*A*) Regular aorta with intact vessel wall. (*B*) Classic aortic dissecting with disruption of medial layer allowing blood propagation with creation of true and false lumens separated by intimal flap. (*C*) Intramural hematoma creating separation between medial layers without intimal tear or blood propagation. (*D*) Penetrating aortic ulcer with disruption of intima and penetration into media. (*E*) Blunt thoracic traumatic aortic injury with disruption of all layers of the vascular wall. (*From* Bossone E, Eagle KA. Epidemiology and management of aortic disease: aortic aneurysms and acute aortic syndromes. Nat Rev Cardiol. May 2021;18(5):331-348. doi:10.1038/s41569-020-00472-6).

tear sometimes occurs, allowing re-entry of blood back into the true lumen from the false lumen. The dissection plane itself can propagate proximally and/or distally and involve branch vessels coming off the aorta. If this occurs, vascular compromise, stenosis, or occlusion with tissue ischemia, and end-organ injury can result.

There are a number of heritable and/or genetic syndromes (**Box 1**) which result in abnormalities to the aortic media and thereby increase the risk of AD; among the most common is bicuspid aortic valve with associated aortopathy, given that bicuspid aortic valve is the most common congenital cardiac abnormality.[5] It is important to identify associated conditions as their presence can inform screening of close relatives; indeed, a family history of AD is a major risk factor for AAS.[2,6] Additionally, nonheritable risk factors which increase wall stress or contribute to compromise in wall integrity can also help precipitate AAS (see **Box 1**). Often, these are associated with increased aortic diameter.[2,7–10] Many are modifiable risk factors which offer therapeutic opportunities for intervention. Clinicians should be cognizant of such associated conditions and risk factors in dealing with patients with suspected AAS. The majority of cases of AD occur in males, with a mean age of 63 year old. Dissections are more common in the morning hours, between 6:00 AM and 12:00 PM, as well as in the winter months, suggesting

that the circadian variation in varying physiologic processes (eg, the morning adrenergic surge) contributes to the development of AD.

Pregnancy represents a uniquely vulnerable period where hormonal and hemodynamic changes increase the susceptibility to AD, especially in women with underlying aortopathy or aortic dilation.[2,11] Dissection can occur anytime throughout pregnancy; however, it most commonly occurs within the third trimester (often Stanford type A) or within the first 12weeks post-partum (often Stanford type B) due to increases in blood volume expansion, heart rate, stroke volume, and neurohormonal activity which peaks during this time period.[11] Prophylactic aortic surgery prior to conception is recommended to decrease the risk of AD in individuals with pre-existing aortopathy and aortic dilation, although size cutoffs vary based on underlying condition.[2]

Aortic dissection (AD) can occur iatrogenically during percutaneous intravascular procedures, where an intimal tear results from procedural manipulation and disruption, often with retorgrade propagation of the dissection plane (eg, proceeding cephalad from femoral access), unlike most spontaneous AD where antegrade blood flow propagates the dissection caudally. Iatrogenic AD is most commonly precipitated by trauma from catheter maneuvering, balloon inflation, contrast injection, and guidewire manipulation.[12] Procedural

---

Box 1
Clinical syndromes associated with increased wall stress or vascular media weakness contributing to acute aortic syndrome

Heritable Conditions Associated with Vascular Wall Abnormalities

- Marfan Syndrome
- Loeys-Dietz Syndrome
- Vascular Form of Ehlers-Danlos Syndrome
- Meester-Loeys Syndrome
- LOX-related Thoracic Aortic Syndrome
- Familial Thoracic Aortic Aneurysm (and dissection) Syndrome
- Bicuspid Aortic Valve (with aortopathy)
- Turner syndrome

Clinical Factors Associated with Vascular Wall Abnormalities

- Rheumatologic and Non-Infectious Inflammatory Conditions
  - Takayasu arteritis
  - Rheumatoid arthritis
  - Temporal arteritis
  - HLA-B27 associated spondyloarthropathies (ankylosing spondylitis, reactive arthritis)
  - Cogan's syndrome
  - Relapsing polychondritis
  - Systemic lupus erythematosus
  - Behçet's disease
  - ANCA-related vasculitis (Polyarteritis Nodosa, Microscopic Polyangiitis, Granulomatosis with Polyangiitis)
  - Juvenile idiopathic (rheumatoid) arthritis
  - Idiopathic aortitis and inflammatory aortic aneurysms
  - Sarcoidosis
  - Giant Cell Arteritis
  - IgG4-related disease
- Infectious Conditions
  - Bacterial aortitis (*Salmonella spp, Staphylococcus spp, S spp*)
  - Syphilitic aortitis
  - Mycobacterial aortitis
  - Fungal aortitis
- Other Clinical Factors Associated with Vascular Wall Abnormalities
  - Atherosclerosis
  - Pregnancy
  - Polycystic kidney disease
  - Chronic steroid use
  - Tobacco use
  - Diabetes

Clinical Factors Increasing Wall Stress

- Hypertension
- Pheochromocytoma
- Use of cocaine or other stimulants
- Vigorous Valsalva maneuvers (eg, weightlifting)
- Trauma, especially deceleration injury
- Aortic coarctation
- Aortic aneurysm

AD is most common during chronic total occlusion (CTO) procedures, in those with history of coronary artery bypass grafting, and during emergency catheterization.[12,13] Overall, procedural AD is rare with a reported incidence of 0.02%.[13] In many cases, procedural AD occurring at the coronary ostia can be managed by coronary stenting to prevent AD extension. However, in those cases where the dissection extends more than 40 cm into the ascending aorta, surgery is often necessary.[12,13] In cases where the patient is hemodynamically stable, the origin is controlled, and the dissection is not expanding, it is reasonable to treat conservatively as the antegrade blood flow will compress the false lumen and help to resolve the hematoma in the setting of retrograde AD.[12]

IMH represents a confined hemorrhage into the wall of the aorta. Classically, it was believed that IMH resulted from hemorrhage from the *vasa vasorum* which had proliferated into an area rich with atherosclerotic plaque.[14–16] Alterations in vascular loading conditions which result in changes in wall stress concentrated at the interface of the media and adventitia have also been postulated as a contributory factor to IMH development.[17] This localized hemorrhage into vascular walls can propagate and develop into overt AD, and IMH can be considered a potential precursor to AD.[18]

Penetrating aortic ulcers result from rupture of an atherosclerotic lesion through the internal elastic lamina and allow for hematoma formation in the vascular wall.[19] There can be varying degrees of compromise to the vessel wall from local penetration of the internal elastic lamina, to medial disruption with formation of IMH and dissection, to compromise of the adventitia and subsequent free rupture of the aorta.[20] However, in isolated PAU, it is speculated that medial fibrosis and chronic atheromatous changes surrounding the lesion limit propagation of blood into the medial layer and prevent hematoma propagation.[21]

BTTAI results from rapid shearing forces exerting differential wall stress on adjacent regions of the aortic wall, most often at the isthmus where the arch becomes the mobile descending thoracic aorta (ie, just distal to the ligamentum arteriosum).[20,22] This most often occurs during rapid deceleration injuries related to automobile crashes. The spectrum of vascular injury can vary from a simple intimal disruption to frank aortic rupture and has historically been associated with a high mortality rate.[20] Therefore, BTTAI arises from a distinct pathophysiological mechanism than other AAS, despite similarities in presentation and treatment.

CLASSIFICATION

AAS are classified based on their anatomic locations and time course. The DeBakey and Stanford classification schema are the most commonly used. The DeBakey system classifies AAS based on origin of the intimal tear and the presence or absence of involvement of the ascending aorta.[4,23] In DeBakey Type I AD, the tear occurs in the ascending aorta and propagates distally to involve the arch extending into the descending aorta. In contrast, in DeBakey Type II AD, the tear and the dissection are confined to the ascending aorta alone. In DeBakey Type III AD, the tear and dissection occur in the descending aorta, with type IIIa having the dissection tear confined to only the descending thoracic aorta, and IIIb having the dissection extend below the diaphragm. The Stanford system classifies AAS based on involvement or lack of involvement of the ascending aorta, regardless of the site of origin. Stanford Type A dissections include all dissections which involve the ascending aorta, regardless of the location of the initial tear, and Stanford Type B dissections are those that do not involve the ascending aorta, including those that involve the aortic arch (**Fig. 2**A).[23] As such, Stanford Type A dissections essentially include both DeBakey Type I and II, and Stanford type B is functionally equivalent to DeBakey type III. IMH and PUD can also be classified using the DeBakey and Stanford systems based on the locations where they occur.[2] BTTAI is classified based on the degree of disruption aorta with Grade I consisting of an intimal tear, Grade II an IMH, Grade III a pseudoaneurysm, and Grade IV a rupture of the aorta itself (**Fig. 2**B).[20] The International Registry of Acute Aortic Dissection (IRAD) classifies AAS based on their time course into 4 distinct periods associated with worsening survival

as time progresses: hyperacute (symptom onset <24 hours), acute (2–7 days of symptoms), subacute (8–30 days of symptoms), and chronic (>30 days of symptoms).[24] Appropriate classification is important, as location and duration of the dissection influence survival and inform treatment strategies, particularly surgical approaches.

EPIDEMIOLOGY AND OUTCOMES OF ACUTE AORTIC SYNDROMES

IRAD data suggest that the majority of patients with AD present with Stanford Type A (67%) rather than Type B (33%) and that the differential type of AD confers different mortality and treatment strategies.[10,25] Acute aortic dissection is highly lethal entity with a mortality of 1% to 2% per hour after symptom onset if it occurs in the ascending aorta, making it perhaps the most acutely life-threatening cause of chest pain.[26] Overall in-hospital mortality has fallen from 31.4% to 21.7% in Type A AD between 1995 to 1999 and 2010 to 2013, respectively, driven primarily by declining surgical mortality with the associated repair.[25] In this same analysis, mortality in Type B AD has remained roughly constant: 12.1% from 1995 to 1999 and 14.1% from 2010 to 2013 despite the greater use of endovascular management during these time periods.

IMH represents a less common cause of AAS. Although some series describe as high as a 10% to 30% incidence, IRAD reports a more conservative incidence of 6.3% in their large series of AAS.[27] IRAD data might represent an underestimation of true IMH incidence as it is gleaned from tertiary referral centers which might not capture IMHs diagnosed at community hospitals and not referred to IRAD centers. Groups in Asia report an incidence of IMH of up to 30%, reflecting heterogeneity in IMH prevalence and reporting between centers.[28] While ADs favor the ascending aorta, IMHs preferentially involve the descending aorta (40% Type A, 60% Type B).[29] IMHs either resorb, evolve into a contained rupture, form an aneurysm, or progress to AD, with older autopsy series noting 13% of patients had ADs that originated from IMHs.[18] Both acute and chronic mortality for IMH are high (14% acutely, 12% over 3 months) and outcome is heavily influenced by maximum aortic diameter with larger maximum aortic diameters (>50 mm) conferring a worse prognosis.[30–32] Similar to IMH, PAUs represent a rare cause of AAS with reports of their incidence ranging from 2% to 11%.[28,33,34] The majority of PAUs are found in the descending thoracic aorta, followed by abdominal aorta, and aortic arch.[35] PAUs also occasionally evolve into AD, with

A

De Bakey	Type I	Type II	Type III
Stanford	Type A	Type A	Type B

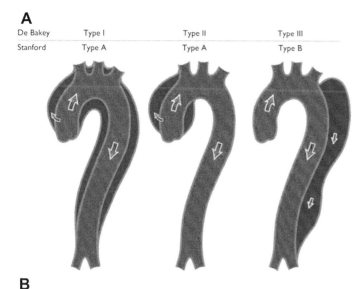

B

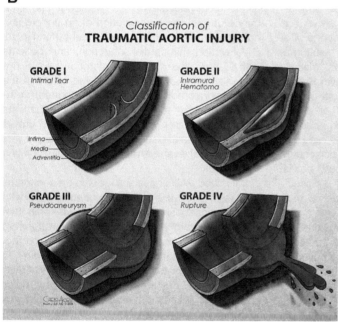

Classification of
TRAUMATIC AORTIC INJURY

GRADE I
Intimal Tear

GRADE II
Intramural Hematoma

Intima
Media
Adventitia

GRADE III
Pseudoaneurysm

GRADE IV
Rupture

Fig. 2. Classification of acute aortic syndromes (A) Classification of aortic dissection, intramural hematoma, and penetrating aortic ulcer are based on the location of pathology. The DeBakey system classifies aortic pathology based on the location of the initial tear. The Stanford classification is based on the involvement of the ascending aorta. Standford A dissections involve the ascending aorta. Standford B dissections do not involve the ascending aorta. DeBakey I dissections involve the ascending aorta and propagate distally. DeBakey II dissections are confined to the ascending aorta. DeBakey III involves the descending aorta. (B) Blunt traumatic thoracic aortic injuries are graded based on degree of compromise to the aorta. Grade I is an intimal tear, Grade II is an IMH, Grade III is a pseudoaneurysm, in Grade IV there is aortic rupture. (From Erbel R, Aboyans V, Boileau C, et al. 2014 ESC Guidelines on the diagnosis and treatment of aortic diseases: Document covering acute and chronic aortic diseases of the thoracic and abdominal aorta of the adult. The Task Force for the Diagnosis and Treatment of Aortic Diseases of the European Society of Cardiology (ESC). Eur Heart J. Nov 1 2014; 35(41):2873-926. doi:10.1093/eurheartj/ehu28. https://doi.org/10.1093/eurheartj/ehu28; and Azizzadeh A, Keyhani K, Miller CC, 3rd, Coogan SM, Safi HJ, Estrera AL. Blunt traumatic aortic injury: initial experience with endovascular repair. J Vasc Surg. Jun 2009;49(6):1403-8. https://doi.org/10.1016/j.jvs.2009.02.234.)

autopsy series documenting that 5% of cases of AD originating from PAUs.[36]

BTTAI is rare, accounting for 1.5% of thoracic trauma cases; however, it remains the second largest traumatic cause of death after head injury.[37] The majority (81%) of BTTAIs occur in the setting of automobile collisions. Despite the increasing use of safety measures such as seatbelts and airbags, there has been no change in the incidence of BTTAI.[38] It remains a highly lethal disease with the vast majority of patients dying before ever reaching a hospital (up to 80%).[37] Traditional BTTAI repair has been with an open surgical approach; however, there has been increasing adoption of thoracic endovascular aortic repair (TEVAR) which has resulted in a reduction in operative mortality (16% surgical mortality with open repair, 9% with TEVAR) with fewer spinal cord injuries.[39] Despite this, in-hospital mortality has remained high, up to 46%.[37]

PRESENTATION AND DIAGNOSIS

The AAS are often described as "great masqueraders" which can present with protean or nonspecific symptoms necessitating a high index of suspicion. Classically, AD presents with chest pain (79%–83% of patients with Type A, 63%–71% of patients with Type B) that is abrupt in onset;

pain often radiates, for example, from the chest to the back.[25,40] However, the presentation can be quite variable—while most patients endorse anterior chest pain or back pain, abdominal pain and migratory pain are also common presenting signs. The pain is typically rated as "severe" or "worst ever" with sharp, tearing, or ripping qualities; pain is often most intense at its onset, and a spontaneous improvement in pain over time can lead to a false sense of security. A minority of patients will present with syncope or cerebrovascular accident, and providers should always suspect AD in patients with "chest pain plus" syndromes involving non-thoracic symptoms plus thoracic pain.

Similarly, physical examination signs characteristic of AD might be subtle or not present at all, and physical examination alone is never sufficient to exclude AD. Patients are often hypertensive on initial evaluation; however, some can be normotensive, in congestive heart failure, in shock, or display tamponade physiology; the presence of a pulse deficit can mask hypertension or result in a blood pressure differential between limbs.[40] However, pulse deficits are found only in fewer than a third of patients and absence of unequal pulses does not exclude AD.[25,40] A murmur of aortic insufficiency (due to dissection into the aortic root disrupting aortic valve coaptation) may be auscultated in patients with Type A dissection (44% of patients in the initial IRAD report) but is much less common in patients with Type B dissection (12% of patients) due to lack of aortic root involvement.[40]

Patients with AD may develop malperfusion syndromes which occur when blood flow is impaired due to expansion of the false lumen and collapse of the true lumen, causing end-organ ischemia.[2] This obstruction can be static or dynamic in nature and can affect all major vascular beds.[41] Therefore, AD with malperfusion syndrome can present with stroke, spinal cord ischemia, paralysis, myocardial ischemia, mesenteric ischemia, renal failure, and/ or limb ischemia that can be persistent or dynamic. One of the most dangerous complications of AD is dissection into the pericardial space, causing hemopericardium and potentially tamponade; AD is important to recognize as a potential cause of pericardial effusion, as acute and rapid drainage can result in hemodynamic collapse.[42] If salvage pericardiocentesis must be performed for emergent stabilization prior to definitive operative management for Type A AD due to shock from cardiac tamponade, it should be done in a careful and controlled manner, withdrawing only 5 to 10 mL at a time and maintaining a systolic blood pressure of 80 to 90 mm Hg (ie, permissive hypotension).[43]

Preliminary basic diagnostic studies in AD frequently yield nonspecific findings and are likewise insufficient to exclude AD except in patients with low pretest probability and a clear alternative diagnosis. Chest roentgenography may show a widened mediastinum, abnormal cardiac or aortic contour, pleural effusions, or a calcified aorta (rarely with evidence of aortic wall calcium displacement). Electrocardiography may show non-specific ST-segment or T-wave abnormalities, left ventricular hypertrophy, myocardial ischemia, or myocardial infarction with or without Q-waves. However, a significant number of patients may have a normal chest film and electrocardiogram (ECG), making these screening tests alone insufficient to rule out AD. Rarely, dissection of the aortic root involving the coronary ostia can result in localized ST-segment elevation on ECG in a coronary distribution, more often involving the right coronary artery with inferior ST-segment elevation.[40,44,45] Notably, the incidence of this rare complication of an uncommon condition is dramatically less frequent than typical ST-elevation myocardial infarction, and patients with ST-elevation myocardial infarction are very unlikely to have AD as the underlying cause in the absence of a predisposing condition. Indeed, the index of suspicion for AD should be low in patients with ST-elevation myocardial infarction unless objective evidence suggesting AD is present (eg, malperfusion), even with severe chest pain radiating to the back.

IMHs and PAUs have similar pain presentations to classic AD. IMHs and PAUs often present with sudden onset, severe chest or back pain that can be migratory in nature.[28] PAUs often are asymptomatic and are incidentally detected. Physical examination findings are even rarer in IMHs and PAUs than in AD as IMHs and PAUs less frequently develop aortic insufficiency, pulse deficits, or ischemic limbs. Likewise, patients with IMHs are even less likely to have abnormalities on chest roentgenography or electrocardiogram than those presenting with AD.

BTTAI is even more challenging to detect as patients with severe polytrauma often present with altered mental status, obtundation, or other distracting injuries.[37] The presence of injuries to the chest wall (eg, sternal fractures, rib fractures, scapular fractures, pneumothoraces, hemothoraces), lung parenchyma (pulmonary contusion), tracheobronchial tree, diaphragm, or esophagus should raise concern for BTTAI. Patients with BTTAI may sometimes present with upper extremity hypertension which occurs due to the development of pseudo-coarctation physiology from an evolving dissection flap at the aortic isthmus, as can occasionally occur with traditional

AD. However, this phenomenon is rare as many of these patients present in shock due to hemorrhage or other injury. Chest roentgenography and focused ultrasonography in trauma (focused assessment with sonography for trauma [FAST] examination) are frequently utilized as initial diagnostic modalities in the primary survey in polytrauma. Simple chest films may show widened mediastinum, loss of the aortopulmonary window, capping of the lung apices from blood products, large pleural effusions from evolving hemothoraces, shift of the mainstem bronchus and trachea, or widening of the paravertebral stripe. Likewise, FAST examination may show hemothoraces or pericardial effusions. However, findings on these diagnostic tests are neither sensitive nor specific for BTTAI and cross-sectional imaging is needed.

In patients where there is suspicion for AD, basic laboratory testing is important in evaluating for alternative etiologies of symptoms as well as determining the presence and extent of end-organ dysfunction (**Table 1**).[4] D-dimer, a degradation product of fibrin cross linking, is often elevated in AD, IMH, and PAU and is a sensitive marker (>95%) for the presence of AAS.[46–48] A cutoff value of less than 500 ng/ml has been proposed to rule out AD within 6 hours of presentation.[46,49] However, while low D-dimer may be sufficiently sensitive to rule out possible AD, it lacks sensitivity for chronic dissections or those with thrombosed false lumens, IMHs, or PAUs. D-dimer also lacks specificity for AAS and can be elevated in other pathologic conditions such as pulmonary embolism, deep vein thrombosis, or disseminated intravascular coagulation where there is increased turnover of cross-linked fibrin.[3,50] A normal D-dimer should only be used to rule out AD in patients in whom there is low clinical suspicion and a clear alternative diagnosis.

Ultimately, definitive diagnosis requires an understanding of aortic anatomy and vascular physiology which includes a complete assessment of the aorta describing the vessel dimensions and concomitant pathology, shape and extent of the dissection flap if present, involvement of branch vessels, compromise of aortic valve, size of the IMH or PAU if present, effects on end-organs, and presence or absence of pericardial effusion or other bleeding (**Box 2**). This is best accomplished with imaging modalities which have high sensitivity and specificity for aortic pathology. Contrast-enhanced, ECG-gated computer tomography (CT) angiography has excellent sensitivity and specificity for the detection of aortic pathology and can be done rapidly making it the preferred diagnostic test for AAS under most circumstances. There are multiple characteristic imaging findings in AD which help distinguish the true from the false lumen. Generally, the true lumen is smaller than the false lumen. Due to slower flow and lower pressures in the false lumen, the convex face of the dissection flap faces toward the false lumen. Often, the lumen that extends more caudally is the true lumen. Despite these generalities, only visualization of the entry flap allows for true determination of the true and false lumens. Multiplanar reconstruction of CT imaging assists with assessment of branch vessel involvement and ECG-gating of CT imaging helps reduce pulsation artifact which may mimic an AD on ungated CT imaging (as is often performed to exclude pulmonary embolism). CT is also helpful in assessing for active hemorrhage or blood collections in the mediastinum, pleura, or pericardium, and for excluding aortic rupture. The "triple-rule out" CT scan can allow for rapid evaluation for the presence of aortic pathology, pulmonary embolism,

Table 1
Basic laboratory evaluation for aortic dissection

Laboratory Test:	Helpful in Screening for:
Hemoglobin	Blood loss, bleeding, anemia
White blood cell count	Infection, inflammation
C-reactive protein	Inflammatory response
Troponin I or T	Myocardial ischemia, myocardial infarction
D-dimer	Aortic dissection, pulmonary embolism, thrombosis
Creatinine	Renal failure (existing or developing)
Aspartate transaminase/ Alanine aminotransferase	Liver ischemia/ liver disease
Lactate	Bowel ischemia, metabolic disorder
Glucose	Diabetes mellitus
Blood gases	Metabolic disorder, oxygenation
PT/INR and PTT, platelet count	Bleeding diathesis

https://doi.org/10.1093/eurheartj/ehu28 From Erbel R, Aboyans V, Boileau C, et al. 2014 ESC Guidelines on the diagnosis and treatment of aortic diseases: Document covering acute and chronic aortic diseases of the thoracic and abdominal aorta of the adult. The Task Force for the Diagnosis and Treatment of Aortic Diseases of the European Society of Cardiology (ESC). Eur Heart J. Nov 1 2014;35(41):2873-926. doi:10.1093/eurheartj/ehu28.

Box 2
Imaging considerations in acute aortic syndromes

Aortic Dissection

- Visualization of the intimal flap
- Extent of the disease according to the aortic anatomic segmentation
- Identification of the false and true lumens (if present)
- Location of entry and re-entry tears (if present)
- Identification of antegrade and/or retrograde aortic dissection
- Identification grading and mechanism of aortic valve regurgitations (if present)
- Involvement of side branch vessels
- Evidence of malperfusion (low flow or no flow)
- Evidence of organ injury (brain, myocardium, bowels, kidneys, etc.)
- Evidence of pericardial effusion and its severity
- Evidence and extent of pleural effusion
- Detection of peri-aortic bleeding
- Signs of mediastinal bleeding

Intramural hematoma

- Localization and extent of aortic wall thickening
- Co-existence of atheromatous disease (calcium shift)
- Presence of small intimal tears

Penetrating aortic ulcer

- Localization of the lesion (depth and length)
- Co-existence of intramural hematoma
- Involvement of the peri-aortic tissue and bleeding
- Thickness of the residual wall

In all cases

- Co-existence of other aortic lesions: aneurysms, plaques, signs of inflammatory disease, etc.

and coronary artery disease with a high negative predictive value in patients presenting with undifferentiated chest pain.[51–53] However, this may not provide optimal aortic imaging when AD is the leading differential diagnosis. For pregnant women with a high index of suspicion for AD, CT imaging can be obtained as for other patients recognizing the high risk of maternal morbidity and mortality with delayed diagnosis and the relatively lower risk of fetal harm with exposure to ionizing radiation during the third trimester (when AD often occur). When there is a lower index of suspicion, the risk/benefit of CT versus alternative imaging tests (which have their own potential risks) should be carefully balanced via shared decision-making.

MRI angiography is also a highly sensitive imaging modality for detection of aortic pathology and allows for visualization of the vessel from the arch to the distal segment, especially when contrast enhancement is used.[54] MRI can effectively visualize the intimal flap in AD and evaluate for aortic regurgitation, pericardial effusion, and involvement of the carotid or proximal coronary vessels.[54–57] However, because MRI cannot be performed as rapidly as a contrast-enhanced computed tomography (CT) scan due to more lengthy scanning time, it should be used with caution in those at risk of deterioration and is typically more appropriate for chronic aortic pathology in a non-emergency setting (particularly for serial imaging).

Ultrasonographic techniques can detect aortic pathology, although these can be notoriously operator-dependent and imaging-dependent. Transesophageal echocardiogram (TEE) has high sensitivity (>95%) in the detection of AAS.[54] Advantageously, TEE can be performed at bedside and does not expose patients to radiation or contrast agents, but has the disadvantage of requiring personnel and conscious sedation which can lead to logistic delays.[58] For patients who are considered too unstable for a CT scan (particularly those who are endotracheally intubated), TEE is preferred if it can be performed expeditiously. TEE also easily provides functional information on cardiac contractility and can detect pericardial effusion, cardiac tamponade, or new valvular regurgitation. Transthoracic echocardiogram (TTE) is not sensitive enough to detect AAS (78% sensitivity in Acute Type A dissection, 40% in Type B) and should not be used to exclude the disease; the presence of a dilated aortic root seen on TTE may increase suspicion for AD in patients with undifferentiated chest pain.[54,58]

Historically, retrograde aortography was the prior gold standard for detection of AAS due to its high sensitivity and specificity.[4] While it does offer the advantage of allowing for assessment of the coronary arteries, the test has fallen out of use due to its invasive nature, time, and cost. However, this may be appropriate for a patient with apparent ST-elevation myocardial infarction when AD must be ruled out (as opposed to creating a potential delay by performing a CT scan).

COMMON PHENOTYPES OF ACUTE AORTIC SYNDROMES

Because AAS can present with heterogeneous signs, symptoms, and result on laboratory testing, prompt diagnosis and initial treatment can be challenging and is often delayed. Effectively diagnosing and managing AAS requires that clinicians first have a high index of suspicion. The authors propose that clinicians assess risk factors and comorbidities, take a focused history, and conduct a limited physical examination and group patients into 1 of 4 common phenotypes that then guide further diagnostic evaluation and treatment:

Phenotype 1: Classic Dissection. In patients presenting with clear signs and symptoms of AAS where the pre-test probability is judged to be high by the evaluating clinician, initiation of empiric treatment is reasonable as described later. These very high-risk patients endorse characteristic "tearing" or "ripping" chest pain and/or have classic physical examination features such as pulse discrepancy, the murmur of acute aortic insufficiency, or end-organ damage concerning for malperfusion, often with 1 or more risk factors. Here, aggressive upfront treatment is warranted prior to and during confirmatory diagnostic testing which typically is with CT angiography, with TEE preferred for unstable patients in whom CT is not feasible. In many cases, early consultation with a surgeon is appropriate.

Phenotype 2: The undifferentiated syndrome. AAS should be considered in patients presenting with acute chest, back, or abdominal pain; syncope; and/or signs and symptoms of malperfusion. Here, clinicians should consider the pre-test probability of AAS (vs other likely alternative diagnoses) as informed by patient risk factors and comorbidities, features of the pain, and high-risk examination features (**Box 3**). The Aortic Dissection Detection Risk Score (ADD-RS) is a highly sensitive and easily calculable score to help guide the workup of the undifferentiated patient with possible AD by providing an estimate of pre-test probability (**Fig. 3**).[59,60] Here, in the absence of an alternative diagnosis, the presence of 1 or more of the high risk features listed in **Box 3** should prompt aggressive evaluation with expedited

---

Box 3
High-risk features for aortic dissection

1. High-risk conditions
   - Marfan syndrome
   - Family history of aortic disease (esp. dissection)
   - Known aortic valve disease
   - Recent Aortic manipulation
   - Known thoracic aortic aneurysm ± bicuspid aortic valve

2. High-risk chest pain features
   - Chest, back, or abdominal pain described as:
     - Abrupt onset
     - Severe intensity
     - Ripping or tearing

3. High-risk examination features
   - Evidence of perfusion deficit
     - Pulse deficit
     - Systolic BP differential
     - Focal neurologic deficit (in conjunction with pain)
   - Murmur of aortic insufficiency (new and with pain)
   - Hypotension or shock state

Adopted from Rogers AM, Hermann LK, Booher AM, et al. Sensitivity of the aortic dissection detection risk score, a novel guideline-based tool for identification of acute aortic dissection at initial presentation: results from the international registry of acute aortic dissection. Circulation. May 24 2011;123(20):2213-8. https://doi.org/10.1161/CIRCULATIONAHA.110.988568.

---

aortic imaging using CT angiography. A low ADD paired with a D-dimer less than 500 ng/mL is very effective in excluding AAS, but D-dimer should not be used when the ADD is not low.[61] In the ADvISED registry, the false-negative rate of an ADD-RS ≤1 combined with a negative D-dimer was 0.3%, suggesting that this strategy might be highly efficacious in ruling out AAS—indeed, this false-negative rate is likely equivalent to a CT scan. For intermediate-risk patients in whom AD is one of multiple potential diagnoses, a "triple-rule-out" CT scan is an efficient way to make a diagnosis. In undifferentiated trauma patients, there must be high suspicion for BTTAI in those with injuries to the chest or with complaints of chest pain and dedicated CT aortic imaging should be obtained expeditiously.[37]

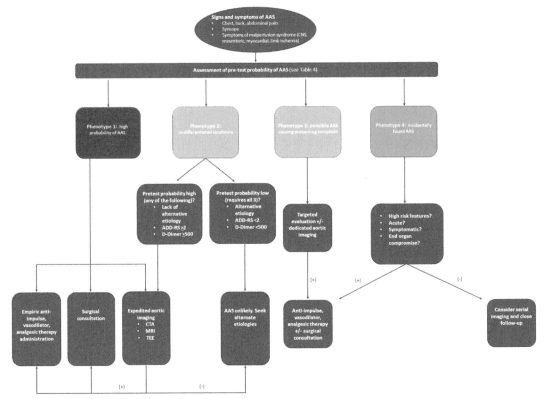

Fig. 3. Evaluation of acute aortic syndrome. Appropriate evaluation and management of acute aortic syndromes involve first considering the pre-test probability based on underlying risk factors and clinical presentation. Patients can then be grouped into 1 of 4 phenotypes with different diagnostic and management strategies.

Phenotype 3: AD as the cause of the presenting illness. Patients may present with non-thoracic conditions where AD is the proximate cause. Here, in the time-limited evaluation of presenting condition, it is important to remain cognizant that AD may be the upstream process responsible. As an example, in a patient presenting with new severe aortic regurgitation or a pericardial effusion, AD should be strongly considered (particularly if there is associated chest pain). Similarly, AD should be considered in patients presenting with mesenteric, limb, spinal cord, or even myocardial ischemia. The clinician must weigh the likelihood of AD being the precipitant of the presenting condition against the time, resources, and risks of further diagnostic testing. Again, expedited CT imaging is often justified.

Phenotype 4: incidentally discovered aortic pathology. In many cases, aortic pathology in the AAS spectrum may be incidentally discovered on cross-sectional imaging performed for some other indication; indeed, the increased use of advanced imaging could potentially be driving an increase in the apparent prevalence of aortic pathology. Here, where the clinical presentation is not due to aortic disease and the patient may even be an asymptomatic outpatient, clinicians are challenged to determine if the aortic pathology is (1) acute or chronic, (2) causative or incidentally found, and (3) needs to be addressed promptly or can be deferred until a later time based on the symptomatology and evidence of vascular compromise or complications. A common example is an asymptomatic patient found to have interval development of AD on surveillance CT scan performed for a different indication.

MANAGEMENT

In all patients presenting with AAS, the initial therapy should be focused on reducing the transmural wall stress of the aorta while proceeding with evaluation for definitive management. The propagation of an evolving AD is dependent on the degree of intimal compromise as well as the rate of change in intraluminal pressure within the vessel from end diastole to systole (dP/dt).[62] Therefore, initial medical therapy is focused on "impulse control" with immediate management focused on a combination of reduction in both the blood pressure and

Table 2
Intravenous antihypertensive pharmacotherapies in acute aortic syndrome

Medication	Bolus	Initial Infusion Rate	Infusion Titration Parameters	Max	Half Life	Notes
Beta-blockers (first-line therapies)						
Esmolol	500 mcg/kg q5min (up to 3 doses)	50 mcg/kg/min	Increase by 50 mcg/kg/min q5 min ×3 (with loading dose) then may increase by 50 mcg/kg/min q15 min thereafter	300 mcg/kg/min	2–5 min	Blood pressure-lowering effects delayed compared with heart rate-lowering effects Bolus and uptitrate infusion q5 min initially up to 3 times
Labetalol	20 mg, followed by 20–80 mg q10 min up to 300 mg total dose	1 mg/min	Increase by 0.5 mg/min q15 min	10 mg/min	3–8 h	Ratio of beta to alpha blocking activity is 7:1 Blood pressure effects greater and heart rate effects less than other listed beta-blockers
Metoprolol	5–10 mg (up to 0.15 mg/kg) initial dose and/or 5 mg q3-5 min for 3–4 doses	n/a	n/a	20–30 mg	3–4 h	More effective for lowering heart rate than blood pressure Higher doses can be used if not meeting heart rate or blood pressure goals, with diminishing returns seen
Vasodilators (add-on therapies)						
Sodium nitroprusside	n/a	0.5–1 mcg/kg/min	Increase by 0.5 mcg/kg/min	2–5 mcg/kg/min (up to 8–10 mcg/kg/min for short term)	2 min	Must monitor closely for cyanide and thiocyanate toxicity with prolonged use or high doses. Doses exceeding 5 mcg/kg/min should only be used for 10 min. Can elevate ICP, decrease cerebral blood flow, and reduce coronary blood flow (coronary steal)

(continued on next page)

Table 2
(continued)

Medication	Bolus	Initial Infusion Rate	Infusion Titration Parameters	Max	Half Life	Notes
Nicardipine	n/a	5 mg/h	Increase by 2.5 mg/hq5min	15 mg/h	3–14 h	Delayed/prolonged effect; higher initial infusion rate (10 mg/h) can be used for up to 30 min as a loading dose. Reduce dose to 2–5 mg/h once BP target is reached
Clevidipine	n/a	1–2 mg/hr	Double dose q2min. As BP approaches target, extend titration interval to 5–10 min.	21 mg/h (up to 32 mg/h for short term)	1 min	Delivered in lipid emulsion. Must check triglycerides and limit to 1000 mL maximum over 24 h
Nitroglycerin	n/a	20 mcg/min (up to 50 mcg/min)	Increase by 20 mcg/min (up to 50 mcg/min) q5min	200 mcg/min (up to 400 mcg/min for short term)	1–4 min	Tolerance (tachyphylaxis) develops over time. Monitor for methemoglobinemia with prolonged or high-dose use
Non-dihydropyridine Calcium channel blockers (alternative first-line therapy)						
Diltiazem	0.25 mg/kg (up to 20 mg), may repeat 0.35 mg/kg (up to 25 mg) after 15 min	5 mg/h	Increase infusion by 2.5 mg/ h q15 min	20 mg/h	3–7 h	Useful for bronchospastic airways disease as an alternative to beta-blocker (or for uncontrolled heart rate). Avoid in decompensated heart failure

heart rate to reduce dP/dt, although no high-quality evidence exists to guide selection of drugs (**Table 2**).

Beta-blockers reduce dP/dt and transmural wall stress through negative inotropic/chronotropic and antihypertensive effects; therefore, intravenous rapid-acting beta blockers such as esmolol, labetalol, or metoprolol are first line for the treatment of AD.[2,4,63] This is true even in pregnancy and the post-partum states where the benefits of impulse control outweigh that of fetal growth restriction.[2] Esmolol is an ultrashort-acting intravenous beta-blocker which is often preferred due to its rapid onset, fast titration (with bolus dosing), and short duration of effect in the event of hemodynamic instability. Labetalol does not always provide maximal heart rate control despite its superior antihypertensive properties versus other intravenous beta-blockers. Patients will often continue to be hypertensive despite maximal beta blocker therapy and so frequently multiple agents are required for blood pressure control. Short-acting, rapidly titratable intravenous vasodilators such as sodium nitroprusside, clevidipine (preferred due to ease of use), or nicardipine can be used as adjuncts to beta-blockade, but should not be started before comprehensive beta-blockade due to reflex tachycardia from sympathetic activation that may increase dP/dt.[2,64–66] Those patients intolerant to beta-blockers (or in whom beta-blockers fail to control the heart rate) can receive non-dihydropyridine calcium channel blockers (eg, diltiazem) for heart rate and blood pressure control.

Although consensus regarding hemodynamic goals does not exist, antihypertensive pharmacotherapies should be generally titrated to a heart rate below 70 beats per minute and a systolic blood pressure less than 120 mm Hg (or to the lowest blood pressure that maintains end-organ perfusion), often justifying placement of an arterial line in a limb without compromised perfusion.[2] Optimal heart rate and blood pressure targets have not been clearly defined in the setting of AAS, and the limb with the highest recorded blood pressure should generally be used for drug titration in patients with pulse deficits or between-limb blood pressure discrepancies. Sympathetic outflow secondary to pain can drive a tachycardiac and hypertensive response and so initiation of appropriate analgesic therapy, often with escalating doses of intravenous opiates, is critical as an early step in management (ie, before aggressive antihypertensive therapy is escalated).

Acute Stanford type A AD represents a surgical emergency and immediate surgical consultation is essential.[2,25,40] The specific surgical techniques are beyond the scope of this review and are tailored to the individual's anatomy and surgeon's expertise. In general, the surgical approach is to prevent extension of the dissection or rupture of the aorta with the specific surgery tailored to the extent of the vascular compromise, anatomy, the patient's signs and symptoms, and complications of vascular compromise the patient is manifesting to restore organ perfusion. Open repair is typical for patients with aortic arch involvement, while endovascular approaches (eg, TEVAR) may be appropriate when AD is isolated to the descending aorta. In pregnant patients, if Type A AD occurs within the first 26 weeks of gestation, emergency aortic surgery is recommended with fetal monitoring, recognizing the potential for fetal loss.[2] When the duration of pregnancy reaches the point where it is associated with high likelihood of independent fetal survival (especially after 28 weeks gestation), then emergency cesarean delivery followed by aortic surgery maximizes both maternal and fetal survival in acute Type A AD.[2]

In uncomplicated Stanford type B AD, medical management with impulse control, blood pressure management, and analgesia is the preferred treatment strategy.[2] However, in those patients who present with or develop complicated Type B AD (ie, with vascular compromise), surgical repair is indicated.[2] Similarly, surgical repair of uncomplicated Type B AD can be considered in situations of high-risk imaging or clinical features (**Box 4**).[2,67–71] Here too, technique of the repair is informed by patient anatomy, signs and symptoms, and extent of the vascular compromise. After acute antihypertensive and anti-impulse therapy, transition to long-acting oral agents is appropriate to maintain adequate hemodynamic control without swings in blood pressure for patients in whom urgent surgical repair is not planned.

IMH and PAU are treated, for the most part, similarly to acute AD. Surgical repair should be undertaken in Type A IMH as well as Type B IMH complicated by high-risk features such as aortic rupture, end-organ malperfusion, periaortic hematoma, pericardial effusion with tamponade, and/or chest pain that is refractory or recurrent.[2] Expectant management is reasonable in uncomplicated Type B IMH as well as Type A IMH with prohibitively high operative mortality and absence of concerning features on imaging. PAUs are managed surgically if they are associated with IMH or aortic rupture.[2]

Initial management of BTTAI should consist of resuscitation and treatment of hemorrhagic shock with hypotension being allowed (permissive hypotension) to prevent propagation of the aortic injury. Like other AAS, impulse control is the preferred

Box 4
Features of type B dissection which would prompt surgical repair

Complicated Type B dissection

- Aortic rupture
- Malperfusion from branch artery occlusion
- Extension of Type B dissection distally or proximally into ascending aorta (retrograde Type A)
- Progressive enlargement of true lumen, false lumen, or both during the acute phase
- Intractable pain
- Uncontrolled hypertension

High-risk clinical features of uncomplicated Type B dissection

- Hypertension refractory to greater than 3 different classes of antihypertensive agents at maximum tolerated doses
- Pain refractory to maximum tolerated doses of pain medications lasting greater than 12 hours
- Need for readmission

High-risk imaging features of uncomplicated Type B dissection

- Maximum aortic diameter greater than 40 mm
- False-lumen diameter greater than 20 to 22 mm
- Entry tear on lesser curvature
- Increase in total aortic diameter greater than 5 mm between serial imaging studies
- Bloody pleural effusion/hemothorax
- Imaging evidence of malperfusion

Adopted from Isselbacher EM, Preventza O, Hamilton Black J, 3rd, et al. 2022 ACC/AHA Guideline for the Diagnosis and Management of Aortic Disease: A Report of the American Heart Association/American College of Cardiology Joint Committee on Clinical Practice Guidelines. Circulation. Dec 13 2022;146(24):e334-e482. https://doi.org/10.1161/CIR.0000000000001106.

initial treatment strategy with short- acting intravenous beta-blockers and vasodilators being used to target systolic blood pressures less than 100 mm Hg and a heart rate of less than 100 beats per minute.[37] Grade I BTTAIs are managed expectantly with medical therapy, unless they progress on serial imaging. Grades III and IV require operative intervention. Grade II BTTAIs can be managed either surgically or with medical therapy and close follow-up.

Management of chronic AD is an evolving area with the increased incidental diagnosis of aortic pathology resulting from expanding use of cross-sectional imaging. In the absence of symptoms or end-organ complications, a non-urgent surgical approach is often appropriate, coupled with aggressive chronic antihypertensive therapy.[2,4] Of note, even with a conservative strategy of "watchful waiting" in patients with a chronic Type A AD below the surgical threshold for intervention (55 mm), the risk of adverse aortic events remains high and increases over time.[72] In cases where the precise timing is unclear but some chronicity is present, expectant management with acute antihypertensive therapy and serial imaging may be appropriate in the absence of complications, with a transition to chronic therapy if no change over time is observed on imaging.

REGIONALIZATION OF CARE

The effective diagnosis and management of AAS often requires multispecialty expertise. While many patients can be effectively managed at the center where they initially present, it is important to recognize that some patients may benefit from expeditious transfer to centers with expertise in managing AAS. This is particularly true for those patients who may need surgery, recognizing that specialty centers with extensive experience managing aortic disease are better equipped to handle the complexity of these cases.[73] Regionalized "Hub and Spoke" networks of care allow for the quick transfer of patients with AAS from sites of initial diagnosis to tertiary or quaternary cardiac intensive care units at high- volume aortic centers.[74] Even in acute Type A AD, where time is precious, acute medical therapy and diagnosis followed by urgent transfer to a high-volume center with subspeciality expertise is safe and has been associated with reductions in operative mortality.[75]

Smoothly and swiftly transitioning patients between facilities requires streamlined performance at multiple levels. First, there needs to be easy access to subspecialty centers without delay in accepting a patient due to bed or transport team availability. Second, frequent bi-directional communication between practitioners at referring centers and those at the receiving center is essential. Third, referring centers should be easily able to provide any imaging or laboratory data that were obtained so that receiving centers do not need to duplicate these studies. Cloud networks can be helpful in data sharing and allow experts at the receiving facilities to review the data while the patient is actively being transported and thereby start formulating a treatment plan.[76] Fourth, a cardiovascular expert at the subspecialty center should be immediately available and in frequent communication with the referral center and transport team. This clinician can mobilize resources at the receiving facility prior to patient arrival, particularly for patients who may need surgery. Lastly, transport teams should be agile with access to a variety of different types of transportation (ground, helicopter, fixed wing aircraft) to accommodate different weather conditions and move the patient as quickly and safely as possible. These teams should be able to initiate treatment and titrate therapies en route to the receiving facility with clear instructions on hemodynamic goals as often blood pressure and heart rate targets are not reached prior to transport.[77]

The authors suggest that when Phenotype 1 patients, where the pretest probability of AAS is high, present to resource-limited facilities, empiric antihypertensive treatment should be initiated and the subspeciality center should be immediately contacted for transfer. Further diagnostic workup can then be done in collaboration with guidance from the subspeciality teams at the accepting facility. This can be particularly challenging at centers who do not have advanced CT angiography capabilities, raising questions about whether a non-dedicated (ie, non-gated) CT scan should be done prior to transfer rather than a dedicated aortic CT angiogram after transfer; many hub centers favor the latter approach to avoid repeating contrast imaging and potential logistical delays. Close collaboration on further workup may help mitigate delays in transport while patient is undergoing imaging testing at the initial facility. Alternatively, if the receiving bed is not ready at the accepting facility, clinicians can discuss when workup can be done where the patient initially presented.

SUMMARY

AAS represent a spectrum of highly lethal diseases that include AD, IMH, PAU, and BTTAI. It is important that clinicians remain vigilant and maintain a high index of suspicion as these diseases often present with non-specific signs and symptoms. To effectively diagnose and treat AAS, clinicians should undertake a prompt targeted evaluation which is informed by pre-test probability and patient risk factors. Clinicians should consider clinical factors which are associated with vascular abnormalities or increase wall stress as well as the characteristics of the presenting pain. It is crucial to be wary of malperfusion syndromes and consider whether upstream AAS is the proximate cause of the presenting end-organ compromise even in patients without chest pain. In those with a high

pre-test probability of AAS, empiric antihypertensive treatment should be initiated before the diagnostic workup is complete (eg, intravenous beta-blockade prior to CT imaging). In patients with an undifferentiated clinical syndrome where AAS is possible, dedicated aortic imaging with CT (including a "triple-rule-out" scan) can be useful to make the diagnosis. In patients with high-pretest probability or confirmed AAS, immediate treatment should be implemented with impulse control aimed at reducing blood pressure and heart rate. Short-acting, rapidly titratable beta-blockers are the mainstay of treatment; however, additional rapidly acting vasodilators may be required to achieve hemodynamic targets. Operative intervention should be informed by the location of the pathology as well as complications and extent of downstream injury, and early surgical consultation is essential. Emergent transfer to subspeciality aortic centers to undergo definitive management is feasible and safe but must be done expeditiously and with close collaboration between the transferring and receiving facility. It is only through clinical vigilance, rapid action, and close coordination across regions and specialties that the care of patients with AAS will improve.

CLINICS CARE POINTS

- AAs classically presents as ripping or tearing pain in the flank, chest, or back that is abrupt in onset and often migratory. However, presentation of this highly lethal syndrome can be variable and masquerade as other common conditions including stroke, syncope, heart failure, tamponade, spinal ischemia, myocardial infarction, mesenteric ischemia, renal failure, limb ischemia, valvular regurgitation, or other end organ hypoperfusion. Clinicians should be wary of 'Chest pain plus' syndromes which involve non-thoracic symptoms plus thoracic pain.

- Heritable conditions and nonheritable risk factors which increase transmural aortic wall stress can compromise vascular integrity and precipitate AAS. Clinicians should consider pre-existing risk factors and maintain a high index of suspicion for AAS.

- Survival worsens as time elapses in AAS and so prompt diagnosis is critical.

- D-Dimer is a sensitive marker for AAS. A cutoff of <500ng/ml has been proposed to rule out AD within 6 hours of presentation. It is not sufficiently sensitive to rule out chronic dissection, IMHs, or PAUs. Therefore, a normal D-Dimer should only be used to rule out

- dissection when there is a low index of suspicion and clear alternative diagnosis.
- CTA, MRI, and TEE are all highly sensitive methods of diagnosing AAS.
- We propose that patients conceptually group patients into four different phenotypes to guide further diagnosis and treatment. In phenotype 1, Classic Aortic Dissection, aggressive immediate treatment is critical both prior to and during diagnostic testing. In phenotype 2, the undifferentiated syndrome, clinicians should maintain a high index of suspicion and use risk scores to guide workup. A low ADD score and D-Dimer <500ng/ml effectively excludes AAS. D-dimer should not be used when ADD is elevated. In Phenotype 3, where AAS is the possible proximate cause of the presenting illness, clinicians should maintain a high index of suspicion for AAS and engage in a targeted workup informed by risk factors and pretest probability. In Phenotype 4, incidentally discovered aortic pathology, clinicians must determine the chronicity, likelihood that the aortic pathology is driving the initial presentation, and need for urgent versus later intervention.

REFERENCES

1. Wheat MW Jr, Palmer RF. Dissecting aneurysms of the aorta. Curr Probl Surg 1971;1–43.
2. Isselbacher EM, Preventza O, Hamilton Black J 3rd, et al. 2022 ACC/AHA guideline for the diagnosis and management of aortic disease: a report of the American heart association/American College of Cardiology Joint Committee on clinical Practice guidelines. Circulation 2022;146(24):e334–482. https://doi.org/10.1161/CIR.0000000000001106.
3. Bossone E, LaBounty TM, Eagle KA. Acute aortic syndromes: diagnosis and management, an update. Eur Heart J 2018;39(9):739–749d. https://doi.org/10.1093/eurheartj/ehx319.
4. Erbel R, Aboyans V, Boileau C, et al. 2014 ESC Guidelines on the diagnosis and treatment of aortic diseases: Document covering acute and chronic aortic diseases of the thoracic and abdominal aorta of the adult. The Task Force for the Diagnosis and Treatment of Aortic Diseases of the European Society of Cardiology (ESC). Eur Heart J 2014;35(41):2873–926. https://doi.org/10.1093/eurheartj/ehu281.
5. Bossone E, Eagle KA. Epidemiology and management of aortic disease: aortic aneurysms and acute aortic syndromes. Nat Rev Cardiol 2021;18(5):331–48. https://doi.org/10.1038/s41569-020-00472-6.
6. Chen SW, Kuo CF, Huang YT, et al. Association of family history with incidence and outcomes of aortic dissection. J Am Coll Cardiol 2020;76(10):1181–92. https://doi.org/10.1016/j.jacc.2020.07.028.
7. Liang KP, Chowdhary VR, Michet CJ, et al. Noninfectious ascending aortitis: a case series of 64 patients. J Rheumatol 2009;36(10):2290–7. https://doi.org/10.3899/jrheum.090081.
8. Slobodin G, Naschitz JE, Zuckerman E, et al. Aortic involvement in rheumatic diseases. Clin Exp Rheumatol 2006;24(2 Suppl 41):S41–7.
9. Gornik HL, Creager MA. Aortitis. Circulation 2008;117(23):3039–51. https://doi.org/10.1161/CIRCULATIONAHA.107.760686.
10. Evangelista A, Isselbacher EM, Bossone E, et al. Insights from the international registry of acute aortic dissection: a 20-Year experience of collaborative clinical Research. Circulation 2018;137(17):1846–60. https://doi.org/10.1161/CIRCULATIONAHA.117.031264.
11. Braverman AC, Mittauer E, Harris KM, et al. Clinical features and outcomes of pregnancy-related acute aortic dissection. JAMA Cardiol 2021;6(1):58–66. https://doi.org/10.1001/jamacardio.2020.4876.
12. Shah P, Bajaj S, Shamoon F. Aortic dissection caused by percutaneous coronary intervention: 2 new case reports and Detailed analysis of 86 Previous cases. Tex Heart Inst J 2016;43(1):52–60. https://doi.org/10.14503/THIJ-14-4585.
13. Dunning DW, Kahn JK, Hawkins ET, et al. Iatrogenic coronary artery dissections extending into and involving the aortic root. Catheter Cardiovasc Interv 2000;51(4):387–93.
14. Sheikh AS, Ali K, Mazhar S. Acute aortic syndrome. Circulation 2013;128(10):1122–7. https://doi.org/10.1161/CIRCULATIONAHA.112.000170.
15. Heistad DD, Armstrong ML. Sick vessel syndrome. Can atherosclerotic arteries recover? Circulation 1994;89(5):2447–50. https://doi.org/10.1161/01.cir.89.5.2447.
16. Sundt TM. Intramural hematoma and penetrating aortic ulcer. Curr Opin Cardiol 2007;22(6):504–9. https://doi.org/10.1097/HCO.0b013e3282f0fd72.
17. Sundt TM 3rd. Residual strain in the aorta. J Thorac Cardiovasc Surg 2006;131(6):1420–1. https://doi.org/10.1016/j.jtcvs.2005.12.070. author reply 1421-2.
18. Wilson SK, Hutchins GM. Aortic dissecting aneurysms: causative factors in 204 subjects. Arch Pathol Lab Med 1982;106(4):175–80.
19. Stanson AW, Kazmier FJ, Hollier LH, et al. Penetrating atherosclerotic ulcers of the thoracic aorta: natural history and clinicopathologic correlations. Ann Vasc Surg 1986;1(1):15–23. https://doi.org/10.1016/S0890-5096(06)60697-3.
20. Azizzadeh A, Keyhani K, Miller CC 3rd, et al. Blunt traumatic aortic injury: initial experience with endovascular repair. J Vasc Surg 2009;49(6):1403–8. https://doi.org/10.1016/j.jvs.2009.02.234.

21. Warner DL, Bhamidipati CM, Abraham CZ. Management of penetrating aortic ulcer and intramural hematoma in the thoracic aorta. Indian J Thorac Cardiovasc Surg 2022;38(Suppl 1):198–203. https://doi.org/10.1007/s12055-022-01332-3.

22. Pearson R, Philips N, Hancock R, et al. Regional wall mechanics and blunt traumatic aortic rupture at the isthmus. Eur J Cardiothorac Surg 2008;34(3):616–22. https://doi.org/10.1016/j.ejcts.2008.03.069.

23. Nienaber CA, Clough RE. Management of acute aortic dissection. Lancet 2015;385(9970):800–11. https://doi.org/10.1016/S0140-6736(14)61005-9.

24. Booher AM, Isselbacher EM, Nienaber CA, et al. The IRAD classification system for characterizing survival after aortic dissection. Am J Med 2013;126(8):730. https://doi.org/10.1016/j.amjmed.2013.01.020. e19-24.

25. Pape LA, Awais M, Woznicki EM, et al. Presentation, diagnosis, and outcomes of acute aortic dissection: 17-Year Trends from the international registry of acute aortic dissection. J Am Coll Cardiol 2015;66(4):350–8. https://doi.org/10.1016/j.jacc.2015.05.029.

26. Tsai TT, Nienaber CA, Eagle KA. Acute aortic syndromes. Circulation 2005;112(24):3802–13. https://doi.org/10.1161/CIRCULATIONAHA.105.534198.

27. Harris KM, Braverman AC, Eagle KA, et al. Acute aortic intramural hematoma: an analysis from the international registry of acute aortic dissection. Circulation 2012;126(11 Suppl 1):S91–6. https://doi.org/10.1161/CIRCULATIONAHA.111.084541.

28. Evangelista A, Maldonado G, Moral S, et al. Intramural hematoma and penetrating ulcer in the descending aorta: differences and similarities. Ann Cardiothorac Surg 2019;8(4):456–70. https://doi.org/10.21037/acs.2019.07.05.

29. Evangelista A, Mukherjee D, Mehta RH, et al. Acute intramural hematoma of the aorta: a mystery in evolution. Circulation 2005;111(8):1063–70. https://doi.org/10.1161/01.CIR.0000156444.26393.80.

30. Evangelista A, Dominguez R, Sebastia C, et al. Prognostic value of clinical and morphologic findings in short-term evolution of aortic intramural haematoma. Therapeutic implications. Eur Heart J 2004;25(1):81–7. https://doi.org/10.1016/j.ehj.2003.10.011.

31. Maraj R, Rerkpattanapipat P, Jacobs LE, et al. Meta-analysis of 143 reported cases of aortic intramural hematoma. Am J Cardiol 2000;86(6):664–8. https://doi.org/10.1016/s0002-9149(00)01049-3.

32. Nienaber CA, Richartz BM, Rehders T, et al. Aortic intramural haematoma: natural history and predictive factors for complications. Heart 2004;90(4):372–4. https://doi.org/10.1136/hrt.2003.027615.

33. Evangelista A, Czerny M, Nienaber C, et al. Interdisciplinary expert consensus on management of type B intramural haematoma and penetrating aortic ulcer. Eur J Cardiothorac Surg 2015;47(2):209–17. https://doi.org/10.1093/ejcts/ezu386.

34. DeMartino RR, Sen I, Huang Y, et al. Population-based assessment of the incidence of aortic dissection, intramural hematoma, and penetrating ulcer, and its associated mortality from 1995 to 2015. Circ Cardiovasc Qual Outcomes 2018;11(8):e004689. https://doi.org/10.1161/CIRCOUTCOMES.118.004689.

35. DeCarlo C, Latz CA, Boitano LT, et al. Prognostication of asymptomatic penetrating aortic ulcers: a modern approach. Circulation 2021;144(14):1091–101. https://doi.org/10.1161/CIRCULATIONAHA.121.054710.

36. Hirst AE Jr, Barbour BH. Dissecting aneurysm with hemopericardium; report of a case with healing. N Engl J Med 1958;258(3):116–20. https://doi.org/10.1056/NEJM195801162580303.

37. Mouawad NJ, Paulisin J, Hofmeister S, et al. Blunt thoracic aortic injury - concepts and management. J Cardiothorac Surg 2020;15(1):62. https://doi.org/10.1186/s13019-020-01101-6.

38. Schulman CI, Carvajal D, Lopez PP, et al. Incidence and crash mechanisms of aortic injury during the past decade. J Trauma 2007;62(3):664–7. https://doi.org/10.1097/TA.0b013e318031b58c.

39. Takagi H, Kawai N, Umemoto T. A meta-analysis of comparative studies of endovascular versus open repair for blunt thoracic aortic injury. J Thorac Cardiovasc Surg 2008;135(6):1392–4. https://doi.org/10.1016/j.jtcvs.2008.01.033.

40. Hagan PG, Nienaber CA, Isselbacher EM, et al. The international registry of acute aortic dissection (IRAD): new insights into an old disease. JAMA 2000;283(7):897–903. https://doi.org/10.1001/jama.283.7.897.

41. Crawford TC, Beaulieu RJ, Ehlert BA, et al. Malperfusion syndromes in aortic dissections. Vasc Med 2016;21(3):264–73. https://doi.org/10.1177/1358863X15625371.

42. Isselbacher EM, Cigarroa JE, Eagle KA. Cardiac tamponade complicating proximal aortic dissection. Is pericardiocentesis harmful? Circulation 1994;90(5):2375–8. https://doi.org/10.1161/01.cir.90.5.2375.

43. Hayashi T, Tsukube T, Yamashita T, et al. Impact of controlled pericardial drainage on critical cardiac tamponade with acute type A aortic dissection. Circulation 2012;126(11 Suppl 1):S97–101. https://doi.org/10.1161/CIRCULATIONAHA.111.082685.

44. Luo JL, Wu CK, Lin YH, et al. Type A aortic dissection manifesting as acute myocardial infarction: still a lesson to learn. Acta Cardiol 2009;64(4):499–504. https://doi.org/10.2143/AC.64.4.2041615.

45. Kawahito K, Adachi H, Murata S, et al. Coronary malperfusion due to type A aortic dissection: mechanism and surgical management. Ann Thorac Surg

2003;76(5):1471–6. https://doi.org/10.1016/s0003-4975(03)00899-3. discussion 1476.

46. Watanabe H, Horita N, Shibata Y, et al. Diagnostic test accuracy of D-dimer for acute aortic syndrome: systematic review and meta-analysis of 22 studies with 5000 subjects. Sci Rep 2016;6:26893. https://doi.org/10.1038/srep26893.

47. Cui JS, Jing ZP, Zhuang SJ, et al. D-dimer as a biomarker for acute aortic dissection: a systematic review and meta-analysis. Medicine (Baltimore) 2015;94(4):e471. https://doi.org/10.1097/MD.0000000000000471.

48. Asha SE, Miers JW. A systematic review and meta-analysis of D-dimer as a rule-out test for suspected acute aortic dissection. Ann Emerg Med 2015;66(4):368–78. https://doi.org/10.1016/j.annemergmed.2015.02.013.

49. Suzuki T, Bossone E, Sawaki D, et al. Biomarkers of aortic diseases. Am Heart J 2013;165(1):15–25. https://doi.org/10.1016/j.ahj.2012.10.006.

50. Gorla R, Erbel R, Kahlert P, et al. Diagnostic role and prognostic implications of D-dimer in different classes of acute aortic syndromes. Eur Heart J Acute Cardiovasc Care 2017;6(5):379–88. https://doi.org/10.1177/2048872615594500.

51. Litmanovich D, Bankier AA, Cantin L, et al. CT and MRI in diseases of the aorta. AJR Am J Roentgenol 2009;193(4):928–40. https://doi.org/10.2214/AJR.08.2166.

52. Johnson TR, Nikolaou K, Wintersperger BJ, et al. ECG-gated 64-MDCT angiography in the differential diagnosis of acute chest pain. AJR Am J Roentgenol 2007;188(1):76–82. https://doi.org/10.2214/AJR.05.1153.

53. Ayaram D, Bellolio MF, Murad MH, et al. Triple rule-out computed tomographic angiography for chest pain: a diagnostic systematic review and meta-analysis. Acad Emerg Med 2013;20(9):861–71. https://doi.org/10.1111/acem.12210.

54. Nienaber CA, von Kodolitsch Y, Nicolas V, et al. The diagnosis of thoracic aortic dissection by noninvasive imaging procedures. N Engl J Med 1993;328(1):1–9. https://doi.org/10.1056/NEJM199301073280101.

55. Sakamoto I, Sueyoshi E, Uetani M. MR imaging of the aorta. Radiol Clin North Am 2007;45(3):485–97. https://doi.org/10.1016/j.rcl.2007.04.007, viii.

56. Wagner S, Auffermann W, Buser P, et al. Diagnostic accuracy and estimation of the severity of valvular regurgitation from the signal void on cine magnetic resonance images. Am Heart J 1989;118(4):760–7. https://doi.org/10.1016/0002-8703(89)90590-5.

57. van Rossum AC, Post JC, Visser CA. Coronary imaging using MRI. Herz 1996;21(2):97–105.

58. Neskovic AN, Hagendorff A, Lancellotti P, et al. Emergency echocardiography: the European association of cardiovascular imaging recommendations. Eur Heart J Cardiovasc Imaging 2013;14(1):1–11. https://doi.org/10.1093/ehjci/jes193.

59. Rogers AM, Hermann LK, Booher AM, et al. Sensitivity of the aortic dissection detection risk score, a novel guideline-based tool for identification of acute aortic dissection at initial presentation: results from the international registry of acute aortic dissection. Circulation 2011;123(20):2213–8. https://doi.org/10.1161/CIRCULATIONAHA.110.988568.

60. Beckmann E, Grau JB, Sainger R, et al. Insights into the use of biomarkers in calcific aortic valve disease. J Heart Valve Dis 2010;19(4):441–52.

61. Nazerian P, Mueller C, Soeiro AM, et al. Diagnostic accuracy of the aortic dissection detection risk score plus D-dimer for acute aortic syndromes: the ADvISED Prospective Multicenter study. Circulation 2018;137(3):250–8. https://doi.org/10.1161/CIRCULATIONAHA.117.029457.

62. van Baardwijk C, Roach MR. Factors in the propagation of aortic dissections in canine thoracic aortas. J Biomech 1987;20(1):67–73. https://doi.org/10.1016/0021-9290(87)90268-5.

63. Braverman AC. Acute aortic dissection: clinician update. Circulation 2010;122(2):184–8. https://doi.org/10.1161/CIRCULATIONAHA.110.958975.

64. Alviar CL, Gutierrez A, Cho L, et al. Clevidipine as a therapeutic and cost-effective alternative to sodium nitroprusside in patients with acute aortic syndromes. Eur Heart J Acute Cardiovasc Care 2020;9(3_suppl):S5–12. https://doi.org/10.1177/2048872618777919.

65. Ulici A, Jancik J, Lam TS, et al. Clevidipine versus sodium nitroprusside in acute aortic dissection: a retrospective chart review. Am J Emerg Med 2017;35(10):1514–8. https://doi.org/10.1016/j.ajem.2017.06.030.

66. Kim KH, Moon IS, Park JS, et al. Nicardipine hydrochloride injectable phase IV open-label clinical trial: study on the anti-hypertensive effect and safety of nicardipine for acute aortic dissection. J Int Med Res 2002;30(3):337–45. https://doi.org/10.1177/147323000203000318.

67. Suzuki T, Mehta RH, Ince H, et al. Clinical profiles and outcomes of acute type B aortic dissection in the current era: lessons from the International Registry of Aortic Dissection (IRAD). Circulation 2003;108(Suppl 1). II312–II317. 10.1161/01.cir.0000087386.07204.09.

68. Estrera AL, Miller CC 3rd, Safi HJ, et al. Outcomes of medical management of acute type B aortic dissection. Circulation 2006;114(1 Suppl):I384–9. https://doi.org/10.1161/CIRCULATIONAHA.105.001479.

69. Umana JP, Lai DT, Mitchell RS, et al. Is medical therapy still the optimal treatment strategy for patients with acute type B aortic dissections? J Thorac Cardiovasc Surg 2002;124(5):896–910. https://doi.org/10.1067/mtc.2002.123131.

70. Schwartz SI, Durham C, Clouse WD, et al. Predictors of late aortic intervention in patients with medically treated type B aortic dissection. J Vasc Surg 2018; 67(1):78–84. https://doi.org/10.1016/j.jvs.2017.05.128.

71. Trimarchi S, Eagle KA, Nienaber CA, et al. Importance of refractory pain and hypertension in acute type B aortic dissection: insights from the International Registry of Acute Aortic Dissection (IRAD). Circulation 2010;122(13):1283–9. https://doi.org/10.1161/CIRCULATIONAHA.109.929422.

72. Kim WK, Park SJ, Kim HJ, et al. The fate of unrepaired chronic type A aortic dissection. J Thorac Cardiovasc Surg 2019;158(4):996–1004 e3. https://doi.org/10.1016/j.jtcvs.2018.11.021.

73. Chikwe J, Cavallaro P, Itagaki S, et al. National outcomes in acute aortic dissection: influence of surgeon and institutional volume on operative mortality. Ann Thorac Surg 2013;95(5):1563–9. https://doi.org/10.1016/j.athoracsur.2013.02.039.

74. Aggarwal B, Raymond C, Jacob J, et al. Transfer of patients with suspected acute aortic syndrome. Am J Cardiol 2013;112(3):430–5. https://doi.org/10.1016/j.amjcard.2013.03.049.

75. Goldstone AB, Chiu P, Baiocchi M, et al. Interfacility transfer of Medicare Beneficiaries with acute type A aortic dissection and Regionalization of care in the United States. Circulation 2019;140(15):1239–50. https://doi.org/10.1161/CIRCULATIONAHA.118.038867.

76. Schoenhagen P, Roselli EE, Harris CM, et al. Online network of subspecialty aortic disease experts: Impact of "cloud" technology on management of acute aortic emergencies. J Thorac Cardiovasc Surg 2016;152(1):39–42. https://doi.org/10.1016/j.jtcvs.2016.02.057.

77. Winsor G, Thomas SH, Biddinger PD, et al. Inadequate hemodynamic management in patients undergoing interfacility transfer for suspected aortic dissection. Am J Emerg Med 2005;23(1):24–9. https://doi.org/10.1016/j.ajem.2004.01.008.

Intermediate-Risk and High-Risk Pulmonary Embolism: Recognition and Management

Cardiology Clinics: Cardiac Emergencies

Drew A. Birrenkott, MD, DPhil[a,b], Christopher Kabrhel, MD, MPH[a,b], David M. Dudzinski, MD[b,c,d],*

KEYWORDS

- Pulmonary embolism • Risk stratification • Thrombolysis • Catheter-directed therapy
- Pulmonary embolism response team (PERT)

KEY POINTS

- Pulmonary embolism risk-stratification is dependent on identifying evidence of right ventricle dysfunction, by imaging and by biomarkers.
- The highest risk PE patients need urgent and definitive therapy to support hemodynamics and to clear the pulmonary artery of clots.
- There are limited randomized and comparative effectiveness data to rigorously choose 1 interventional PE therapy over another.
- Intermediate risk PE patients represent a management challenge, in that some of these patients will experience clinical deterioration, and the ultimate hope is to identify such patients and consider definitive PE therapy early.
- Pulmonary embolism response teams (PERT) are essential in contemporary practice to individualize care and decision-making, by marshaling the combined experiences of clinicians with specialized expertise in PE.

INTRODUCTION AND NATURE OF THE PROBLEM OF PULMONARY EMBOLISM

Pulmonary embolism (PE) remains both difficult to diagnose and complex to treat despite over 50 years of recognition as a cause of significant morbidity and mortality.[1] Behind ischemic heart disease and stroke, PE is the third leading cause of cardiovascular death worldwide.[2,3]

The estimated annual population incidence of venous thromboembolism (VTE), including PE, ranges from 0.2 to 1.1 per 1000.[4–7] While the incidence of PE is low in younger populations, the incidence increases approximately 8-fold between the fourth decade and the eighth decade of life.[8,9] In addition, longitudinal data suggest that the annual incidence of PE is increasing, and the 1% to 3% of hospitalized patients with PEs who are in shock or ventilator-dependent have approximately 10-fold higher case fatality rates.[10–14] While not completely explained, this observed increase is likely multifactorial, including more

[a] Department of Emergency Medicine, Massachusetts General Hospital, 55 Fruit Street, Boston, MA 02114, USA; [b] Center for Vascular Emergencies, Massachusetts General Hospital, 55 Fruit Street, Boston, MA 02114, USA; [c] Division of Cardiology, Massachusetts General Hospital, 55 Fruit Street, Boston, MA 02114, USA; [d] Cardiac Intensive Care Unit, Massachusetts General Hospital, 55 Fruit Street, Boston, MA 02114, USA
* Corresponding author. Division of Cardiology, Massachusetts General Hospital, 55 Fruit Street, Boston, MA 02114.
E-mail address: ddudzinski@partners.org

Cardiol Clin 42 (2024) 215–235
https://doi.org/10.1016/j.ccl.2024.02.008

sensitive imaging modalities (computed tomographic pulmonary angiography [CTPA]), and an increase in the number of individuals with severe comorbidities associated with developing PEs.[10,15–19]

The spectrum in PE ranges from asymptomatic to hemodynamic instability and right-sided heart failure.[20] PE represents obstruction of the pulmonary artery, and can be caused by multiple sources including tumors, fat, air, amniotic fluid, and septic emboli, though the vast majority are thromboembolic—the focus of this review.[21] VTE, including PE, develop secondary to factors known as Virchow triad: stasis in blood flow, endothelial injury, and hypercoagulability, either inherited or acquired.[22] The majority of PEs are caused by embolization of a deep venous thrombosis (DVT).[9] Acute PE results in abnormal gas exchange and circulation whereas mortality in PE is caused by increased right ventricular (RV) afterload causing a cascade leading to obstructive shock and death.[10]

Acute PE has been stratified into 3 categories: high-risk (formerly massive), intermediate-risk (formerly submassive), and low-risk based on both imaging findings and patient characteristics. High-risk PE is defined by sustained hypotension (systolic blood pressure [SBP] < 90 mm Hg) for at least 15 minutes or a vasopressor requirement where there is no other reasonable explanation for shock.[23,24] Intermediate-low risk PE is defined by evidence of imaging RV dysfunction or biomarker evidence (myocardial necrosis or chamber dilatation) in the absence of sustained hypotension.[10,24] A subcategory of intermediate-high risk PE features patients with both imaging *and* biomarker evidence of RV dysfunction. Low-risk PE does not meet the classification criteria for a high-risk or intermediate-risk PE.[10,24]

The goal of this review is to outline recent advances in the recognition and management of the intermediate-risk and high-risk PEs.

RECOGNITION: DIAGNOSIS AND PROGNOSIS

PE represents the double-edged sword of being a clinical diagnosis that is over-tested yet often missed. One study found that 5.3% of all emergency department (ED) patients had a diagnostic study for PE.[25,26] Despite this, in a systematic review of diagnostic errors, PE was found to be the second highest missed diagnosis behind cancer.[27] Another systematic review characterizing the missed diagnosis of PE found that 27.5% of the ED patients and 53.6% of the hospital inpatients with PE were misdiagnosed with other medical conditions including respiratory infections,

heart failure, and acute coronary syndrome.[28] Furthermore, it was found that 37.9% of the patients who die in the intensive care unit and subsequently undergo autopsy had PEs.[28] This paradox in the clinical recognition of PE largely stems from the broad spectrum of clinical presentations ranging from asymptomatic to obstructive shock and protean symptomatology that mimics other cardiopulmonary pathologies.

History and Physical Examination

Diagnostic assessment of PE should focus on determining pre-test probability, to determine if further objective testing for PE is warranted. Accurate assessment of pre-test probability for PE relies on patient's risk factors, predisposing conditions, and the physical examination.

Approximately 60% of patients who present with VTE have a known predisposing factor.[10,29] The strongest predisposing factors include prior VTE, lower limb fractures, hip or knee replacements, major trauma, history of myocardial infarction in the last 3 months, or hospitalization for atrial dysrhythmia or heart failure within the last 3 months.[10,30–32] There are many moderate risk factors including history of cancer, obesity, diabetes mellitus, pregnancy, oral contraceptive therapy, bed rest > 3 days, and prolonged immobilization.[10,30–32] Overall incidence of VTE is higher in men compared to women. However, women under 45 and over 80 years of age are more likely to develop VTE compared to men in the same age categories. It is hypothesized that these trends are most likely secondary due to increased VTE risk with oral contraception use and pregnancy in younger women and the overall increased life expectancy for women compared to men.[9,33]

The most common signs and symptoms of PE include dyspnea (with or without exertion), pleuritic chest pain, cough, lower extremity swelling, tachypnea, and tachycardia (**Table 1**).[34] Dyspnea, chest pain, and hemoptysis—considered a classic triad of PE symptoms—occur in only 5% to 7% of patients with PE.[35]

In 67% of cases, onset of PE-related dyspnea occurs within seconds to minutes.[34] One of the more challenging symptoms associated with PE is syncope. One study estimated the prevalence of PE in hospitalized patients with first-time syncope to be as high as 17.3%, while a subsequent study found the prevalence of all VTEs in patients with first-time syncope admitted to the hospital to be only 1.4%.[36,37] Furthermore, a study of patients presenting to the ED with first time-syncope, regardless of hospitalization, found the prevalence of PE to range from 0.06% to

Table 1
Signs and symptoms of pulmonary embolism[34]

Symptoms	
Dyspnea	79%
Pleuritic Chest Pain	47%
Cough	43%
Calf or Thigh Swelling	39%
Wheezing	31%
Non-pleuritic Chest Pain	17%
Calf or Thigh Pain	16%
Signs	
Tachypnea (≥20/min)	57%
Tachycardia (>100/min)	26%
Decreased Breath Sounds	21%
Rales (Crackles)	21%
Increased P2 Heart Sound	15%
Jugular Venous Distension	13%

0.55%.[38] While syncope is not a common presenting symptom, PE should be considered in patients with syncope, and it may be a marker of higher PE risk.

Other manifestations like cough, fever, or diaphoresis may represent sequelae of pulmonary infarction with pleuritis.[39,40]

Clinical Decision Rules and Algorithms

While experienced clinicians have been shown to be effective at determining a patient's pre-test probability for PE based on history, presentation, and laboratory findings alone, clinical decision rules derived from large patient cohorts have supplanted clinical gestalt, and can help inform the need for more testing.[41] The most commonly used and most widely tested PE clinical decision rules include the Wells' Criteria, the YEARS Algorithm, the Revised Geneva Score, and the Pulmonary Embolism Rule out Criteria (PERC) Rule.[42–45]

The Wells' Criteria is a points-based algorithm which assigns patients into 3 probability groups.[46] In an ED population, the incidence of PE was 1.3% in the low probability group, 16.2% in the medium probability group, and 40.6% in the high probability group.[42] In patients with low Wells' pre-test probability, a negative D-dimer assay effectively rules out PE but a positive D-dimer requires definitive diagnostic imaging. All patients with medium or high pre-test probability of PE require definitive diagnostic imaging without consideration of a D-dimer assay.[42] The Wells' Criteria has been well-validated and has several validated variations including the simplified Wells' Criteria.[47–49]

The YEARS Algorithm is a 2-step algorithm that requires consideration of pre-test probability for PE and D-dimer testing. The pre-test probability for PE is based on 3 clinical features: clinical signs of a DVT, hemoptysis, and PE as the most likely diagnosis. If none of these features are present and the patient's D-dimer is <1000 ng/mL, PE can be excluded. If any of these features are present and the patient's D-dimer is <500 ng/mL, PE can also be excluded. If neither of these scenarios is true, the patient requires definitive diagnostic imaging.[45] In this study, PE was detected in 3.2% of the patients with 0 YEARS criteria and 23% of patients with 1 or more YEARS criteria. When the YEARS algorithm was applied in the initial study set, 48% of the patients could be ruled out for PE without definitive diagnostic imaging compared to 34% of the same population when the Wells' Criteria was applied.[45] Performance of the YEARS algorithm has been well-validated.[50,51] More recent work has attempted to adapt the YEARS Algorithm for pregnant patients, a population which has been previously excluded from all PE clinical decision rules.[52]

The revised Geneva Score is a modified version of the Geneva Score, which does not require evaluation with arterial blood gas or chest x-ray prior to determining pre-test probability for PE.[43,53] Unlike the Wells' Criteria and YEARS Algorithm, the revised Geneva Score does not incorporate subjective measurements such as the clinical gestalt of likelihood of PE as a diagnosis. Within a validation cohort, 7.9% of the patients had a PE in the low probability group, 28.5% in the intermediate probability group, and 73.7% in the high probability group.[43] Patients in the low and moderate probability groups had D-dimer testing which ruled out PE if the value was < 500 ng/mL and was followed by definitive diagnostic imaging if the value was ≥500 ng/mL. Patients in the high probability group received definitive diagnostic imaging.[43] The revised Geneva score has been well-validated through several trials; however, a study has shown that clinical gestalt alone is superior.[48,54,55]

Unlike the Wells' Criteria, YEARS Algorithm, and revised Geneva Score, the PERC rule aims to rule out PE without any diagnostic testing if 8 binary features are all negative.[11,56–58] A variation on the PERC rule for patients presenting at altitudes > 4000 ft (1219 m) where the O_2 saturation cut-off is decreased from < 95% to <90% had a slightly decreased sensitivity.[59,60]

These prediction rules are likely most helpful for excluding PE, including low-risk, while high-risk PE will be clinically overt, and in contemporary EDs, the patient with protean cardiopulmonary symptoms will likely already have had biomarkers and electrocardiogram done before being fully evaluated by an ED physician.

Laboratory Studies

Laboratory testing in the diagnosis of PE primarily focuses on the quantitative D-dimer. The D-dimer molecule is generated alongside the coagulation cascade as breakdown product of fibrin in fibrinolysis.[61] Thus, presence of D-dimer in the bloodstream can indicate the presence of intravascular coagulation and conversely low D-dimer levels are suggestive of the absence of DVT and PE.[61] The D-dimer assay is highly sensitive, but poorly specific, using the Food and Drug Administration D-dimer cut-off of 500 ng/mL. Based on this cut-off, PE can be ruled out in patients with a probability < 2% with an already low pre-test probability based on a clinical decision rule.[62] More recently, an age-adjusted D-dimer cut-off has been established where the age-specific D-dimer cut-off is age multiplied by 10 ng/mL when age > 50, or 500 ng/mL for age < 50.[63,64] The use of the age-adjusted D-dimer has been validated for use in conjunction with the Wells' Criteria, YEARS Algorithm, and the revised Geneva Score for determining pre-test probability.[51,65]

In addition to D-dimer, other laboratory tests including arterial blood gas, lactate, cardiac troponins, and brain natriuretic peptide have been studied as possible markers of PE. While none of these are diagnostically useful, they can potentially serve as markers of prognosis and risk-stratification.[10,53,66–87]

Electrocardiogram

The EKG is neither sensitive nor specific for the diagnosis of PE.[72,73] and over one-quarter of patients with PE may have no EKG changes.[74] EKG changes seen in PE occur secondary to the development of acute RV dysfunction meaning any condition that can cause acute RV dysfunction can mimic EKG patterns associated with PE. EKG findings that have been associated with PE include tachyarrhythmias (sinus tachycardia, atrial fibrillation), right bundle branch block (RBBB), right-sided axis deviation, nonspecific ST changes, T-wave inversions (in particular in early precordial or less commonly inferior leads), and the $S_1Q_3T_3$ sign, among others.[75–86] However, only sinus tachycardia and an incomplete RBBB were found to be statistically significantly more likely in patients diagnosed with PE.[72] EKG indicia of right heart strain may be considered with biomarker and imaging data as evidence toward intermediate-risk stratification.[24,73]

Imaging

Diagnostic imaging is the primary means of both diagnosing PE and determining its severity.[24,72,88] The definitive diagnosis of PE is contemporarily made using either CTPA, with other modalities like ventilation/perfusion (V/Q) lung scintigraphy less commonly used if for example, renal dysfunction precludes iodinated contrast. Transthoracic echocardiography (TTE) has insufficient sensitivity for excluding PE, but is essential in risk-stratification; TTE may have roles as an adjunct diagnostic in patients with renal dysfunction or critically ill patients who cannot travel to a CT scanner. In this manner, leg ultrasound has positive predictive value when a DVT is identified in a patient with high pre-test probability of PE. Chest radiograph (CXR), while not diagnostically useful in ruling in a PE can be critical in ruling out other causes of PE-like symptoms. Finally, magnetic resonance angiography (MRA), while not yet clinically validated for diagnosing PE, has shown promise in some investigations, though the duration of the study may preclude patients with possible instability.

Transthoracic echocardiography

Due to increased pulmonary vascular resistance (PVR), echocardiographic signs of RV overload and dysfunction can manifest in acute PE.[10,24,87] Due to complex 3D RV geometry and retrosternal location, no single echocardiographic measure of RV function has been found to be reliable in isolation.[10] The most commonly described ultrasonographic measures for evaluating RV overload and dysfunction include increased RV to left ventricle (LV) linear ratio,[88] abnormal septal wall motion (flattening or bowing of the RV into the LV), McConnell sign (diffuse RV hypokinesis with apical sparing), tricuspid regurgitation (TR), decreased tricuspid annular plane systolic excursion (TAPSE), decreased systolic excursion velocity of the RV basal free wall (S'), pulmonary artery Doppler systolic notching, and decreased RV free wall strain.[89,91] A systematic review found that measures of RV strain are generally specific, with no sign having a specificity < 80%, though some signs are seen with acute RV myocardial infarction. As signs are poorly sensitive, these ultrasonographic findings should be considered "rule in" tests as opposed to PE "rule out" tests.[92]

Finding clot-in-transit (CIT) virtually confirms pulmonary VTE; however, this finding is relatively rare in all PE patients (~4-8%).[93,94] In patients with PE, CIT is associated with increased morbidity and mortality with morality rates ranging from 80% to 100% if left untreated.[94–97]

The overall sensitivity for PE diagnosis by TTE is approximately 50% to 70%, and some of the markers above which are mainly for prognosis can be marshaled to not only assist in diagnosis by suggesting that a presenting syndrome is due to PE rather than another pulmonary or left heart cause including cardiac tamponade, hypovolemia, acute valvular dysfunction, aortic dissection, and LV dysfunction, but also quickly evaluate for evidence of significant right heart dilatation and dysfunction.[10]

TTE remains important in contemporary PE-risk stratification by sorting patients among intermediate-high, intermediate-low, and low-risk.[10] Normotensive acute PE with echocardiographic evidence of RV dysfunction would meet classification as an intermediate-risk PE.[24,98–100] Evolving metrics of ventricular-vascular uncoupling, including a ratio describing RV-pulmonary artery coupling (such as TAPSE/Pulmonary Arterial Systolic Pressure (PASP)), are showing promise not only in PE but also in other states of RV afterload.[101] One caveat when using TTE, or any modality, is that the chronicity of findings is unknown, and that chamber dilatation, TR, elevated RV systolic pressure, or chamber dysfunction could be chronic and secondary to intrinsic heart disease or chronic lung disease.[71,102]

Additionally, in patients with a high-probability of PE who are unstable and where CTPA is unattainable, TTE demonstrating signs of RV pressure overload without other obvious cause of RV overload should be considered for reperfusion therapy.[10,90,103,104]

Chest radiograph
Overall, changes in the CXR due to PE are both poorly sensitive and specific and are not routinely required specifically for the diagnosis of PE.[52,105,106] Previous work has found that the CXR is normal in 25% of patients with PE, with the 3 most common abnormal radiograph findings: cardiomegaly (27%), pleural effusion (23%), and elevated hemidiaphragm (20%).[106] Additionally, several CXR findings can be seen due to pulmonary infarct from PE: Hampton hump (a dome-shaped pleural opacification), Westermark sign (peripheral oligemia, due to pulmonary artery obstruction), atelectasis, and pleural effusion.[105,107–109] Of course, all of these findings are better evaluated with CT.[105,110] CXR still however has value in the urgent evaluation: first, for diagnosing alternative causes of symptoms including pneumothorax, pneumonia, and heart failure,[111] and second, a normal CXR is useful in assessing the utility of ventilation/perfusion (V/Q) scanning.

V/Q scanning is a reasonable alternative to CTPA when the CXR is normal, but when the CXR is abnormal, V/Q is inferior to CTPA.[111]

Computed tomographic pulmonary angiogram
The gold standard for diagnosis of PE is contrast-enhanced multidetector CTPA.[10] In most cases, CTPA is able to evaluate for evidence of PE to the level of the subsegmental pulmonary vessels.[10,112] The Prospective Investigation of Pulmonary Embolism Diagnosis II (PIOPED-II) trial found that the sensitivity and specificity for PE in a multidetector CTPA was 83% and 96%, respectively,[113] though the sensitivity value has only increased over time with advances in CT technology. When considering low and intermediate pretest probability for PE, the negative predictive value (NPV) for PE was 96% and 89%, respectively, while the positive predictive value (PPV) was 58% and 92%, respectively. This is compared to a high pre-test probability where the NPV is 60% and the PPV is 96%.[113] These data suggest that a negative CTPA in a low-risk and intermediate-risk patient essentially rules out PE while a negative CTPA in patient with high pre-test probability or high clinical suspicion may warrant additional evaluation.[113]

In addition to its front-line diagnostic role, CTPA may be simultaneously useful in risk-stratifying for intermediate-risk PE.[24] CTPA may manifest signs analogous to echocardiography including chamber dilatation, interventricular septal bowing, and contrast reflux to the inferior vena cava (suggesting substantial TR). TTE may have better test characteristics for signs of RV dysfunction and strain, with CT similarly sensitive, though less specific.[114,115] Evidence of RV strain on CTPA confers an increased risk for short-term adverse outcomes.[114,116,117] When coupled with TTE, the predictive value for negative outcomes from CTPA increases, suggesting that when evaluating for RV strain, CTPA with TTE is possibly useful for guiding treatment decisions.[114]

Multiple investigations have also assessed metrics of CTPA "clot burden" to predict PE severity; however, these in general do not correlate with the hemodynamic and cardiopulmonary sequelae of PE, and can be cumbersome to calculate in clinical use.

Ventilation/perfusion lung scintigraphy
Using inhaled radioactive tracers, ventilation/perfusion lung scintigraphy (V/Q scan) assesses ventilation and perfusion mismatch, which gives evidence of pulmonary artery obstruction.[10] A primary benefit of V/Q scanning is that it does not require iodinated contrast media and therefore

offers a method to evaluate for PE in patients with anaphylaxis to contrast media or renal failure.[10,118,119] A study comparing CTPA and V/Q scan found both to be equivalent in ruling out clinically significant PE; however, it also found that CTPA diagnosed more PEs.[120] Notably, results of the V/Q scan are reported as positive, negative, and non-diagnostic.[121] One of the challenges of V/Q scanning is that up to 50% of studies are reported as inconclusive or non-diagnostic, thus requiring further diagnostic evaluation.[10] In addition, unlike CTPA, V/Q scanning is less readily available and has higher interobserver interpretation variability.[10] This modality has now been mostly replaced by CTPA except in select instances, such as pregnant women.

Magnetic resonance angiography

The possibility of magnetic resonance angiography (MRA) for PE diagnosis is of interest as there is no associated radiation exposure and it uses gadolinium-based contrast instead of iodinated contrast.[122] However, in several studies, MRA has generally been shown to have a large number of inconclusive or inadequate studies (up to 25%), and low sensitivity,[123,124] with higher sensitivity for proximal PE but more inconclusive for distal PE.[123] Nevertheless, among patients who were evaluated with MRA for PE, a study found that the NPV of 97% and 96% at 3 month and 1 year, respectively, was equivalent with CTPA.[125] While this suggests that MRA may be less effective at evaluating for distal PEs, these may not be a clinically significant finding; however, at present, MRA is not used in the contemporary evaluation of PE.

MANAGEMENT OF INTERMEDIATE-HIGH AND HIGH-RISK PULMONARY EMBOLISM
Delineating Intermediate-Risk and High-Risk Pulmonary Embolism

The management and appropriate therapeutic strategy for diagnosed acute PE depends on severity. Risk-stratification is thus essential to align treatments with clinical scenarios, in order to properly balance PE risk with expected treatment benefits and risk.

High-risk PE includes those with sustained hypotension or vasopressor requirements, as well as those with cardiac arrest or severe arrhythmia, or rapid respiratory failure; such patients generally are clinically manifest, without the need for specific rules or other prognostic information.[88,94] These are the rarest presentations of PE but mandate emergent response in terms of cardiopulmonary stabilization and clearing of PE from the pulmonary arterial tree, which can include considerations like extracorporeal

membrane oxygenation (ECMO) and surgical and percutaneous thrombectomy.[10,24,87]

Low-risk PE represents the most common PE phenotype, and a class of patients that generally experiences good outcomes with anticoagulation alone.

The intermediate-risk PE category, those patients without vital sign instability, but varying levels of imaging evidence of RV dysfunction, or biomarkers indicating myocardial necrosis or chamber dilatation, represent a clinical conundrum in contemporary care.[23,24] The intermediate-low risk stratum, akin to lower-risk PE, generally do well with anticoagulation. However, of normotensive PE patients with the highest evidence of PE-related RV dysfunction by biomarkers and imaging (intermediate-high risk), approximately 10% will experience cardiopulmonary deterioration and thereby require more emergent, and advanced PE-debulking therapies. Identifying these intermediate-risk PE patients who are in jeopardy of deterioration is the "holy grail" of modern risk stratification, so that the inherent risks of interventional PE therapy can be juxtaposed with and balanced judiciously with the potential benefits.[24,87,126]

High-index of suspicion is always required, as one-third of all intermediate-risk PE patients in a contemporary PE registry had depressed cardiac index ("normotensive shock").[127]

In addition to guideline-based definitions of intermediate-risk and high-risk PEs, substantial work has been invested to create quantitative metrics of PE severity, including the Pulmonary Embolism Severity Index (PESI), simplified PESI (sPESI), and Bova score for PE complications.[128–130] Of these scores, the PESI score is the most widely validated.[131,132] The PESI score, based on 11 patient characteristics encompassing both PE severity and known comorbidities (**Table 2**), segregates PE patients into 5 severity classes based on predicted 30-day mortality.[129] Points are added for PESI factors that are present, along with the patient's age, and the combined score translates into a risk prediction class (see **Table 2**).

A simplified version, sPESI, has also been well-validated in observation cohort studies and only requires 6 features including age > 80, history of cancer, history of cardiopulmonary disease, tachycardia ($\geq$110 bpm), tachypnea ($\geq$30 bpm), hypotension (SBP < 100 mm Hg), and oxygen saturation (SpO_2 < 90%).[130,133] Presence of any parameter accrues 1 point, and an sPESI of 0 reflects 30-day low risk (1.1% mortality), while a score $\geq$1 represents high risk (30 day 8.9% mortality).

The 2019 European Society of Cardiology (ESC) guidelines for acute PE recommend considering

Table 2
Pulmonary embolism severity index criteria and interpretation

Pulmonary Embolism Severity Index Clinical Criteria		Points	In simplified Pulmonary Embolism Severity Index?
Age	Years	Years	✓
Sex	Female	Male+10	
Altered Mental Status	No	Yes+60	
Systolic Blood Pressure (BP) <100 mm Hg	No	Yes+30	✓
History of Cancer	No	Yes+30	✓
Temperature <36 °C	No	Yes+20	
Heart Rate ≥110 bpm	No	Yes+20	✓
Respiratory Rate ≥30	No	Yes+20	
Oxygen Saturation <90%	No	Yes+20	✓
History of Heart Failure	No	Yes+10	✓
History of Chronic Lung Disease	No	Yes+10	✓

PESI Score	Class	Risk Profile	30-d Mortality
0–65	I	Very-low risk	0.0%–1.6%
66–85	II	Low-risk	1.7%–3.5%
86–105	III	Intermediate-risk	3.2%–7.1%
106–125	IV	High-risk	4.0%–11.4%
≥125	V	Very high-risk	10%–24.5%

incorporating PESI or sPESI and evidence of RV strain via imaging or biomarkers when considering PE severity (Class IIa recommendation, **Table 3**).[10] Interestingly, while the use of mortality risk scores has been increasingly recommended in evaluation of PE, a recent review found that the PESI, sPESI, Bova, and the recommended 2019 ESC guideline approach had limited model discrimination of patients with low-mortality versus high-mortality risk and poor inter-model correlation.[134]

Pulmonary Embolism Response Team

The depth of expertise required and the need for improvement in PE outcomes have propelled the growth of hospital-based PE Response Teams (PERTs).[24,135] The PERT concept borrows from contemporary best-practice concepts of Heart Teams and Rapid Response teams, and thereby allows for the diagnosing clinician ("afferent arm") to quickly respond to PE patients at risk and to trigger a multi-disciplinary response (efferent arm) to collaboratively evaluate a patient, and determine and implement the best treatment strategy.[135–137] The PERT incorporates experts from several specialties including cardiovascular medicine and surgery, emergency medicine, hematology, pulmonary/critical care, cardiac imaging (radiology and echocardiography), vascular medicine and intervention, and interventional radiology, with differences across centers.[135]

Initial 30-month evaluation at the Massachusetts General Hospital (MGH) found rapid growth in activations by 16% every 6 months with 72% of all activations for intermediate-risk and high-risk PEs, and extrapolation across the United States and world.[138,139] MGH also reported approximately 17% of patients received an advanced reperfusion therapy (catheter or systemic thrombolysis or thrombectomy), but overall similar bleeding risk in patients treated with catheter-directed modalities versus anticoagulation alone.[138] Cleveland Clinic reported their retrospective implementation analysis showed approximately 33% received an advanced reperfusion therapy, with no bleeding events in patients receiving systemic thrombolysis.[140]

Data on the effectiveness of PERTs are emerging,[139,141–144] some showing improvements in PE-related outcomes and mortality. Current ESC guidelines give a class IIa recommendation to set-up of PERT teams to manage intermediate-risk and high-risk PE, depending on the needs and capabilities of the hospital.[10] The mechanisms of benefit of PERT may be multifactorial, and

Table 3
Guidelines-based classification of pulmonary embolism severity[10,24]

			Indicators of Risk		
Early Mortality Risk		Hemodynamic Instability	Clinically Severe Pulmonary Embolism, PESI Class III–V, or sPESI ≥1	RV Dysfunction Transthoracic echocardiography or computed tomographic pulmonary angiography (CTPA)	Elevated Cardiac Troponin Levels
High		(+)	(+)	(+)	(+)
Intermediate	Int.-High	-	+	+	+
	Int.-Low	-	+	One (or none) positive	
Low		-	-	-	-

include protocolization of care, democratization and access to specialists, consensus evaluation of risk, iterative assessment of acute PE patients, more rapid deployment of therapies, PERT-based follow-up, and quality improvement.[24,135,140] PERT teams should work to provide hub-and-spoke service within a network, to facilitate an organized approach to interhospital transfer in particular of critically ill PE patients and those who require advanced reperfusion therapies.[145]

Respiratory and Hemodynamic Support

The key tenet of initial management of intermediate-risk and high-risk PE is to provide hemodynamic and pulmonary support. PE causes RV obstruction, increased PVR, ventilation-perfusion mismatch, and possibly right to left shunting.[146] Hypoxemia must be addressed and treated, ideally achieving oxygen saturation ≥ 90%. Goal blood pressure, while not specifically defined, is targeted to avoid signs of malperfusion, such as altered mental status or decreased urine output, though some authors suggest an optimal mean arterial pressure between 80 and 90 mm Hg for intermediate-risk and high-risk PE.[10,147] Of course, blood pressure goals must always be individualized relative to the patient's baseline blood pressure: clinicians should be cautious about absolute blood pressure cut-offs (including those that are used to define high-risk PE), if for example, the patient has a decline in blood pressure compared to baseline.

Respiratory support

The mainstay of respiratory support patients with intermediate-risk and high-risk PE with hypoxia is supplemental oxygen (O_2). This can be delivered with a nasal cannula, simple facemask, or non-rebreather facemask which is sufficient for the majority of patients.[148] In instances where this is insufficient, a high-flow nasal cannula is preferred over positive-pressure modes of ventilation such as continuous positive airway pressure (CPAP) or biphasic positive airway pressure. This is because increased positive intrathoracic pressure reduces venous return, and contributes to RV afterload.[146,148,149] If positive end-expiratory pressure, either invasive or non-invasive, is necessary, caution is required to keep tidal volumes and plateau pressures low (~6 mL/kg of lean body weight and < 30 cmH_2O, respectively).[10,150] Hypotension and cardiovascular collapse can occur as a result of increased intrathoracic pressure increasing RV afterload, and decreasing preload by limiting blood return.

Additionally, if patients require intubation for respiratory support, there is significant risk of hypotension in patients with RV failure during induction of anesthesia. Given this, anesthetic agents that cause hypotension should be avoided and clinicians should be prepared to provide additional urgent hemodynamic support when using anesthetic agents in patients with acute significant PE.[10]

Supplemental oxygen itself is being re-evaluated as a "drug" in acute PE to improve outcomes. The Air versus Oxygen for Intermediate-Risk Pulmonary Embolism (AIRE) trial (https://classic.clinicaltrials.gov/ct2/show/NCT04003116) was a pilot study that, though being underpowered, found a borderline association between supplemental oxygen therapy and reduced RV dilatation, compared to ambient air.[151] Additional studies examining the mechanism of supplemental oxygen in patients with PE are underway, including Supplemental Oxygen in Pulmonary Embolism (SO-PE) (https://classic.clinicaltrials.gov/ct2/show/NCT05891886).

Hemodynamic support

The etiology of shock in PE is secondary to increased RV afterload as a result of obstruction in the pulmonary vessels as well as secondary effects including vasoconstriction from hypoxia and acidosis.[152] This pathophysiology leads to RV dilation, hypokinesis, tricuspid regurgitation, and RV failure.[153] Further increased RV dilatation, subject to ambient pericardial restraint, impairs LV filling and stroke volume from leftward deviation of the interventricular septum.[153]

A reasoned judicious approach to hemodynamic support for PE with malperfusion, as part of the definitive management strategy, is crucial. While volume resuscitation is standard in many etiologies of shock, its use for managing hypotension and shock in PE is controversial, though most expert authors agree that a small fluid challenge may be appropriate.[10,152–154] A small study giving 500 mL fluid boluses to PE patients found a substantial increase in cardiac output in 12 out of 13 patients.[154] The difficulty is supporting RV preload while avoiding RV overdistention with adverse Frank–Starling consequences[10,146,154]; unfortunately, there is no optimal marker of volume-responsiveness in acute PE. Patients with low central venous pressure or with a small, collapsible IVC may be most likely to benefit from fluid challenge.[10,153] However, volume resuscitation with large fluid boluses is likely to cause RV overdistension and ultimately reduce cardiac output. In fact, there is consideration that *diuresis* may actually be helpful to a failing RV, reducing its distention and wall stress, and relieving impingement of the interventricular septum on the LV.[146] Of course, bolus diuretic can directly cause hypotension, and may impair RV preload; navigating these quandaries requires expert assessment and re-assessment at bedside, with attention to individualization of interventions.

Given the difficulties with fluid assessment and balance in acute PE, vasopressors are a mainstay for hemodynamic support. Ideally, the optimal vasopressor in RV failure should increase RV contractility and systemic arterial pressure while not increasing PVR.[153] The optimal vasopressor for RV failure in PE has not been identified, though norepinephrine seems to be a preferred first-line agent, with its mix of alpha and beta agonism, supporting mean arterial pressure without increasing PVR. Vasopressin is a non-catecholamine that should increase systemic arterial pressure also without increasing PVR.

Parenteral inotropes including epinephrine, dobutamine, and dopamine may have a role when there is insufficient cardiac output, though tachycardia and tachyarrhythmia can occur, which may adversely influence cardiac output.[153,155,156]

The nitric oxide pathway has been considered another possible target intervention, in that this small molecule is a potent, reversible, and selective pulmonary vasodilator. The Inhaled nitric oxide for PE (iNOPE) trial investigated inhaled nitric oxide in intermediate-risk PE, and found that more patients achieved a prespecified secondary endpoint of normalization of RV echocardiographic parameters.[18,157] Nitric oxide has also been evaluated as salvage therapy in high-risk PE but the numbers of studied patients are quite small and do not permit firm conclusions.[158] Analogously, sildenafil, a phosphodiesterase-5-inhibitor, which increases cyclic GMP (the action downstream of nitric oxide) did not improve cardiac index in intermediate-high risk PE, and instead caused hypotension.[159] Overall, treatments of PE with pulmonary vasodilators remain speculative.

Extracorporeal membrane oxygenation

High-risk PE patients with hemodynamic instability despite optimal pharmacologic interventions should be considered for mechanical circulatory support. The most common of these strategies is ECMO, for which there are case studies and case series in highest risk PE, but no randomized control trials. ECMO receives a Class IIb recommendation for acute PE with "refractory circulatory collapse or cardiac arrest" in 2019 ESC guidelines.[10,160,161] The primary goal of ECMO in treating PE is to serve as a bridge to definitive therapy by providing cardiopulmonary support.[162] While there have been rare cases of veno-venous (VV) ECMO used in high-risk PE, it is largely accepted that veno-arterial (VA) ECMO is the optimal modality as it provides both ventilatory and hemodynamic support, whereas VV ECMO only delivers oxygenated blood to the right heart, and does not provide circulatory support.[160,161] Importantly, peripheral VA ECMO bypasses the obstruction of the pulmonary vascular bed, removing blood from the venous system and re-routing it to the femoral artery after oxygenation.[162] Anticoagulation is required for ECMO and thus any patients who cannot be anticoagulated may not be a candidate for ECMO; importantly, this anticoagulation provides treatment of the PE. Other contraindications to ECMO include poor functional status, advanced age, morbid obesity, neurologic dysfunction, chronic organ dysfunction, and prolonged CPR.[162] One systematic review of cases where ECMO was used for high-risk PE found a survival rate of 78% but notes that this survival rate is higher than in many previous studies.[160] Additionally, 2 systematic reviews of patients on ECMO found that they received varied definitive interventions either in isolation or combination including systemic thrombolysis, catheter-guided thrombolysis, and surgical embolectomy.[160,161] A review of the use of ECMO in patients with high-risk PE who have cardiopulmonary arrest found a 61% survival rate for patients who were cannulated for ECMO either during cardiac arrest or after Return of Spontaneous Circulation (ROSC) was achieved.[163] The study did find that mortality was higher in patients who were cannulated during arrest and for patients over age 65.[163] Overall hospital systems should work on optimization of channels and transitions of care, including mobile ECMO and coordination of transfer of ECMO patients to tertiary centers.[145]

There is a small, growing literature on the use of percutaneous RV assist devices in high-risk PE. These devices generally require access to the pulmonary artery, which may be difficult if not contraindicated in acute PE, and they do not directly provide support for ventilation and oxygenation in contrast to VA ECMO.[87]

Reperfusion and Pulmonary Embolism-Debulking Therapies Anticoagulation

The initial treatment of PE, including intermediate-high and high-risk, is anticoagulation. ESC guidelines give a class I recommendation: "initiation of anticoagulation is recommended without delay in patients with high or intermediate clinical probability of PE, while diagnostic workup is in progress."[10,24] This must be considered in terms of certainty of the diagnosis (pre-test probability, to avoid exposing non-PE patients to bleeding risk), stability of the patient, comorbidities and bleeding risk, and delay until definitive diagnosis can be made (eg CTPA). Data support the correlation between early initiation of anticoagulation and

decreased overall mortality.[164] For intermediate-high and high-risk PE, initial anticoagulation is most often achieved with subcutaneous low-molecular weight heparin (LMWH), fondaparinux, or unfractionated heparin (UFH). When not contraindicated, recent data have suggested superiority in using either LMWH or fondaparinux for initial anticoagulation as it decreases both bleeding risk and development of heparin-induced thrombocytopenia.[165,166] However, in high-risk patients where definitive reperfusion and interventional therapy may be needed, UFH may be preferred due to shorter half-life (0.5 - 1.5 hrs) compared to LMWH (3 - 6 hrs) and fondaparinux (17 - 21 hrs).[167] UFH is also preferred in patients with renal dysfunction.[10] In general, contraindications to empiric anticoagulation should be considered in all patients.[10]

Systemic thrombolysis

In addition to anticoagulation, systemic thrombolysis is recommended by both the American College of Chest Physicians guidelines and the ESC guidelines for patients with high-risk PE (hemodynamically unstable patients with a PE, without contraindications to thrombolysis).[10,168] While there is a demonstrated hemodynamic benefit of thrombolysis in intermediate-high risk PE, in terms of hemodynamic deterioration, there is no overall difference in all-cause mortality; benefits of systemic thrombolysis are offset by increased bleeding risk and so thrombolysis is only recommended if patients with intermediate-high risk PE progress to hemodynamic instability.[10,87,168–171]

Both relative and absolute contraindications to systemic thrombolysis must be considered prior to administration (**Table 4**).[172 87,] Some 50% of patients have a contraindication to systemic thrombolysis, limiting its applicability. Additionally, the risk of intracranial or fatal hemorrhage due to

---

Table 4
Major and Minor contraindications to systemic thrombolysis[87,172]

Major Contraindications	Minor Contraindications
Structural intracranial disease	Prolonged cardiopulmonary resuscitation
Intracranial neoplasm	Systolic BP >180 mm Hg
Previous intracranial hemorrhage	Diastolic BP >110 mm Hg
Ischemic stroke (within 3 mo)	Recent non-intracranial bleeding (within 2–4 wk)
Recent brain or spinal surgery (within 3 mo)	Recent surgery (within 2 wk)
Any known bleeding diathesis or internal bleeding	Recent invasive procedure (within 1 mo)
	Ischemic stroke (>3 mo ago)
	Coagulopathy, thrombocytopenia, oral anticoagulant
	Age <18 y or >75y
	Pregnancy (current, or birth within 1 wk)

thrombolysis leads to underuse, even in the most severe PE.

The ESC guideline-recommended regimens for systemic thrombolysis include recombinant tissue-type plasminogen activator (rtPA).[10] Importantly, UFH can be continued if administering rtPA (but must be stopped if administering first-generation thrombolytics, strepokinase and urokinase).[10,173] While several meta-analyses have found tenecteplase to be safe and effective, there are no head-to-head trials comparing it to other thrombolytics, and it is not yet recommended in the ESC guidelines. The American College of Chest Physicians does not offer specific guidance on optimal thrombolytic choice.[10,168,174–176] Notably, there is a small portion of patients who receive systemic thrombolysis who do not respond, with some estimates as high as 8%.[177] Such patients must be carefully evaluated for rescue therapies, including ECMO or an embolectomy procedure.[24,87]

Catheter-directed therapies
Significant work has been conducted on the use of percutaneous catheter-based modalities for clot thrombolysis or evacuation. While the standard of care for hemodynamically unstable patients with high-risk PE remains systemic thrombolysis, catheter-directed modalities have been studied as adjuncts to or second-line therapies for high-risk PE as well as possible first-line treatment for intermediate-high risk PE.[178,179] There are several modalities for catheter-directed treatment of PE including standard catheter-directed thrombolysis (CDT), ultrasound-assisted CDT, fragmentation, and catheter-directed embolectomy.[178]

Catheter-directed thrombolysis An overall theme and goal of catheter-directed thrombolysis is to achieve the benefits of systemic thrombolysis without the same bleeding risk, by using lower doses of locally delivered thrombolytic via a catheter.[24,87,179,180] Ultrasound-assisted CDT (USCDT) operates on the same principle but additionally utilizes high-frequency, low-power ultrasound waves (from a 5F combined ultrasound and thrombolytic infusion catheter) to assist in fibrinolysis by unwinding fibrin strands to unlock thrombolytic binding sites.[87,179] Many of the trials of these devices are based on surrogate PE-endpoints like ventricular size ratio Ultrasound Accelerated Thrombolysis of PE (ULTIMA[181])trail and PASP, and several are a prospective, Single-arm, Multi-center Trial of EkoSonic(R) Endovascular System and Activase for Treatment of Acute Pulmonary Embolism (Seattle II).[182] ULTIMA randomized intermediate-risk PE patients to USCDT

versus anticoagulation, and found that the primary endpoint, 24 h reduction in the dimensionless RV:LV ratio was-0.30 compared to-0.03 with anticoagulation alone. There were no episodes of hemodynamic decompensation or instances of major bleeding events at 90 days in either group.[182] The OPTALYSE PE trial investigated the lower thrombolytic doses and shorter duration of thrombolytic infusions for intermediate-risk PE, and found comparable surrogate outcome (RV:LV ratio) results with lower doses (4 mg per lung similar to 12 mg) and reduced times (2 hours similar to 6 hours).[183-185] While randomized, OPTAYLSE had no control arm, so we cannot compare the RV:LV ratio to a no-treatment or anticoagulation-arm. A meta-analysis of 8 studies comparing CDT and USCDT (7 observational and 1 randomized) showed no overall difference in length of stay, bleeding, or surrogate PE-related measures (though the CDT group had a statistically better reduction in mean pulmonary artery pressure).[184] However, the trials included may have used higher thrombolytic doses with USCDT, and thus not shown a benefit of USCDT on lesser bleeding outcomes. Because the question of whether CDT and USCDT are truly of benefit over anticoagulation alone, there are several ongoing investigations including PE-TRACT (https://www.clinicaltrials.gov/study/NCT05591118) and HI-PEITHO (https://www.clinicaltrials.gov/study/NCT04790370). These trials aim to compare the use of CDT and USCDT, respectively, in intermediate-risk PEs to anticoagulation alone.

Catheter-directed embolectomy Suction embolectomy was first pioneered more than 50 years ago.[87] A large-bore aspiration system (AngioVac) was developed to aspirate intravascular materials with a veno-venous bypass system and filtering mechanism, and has been used for extraction of vena cava and peripheral venous thrombi, right heart vegetations, right heart CIT, and sometimes PE, though the large bore can be difficult to steer in the pulmonary artery. A next generation device (AlphaVac) is being assessed in a single-arm study of intermediate risk PE (APEX-PE, https://classic.clinicaltrials.gov/ct2/show/NCT05318092).

Multiple new catheter-directed embolectomy (CDE) platforms have proliferated in the 2010s. The FlowTriever is a 16, 20, or 24 French catheter for aspiration that also features 3 nitinol-discs that can self-expand and trap thrombus. FlowTriever received approval in 2018 based on the single-arm Flowtriever Pulmonary Embolectomy (FLARE) study showing improved RV:LV ratio in intermediate-risk PE.[24,87,186] Interestingly in practice, the nitinol-discs are not always used relative to the aspiration functionality; aspiration can be repeated as needed to clear the pulmonary artery. Two lines of investigation on FlowTriever were presented in 2023. FlowTriever All-Comer Registry for Patient Safety and Hemodynamics (FLASH)[187,188] is a real-world analysis of intermediate-risk (77%) and high-risk (8%) PE patients of whom one-third had a contraindication to thrombolysis. FlowTriever resulted in immediate 8 mm Hg decline (−23%) in mean pulmonary arterial pressure and increased cardiac index 0.3 L/min/sqm (+19%). Thirty-day mortality was 0.8%. FlowTriever for Acute Massive Pulmonary Embolism was presented at American College of Cardiology March 2023, detailing a prospective observational cohort of high-risk PE (hypotension, vasopressor use, arrest); in-hospital mortality was < 2% compared to > 28% in both a literature-based historical goal and a "context" arm which included ∼70% systemic thrombolysis (https://clinicaltrials.gov/ct2/show/NCT04795167). Rescue therapy, clinical deterioration, and major bleeding were all lower with FlowTriever. The Indigo aspiration catheter is smaller-bore (eg 6F-12F) and may be able to better navigate the pulmonary arterial tree, but it has less cross-sectional area and capacity for clot extraction; single-arm surrogate-endpoint data has studied this device.[189]

Percutaneous devices comparison The 2 major paradigms of percutaneous therapies are CDT and CDE, but comparisons among these are few. One such study from 2016 to 2019 from the Nationwide Readmission Database propensity matched about 800 high-risk PE patients who received CDE and CDT.[189] The cohort featured 75% mechanically ventilated patients, 15% on vasopressors, 12% who required mechanical circulatory support, and 13% who received systemic thrombolysis. There was no difference in all-cause mortality or major bleeding, but this was a retrospective analysis dependent on administrative coding data, and biases for or against a certain

treatment modality cannot be assessed. PEER-LESS (https://classic.clinicaltrials.gov/ct2/show/NCT05111613) is a randomized trial of FlowTriever CDE versus any modality of CDT in intermediate-risk PE, designed to assess a composite win-ratio endpoint based on mortality, bleeding, and deterioration or treatment escalation. A 2024 analysis of real-world data comparing USCDT and CDE showed higher overall major bleeding by International Society for Thrombosis and Hemostasis criteria (11.0% versus 17.3%, p=0.0002). There was also less intracranial hemorrhage in the USCDT group compared to CDE (0.4% versus 1.4%, p=0.015). Selection-biases and confounding cannot be excluded. However, this type of big-data approach, with real-world patients, may provide insights not available in clinical trials, where there are many exclusion criteria. If validated, the result may also suggest that there are unappreciated harms to CDE, or may bear on the skill level or expertise required to conduct CDE. (https://www.jscai.org/article/S2772-9303(23) 01194-8/fulltext).

Where does this leave the practicing clinician faced with an intermediate-high or high-risk PE? First, each institution and center likely will develop expertise in a certain selection of percutaneous devices, and there is likely a volume-quality relationship in employing interventional therapeutics. Second, we can appreciate some differences between CDE and CDT (**Table 5**). There does seem to be a secular evolution in therapy toward CDE, given immediate debulking of PE and reperfusion of the pulmonary arterial tree. Akin to the history of reperfusion therapy for myocardial infarction, evolving from thrombolysis to primary percutaneous coronary intervention to open the coronary artery, we may be on the precipice of moving treatment of advanced, central PE from a pharmacologic (or combined pharmaco-mechanical CDT paradigm) to a CDE paradigm to open the pulmonary artery. Before standards of care change, however, additional comparative and randomized data will be required to fully define

Table 5
Comparison of Catheter-directed thrombolysis and catheter-directed embolectomy

Catheter-directed thrombolysis	Catheter-Directed Embolectomy
Smaller bore devices	Larger devices, less navigable, learning curve
Able to reach distal pulmonary vasculature	Generally treats proximal PE
	Mechanical embolectomy only
Pharmaco-mechanical strategy	Embolectomy has immediate effect
Thrombolytic action takes time	More suited to central PE
Perhaps better for peripheral PEs	Access site risks, risks of injury to pulmonary artery
Bleeding risk (local and systemic)	
Typically performed by interventional cardiologist or interventional radiologist	Typically performed by interventional cardiologist or interventional radiologist

outcomes and risks, and understand the role for each modality.

Overall, ESC guidelines do not recommend the routine use of percutaneous catheter-directed treatments, but do offer a Class IIa consideration for high-risk PE patients in which thrombolysis has failed or is contraindicated.[10]

Surgical thromboembolectomy

The concept of surgical thromboembolectomy for PE was first described in the early twentieth century.[190] Surgical thromboembolectomy is a highly invasive procedure and requires midline sternotomy and cardiopulmonary bypass.[191,192] Surgical thromboembolectomy had most often been reserved as a salvage procedure when other treatment options have failed; however, there is some evidence to support its use in patients with an extensive proximal thrombus burden such as CIT and impending paradoxic embolism.[190,191,192,193] Traditionally, the mortality of patients undergoing surgical thromboembolectomy has been high—a nationwide sample of patients undergoing surgical thromboembolectmy between 1999 and 2008 found a mortality rate of 27.2%, but this was likely due to selection bias and its use as a salvage procedure.[190] Recent data demonstrate an in-hospital mortality rate in high-risk and intermediate-risk PE patients undergoing surgical thromboembolectomy between 6.6% and 11.7%.[191,194,195] Some authors argue that surgical thromboembolectomy should be considered in the treatment algorithm for intermediate-high and high-risk PE, for example, in central emboli or clot-in-transit.[190] A single-center retrospective study of 55 patients with intermediate-risk PE, high-risk PE without cardiac arrest, and high-risk PE with cardiac arrest found a 93% in-hospital survival rate, in-line with other recent data, but found that in-hospital survival in the intermediate-risk group was 100% compared to 88% and 78% in the high-risk PE without and with cardiac arrest, respectively.[196] Despite this, there are no trials directly comparing surgical thromboembolectomy to medical therapies alone.[196] Current ESC guidelines give a Class I recommendation of surgical thromboembolectomy in high-risk PE patients where thrombolysis (or CDT) is contraindicated or has failed.[10,24] Preoperative thrombolysis increases risk of bleeding, but is not an absolute contraindication.

SUMMARY

While the overall incidence of PE is increasing, the incidence of high-risk PE and mortality from PE is decreasing. This trend suggests that both the recognition of PE generally and the recognition of intermediate-risk and high-risk PE is of paramount importance. Clinicians must remember the protean manifestations of PE and its broad range of presentations. Validated scores for diagnosis and prognosis can guide the clinician. In modern practice, the vast majority of PEs are diagnosed by CTPA. Imaging, in particular TTE, and biomarkers are vital adjuncts to prognosis, but no 1 marker or set of markers is superior, and clinical intuition and individualization are essential.

Respiratory and hemodynamic support, attention to volume status, anticoagulation, and consideration for systemic thrombolysis represent the primary management aims of intermediate-high and high-risk PE. There are growing data on CDT and CDE modalities, while surgical thromboembolectomy may also have a role in the initial treatment approach. Because these technologies and therapeutics cross multi-disciplinary lines, and there is equipoise (or lack of data) in preferring 1 advanced PE therapy over another, PERTs can assist the clinician with decision-making and implementation of a treatment plan.

While this review provides a broad overview of the recognition and treatment of intermediate-risk and high-risk PE, it does not provide important context for the treatment of special populations with PE including patients who are pregnant, have history of heparin-induced thrombocytopenia, have inherited thrombophilias, or have sickle cell disease.

CLINICS CARE POINTS

- PE is a great masquerader, and must be considered as a cause of protean cardiopulmonary symptoms and signs, and by every specialty of medicine.

- PE risk factors from the history and examination can increase the pre-test probability of diagnosing PE. Several validated prediction rules are available to assist the clinician.

- Electrocardiography and echocardiography can show evidence of RV dilatation and dysfunction. Echocardiography can also inform the differential diagnosis, and quantify effects on pulmonary arterial pressures. Biomarkers like troponin and natriuretic peptide provide evidence of RV myocardial necrosis and chamber distention, respectively.

- Risk stratification in PE depends on validated prognostic rules (PESI, sPESI), biomarkers, and echocardiography.

- Therapeutic anticoagulation is the backbone of PE therapy regardless of risk profile.
- The highest risk PE patients require urgent and definitive therapy to support hemodynamics and to clear the pulmonary artery of clots.
- Hemodynamic support for the most severe PE includes VA ECMO, for which there are the most available data; VA ECMO be considered for shock (refractory to parenteral vasoactives), cardiac arrest, and pulmonary collapse.
- Systemic thrombolysis is typically the first treatment considered, though many patients have contraindications, and there is a fear of using this therapy due to intracranial hemorrhage (ICH) risk.
- There are limited randomized and comparative effectiveness data to rigorously choose 1 interventional PE therapy over another. CDE and CDT each have advantages, but there is a possible trend toward first-line use of an embolectomy strategy.
- Intermediate-risk PE patients represent a true contemporary management challenge. Most of these patients will do well, and exposing these patients to the risks of advanced therapies is not justified on a large scale. However, some of these intermediate-risk patients will experience clinical deterioration, and require definitive PE therapy early.
- PERTs are essential in to individualize care and decision-making, by marshaling the combined experience of clinicians with expertise in PE, to help match patient risk to appropriate treatment. PERTs can also help with diagnosis.

DISCLOSURE

Dr. Drew Birrenkott has no disclosures. Dr. Dudzinski has no disclosures. Dr. Kabrhel reports Grants (paid to my institution): Grifols, Diagnostica Stago Consulting/Advisory Boards: Siemens, BMS/Pfizer, Abbot Equity: Insera Therapeutics.

REFERENCES

1. Coon WW, Willis PW. Deep venous thrombosis and pulmonary embolism: prediction, prevention and treatment. Am J Cardiol 1959;4:611–21.
2. Goldhaber SZ, Bounameaux H. Pulmonary embolism and deep vein thrombosis. Lancet 2012; 379(9828):1835–46.
3. Raskob GE, Angchaisuksiri P, Blanco AN, et al. Thrombosis: a major contributor to global disease burden. Arterioscler Thromb Vasc Biol 2014; 34(11):2363–71.
4. Tagalakis V, Patenaude V, Kahn SR, Suissa S. Incidence of and mortality from venous thromboembolism in a real-world population: the Q-VTE Study Cohort. Am J Med 2013;126(9):832.e13–21.
5. Wendelboe AM, Raskob GE. Global burden of thrombosis: Epidemiologic Aspects. Circ Res 2016;118(9):1340–7.
6. Silverstein MD, Heit JA, Mohr DN, Petterson TM, O'Fallon WM, Melton LJ III. Trends in the incidence of deep vein thrombosis and pulmonary embolism: a 25-year population-based study. Arch Intern Med 1998;158(6):585–93.
7. Huang W, Goldberg RJ, Anderson FA, Kiefe CI, Spencer FA. Secular trends in occurrence of acute venous thromboembolism: the Worcester VTE study (1985-2009). Am J Med 2014;127(9):829–39.e5.
8. Stein PD, Matta F. Epidemiology and incidence: the Scope of the Problem and risk factors for development of venous thromboembolism. Clin Chest Med 2010;31(4):611–28.
9. Duffett L, Castellucci LA, Forgie MA. Pulmonary embolism: update on management and controversies. BMJ 2020;370:m2177.
10. Konstantinides SV, Meyer G, Becattini C, et al. 2019 ESC Guidelines for the diagnosis and management of acute pulmonary embolism developed in collaboration with the European Respiratory Society (ERS). Eur Heart J 2020;41(4):543–603.
11. Keller K, Hobohm L, Ebner M, et al. Trends in thrombolytic treatment and outcomes of acute pulmonary embolism in Germany. Eur Heart J 2020;41(4):522–9.
12. Lehnert P, Lange T, Møller CH, Olsen PS, Carlsen J. Acute pulmonary embolism in a national Danish cohort: increasing incidence and decreasing mortality. Thromb Haemost 2018;118(3):539–46.
13. Dentali F, Ageno W, Pomero F, Fenoglio L, Squizzato A, Bonzini M. Time trends and case fatality rate of in-hospital treated pulmonary embolism during 11 years of observation in Northwestern Italy. Thromb Haemost 2016;115(2):399–405.
14. de Miguel-Díez J, Jiménez-García R, Jiménez D, et al. Trends in hospital admissions for pulmonary embolism in Spain from 2002 to 2011. Eur Respir J 2014;44(4):942–50.
15. Weiner RS. Finding the path back to patient-oriented research in American Medical Academia. Clin Transl Sci 2011;4(1):7.
16. Barco S, Mahmoudpour SH, Valerio L, et al. Trends in mortality related to pulmonary embolism in the European Region, 2000–15: analysis of vital registration data from the WHO Mortality Database. Lancet Respir Med 2020;8(3):277–87.
17. Smith SB, Geske JB, Kathuria P, et al. Analysis of national trends in admissions for pulmonary embolism. Chest 2016;150(1):35–45.

18. Kline JA, Hernandez J, Garrett JS, Jones AE. Pilot study of a protocol to administer inhaled nitric oxide to treat severe acute submassive pulmonary embolism. Emerg Med J 2014;31(6):459–62.

19. Stein PD, Matta F, Alrifai A, Rahman A. Trends in case fatality rate in pulmonary embolism according to stability and treatment. Thromb Res 2012;130(6): 841–6.

20. Andersson T, Söderberg S. Incidence of acute pulmonary embolism, related comorbidities and survival; analysis of a Swedish national cohort. BMC Cardiovasc Disord 2017;17(1):155.

21. McCabe BE, Veselis CA, Goykhman I, Hochhold J, Eisenberg D, Son H. Beyond pulmonary embolism; nonthrombotic pulmonary embolism as diagnostic challenges. Curr Probl Diagn Radiol 2019;48(4): 387–92.

22. Kumar DR, Hanlin E, Glurich I, Mazza JJ, Yale SH. Virchow's contribution to the understanding of thrombosis and Cellular Biology. Clin Med Res 2010;8(3–4):168–72.

23. Jaff MR, McMurtry MS, Archer SL, et al. Management of massive and submassive pulmonary embolism, Iliofemoral deep vein thrombosis, and chronic thromboembolic pulmonary Hypertension. Circulation 2011;123(16):1788–830.

24. Rivera-Lebron B, McDaniel M, Ahrar K, et al. Diagnosis, treatment, and Follow up of acute pulmonary embolism: consensus practice from the PERT Consortium. Clin Appl Thromb Hemost 2019;25:1–16.

25. Kline JA, Garrett JS, Sarmiento EJ, Strachan CC, Courtney DM. Over-testing for suspected pulmonary embolism in American emergency departments: the continuing Epidemic. Circ Cardiovasc Qual Outcomes 2020;13(1):e005753.

26. Robin ED. Overdiagnosis and overtreatment of pulmonary embolism: the emperor may have no clothes. Ann Intern Med 1977;87(6):775–81.

27. Gunderson CG, Bilan VP, Holleck JL, et al. Prevalence of harmful diagnostic errors in hospitalised adults: a systematic review and meta-analysis. BMJ Qual Saf 2020;29(12):1008–18.

28. Kwok CS, Wong CW, Lovatt S, Myint PK, Loke YK. Misdiagnosis of pulmonary embolism and missed pulmonary embolism: a systematic review of the literature. Health Sciences Review 2022;3:100022.

29. White RH. The epidemiology of venous thromboembolism. Circulation 2003;107(23 Suppl 1):I4–8.

30. Kline JA, Kabrhel C. Emergency evaluation for pulmonary embolism, Part 1: clinical factors that increase risk. J Emerg Med 2015;48(6):771–80.

31. Casazza F, Becattini C, Bongarzoni A, et al. Clinical features and short term outcomes of patients with acute pulmonary embolism. The Italian Pulmonary Embolism Registry (IPER). Thromb Res 2012; 130(6):847–52.

32. Anderson FA, Spencer FA. Risk factors for venous thromboembolism. Circulation 2003;107(23_suppl_1):I–9.

33. Barco S, Valerio L, Ageno W, et al. Age-sex specific pulmonary embolism-related mortality in the USA and Canada, 2000–18: an analysis of the WHO Mortality Database and of the CDC Multiple Cause of Death database. Lancet Respir Med 2021;9(1): 33–42.

34. Stein PD, Beemath A, Matta F, et al. Clinical characteristics of patients with acute pulmonary embolism: data from PIOPED II. Am J Med 2007;120(10): 871–9.

35. Bělohlávek J, Dytrych V, Linhart A. Pulmonary embolism, part I: epidemiology, risk factors and risk stratification, pathophysiology, clinical presentation, diagnosis and nonthrombotic pulmonary embolism. Exp Clin Cardiol 2013;18(2):129–38.

36. Prandoni P, Lensing AWA, Prins MH, et al. Prevalence of pulmonary embolism among patients hospitalized for syncope. N Engl J Med 2016;375(16): 1524–31.

37. Verma AA, Masoom H, Rawal S, Guo Y, Razak F. For the GEMINI Investigators. Pulmonary embolism and deep venous thrombosis in patients hospitalized with syncope: a multicenter cross-sectional study in Toronto, Ontario, Canada. JAMA Intern Med 2017;177(7):1046–8.

38. Costantino G, Ruwald MH, Quinn J, et al. Prevalence of pulmonary embolism in patients with syncope. JAMA Intern Med 2018;178(3):356–62.

39. Bell WR, Simon TL, DeMets DL. The clinical features of submassive and massive pulmonary emboli. Am J Med 1977;62(3):355–60.

40. Chengsupanimit T, Sundaram B, Lau WB, Keith SW, Kane GC. Clinical characteristics of patients with pulmonary infarction – a retrospective review. Respir Med 2018;139:13–8.

41. Value of the ventilation/perfusion scan in acute pulmonary embolism: results of the prospective investigation of pulmonary embolism diagnosis (PIOPED). JAMA 1990;263(20):2753–9.

42. Wells PS, Anderson DR, Rodger M, et al. Excluding pulmonary embolism at the bedside without diagnostic imaging: management of patients with suspected pulmonary embolism presenting to the emergency department by using a simple clinical model and D-dimer. Ann Intern Med 2001;135(2):98–107.

43. Le Gal G, Righini M, Roy PM, et al. Prediction of pulmonary embolism in the emergency department: the revised Geneva score. Ann Intern Med 2006;144(3):165–71.

44. Kline JA, Mitchell AM, Kabrhel C, Richman PB, Courtney DM. Clinical criteria to prevent unnecessary diagnostic testing in emergency department patients with suspected pulmonary embolism. J Thromb Haemost 2004;2(8):1247–55.

45. van der Hulle T, Cheung WY, Kooij S, et al. Simplified diagnostic management of suspected pulmonary embolism (the YEARS study): a prospective, multicentre, cohort study. Lancet 2017; 390(10091):289–97.

46. Wells PS, Anderson DR, Rodger M, et al. Derivation of a simple clinical model to categorize patients probability of pulmonary embolism: increasing the models utility with the SimpliRED D-dimer. Thromb Haemost 2000;83(03):416–20.

47. Gibson NS, Sohne M, Kruip MJHA, et al. Further validation and simplification of the Wells clinical decision rule in pulmonary embolism. Thromb Haemost 2008;99(1):229–34.

48. Ceriani E, Combescure C, Le Gal G, et al. Clinical prediction rules for pulmonary embolism: a systematic review and meta-analysis. J Thromb Haemost 2010;8(5):957–70.

49. Wolf SJ, McCubbin TR, Feldhaus KM, Faragher JP, Adcock DM. Prospective validation of Wells criteria in the evaluation of patients with suspected pulmonary embolism. Ann Emerg Med 2004;44(5): 503–10.

50. Kabrhel C, Van Hylckama Vlieg A, Muzikanski A, et al. Multicenter evaluation of the YEARS criteria in emergency department patients evaluated for pulmonary embolism. Acad Emerg Med 2018; 25(9):987–94.

51. Freund Y, Chauvin A, Jimenez S, et al. Effect of a diagnostic strategy using an elevated and age-adjusted D-dimer threshold on thromboembolic events in emergency department patients with suspected pulmonary embolism: a randomized clinical trial. JAMA 2021;326(21):2141–9.

52. van der Pol LM, Tromeur C, Bistervels IM, et al. Pregnancy-adapted YEARS algorithm for diagnosis of suspected pulmonary embolism. N Engl J Med 2019;380(12):1139–49.

53. Wicki J, Perneger TV, Junod AF, Bounameaux H, Perrier A. Assessing clinical probability of pulmonary embolism in the emergency ward: a simple score. Arch Intern Med 2001;161(1):92–7.

54. Klok FA, Kruisman E, Spaan J, et al. Comparison of the revised Geneva score with the Wells rule for assessing clinical probability of pulmonary embolism. J Thromb Haemost 2008;6(1):40–4.

55. Penaloza A, Verschuren F, Meyer G, et al. Comparison of the unstructured clinician gestalt, the wells score, and the revised Geneva score to estimate pretest probability for suspected pulmonary embolism. Ann Emerg Med 2013;62(2):117–24.e2.

56. Kline JA, Courtney DM, Kabrhel C, et al. Prospective multicenter evaluation of the pulmonary embolism rule-out criteria. J Thromb Haemost 2008;6(5): 772–80.

57. Penaloza A, Soulié C, Moumneh T, et al. Pulmonary embolism rule-out criteria (PERC) rule in European patients with low implicit clinical probability (PER-CEPIC): a multicentre, prospective, observational study. The Lancet Haematology 2017;4(12): e615–21.

58. Crane S, Jaconelli T, Eragat M. Retrospective validation of the pulmonary embolism rule-out criteria rule in 'PE unlikely' patients with suspected pulmonary embolism. Eur J Emerg Med 2018;25(3): 185.

59. Wolf SJ, McCubbin TR, Nordenholz KE, Naviaux NW, Haukoos JS. Assessment of the pulmonary embolism rule-out criteria rule for evaluation of suspected pulmonary embolism in the emergency department. Am J Emerg Med 2008;26(2):181–5.

60. Madsen T, Jedick R, Teeples T, Carlson M, Steenblik J. Impact of altitude-adjusted hypoxia on the pulmonary embolism rule-out criteria. Am J Emerg Med 2019;37(2):281–5.

61. Johnson ED, Schell JC, Rodgers GM. The D-dimer assay. Am J Hematol 2019;94(7):833–9.

62. Kabrhel C, Mark Courtney D, Camargo CA, et al. Potential impact of adjusting the threshold of the quantitative D-dimer based on pretest probability of acute pulmonary embolism. Acad Emerg Med 2009;16(4):325–32.

63. Douma RA, le Gal G, Söhne M, et al. Potential of an age adjusted D-dimer cut-off value to improve the exclusion of pulmonary embolism in older patients: a retrospective analysis of three large cohorts. BMJ 2010;340:c1475.

64. Schouten HJ, Geersing GJ, Koek HL, et al. Diagnostic accuracy of conventional or age adjusted D-dimer cut-off values in older patients with suspected venous thromboembolism: systematic review and meta-analysis. BMJ 2013; 346:f2492.

65. Righini M, Van Es J, Den Exter PL, et al. Age-adjusted D-dimer Cutoff levels to rule out pulmonary embolism: the ADJUST-PE study. JAMA 2014;311(11):1117–24.

66. Meyer G, Roy PM, Sors H, Sanchez O. Laboratory tests in the diagnosis of pulmonary embolism. Respiration 2003;70(2):125–32.

67. Dieter RS, Ernst E, Ende DJ, Stein JH. Diagnostic utility of cardiac troponin-I levels in patients with suspected pulmonary embolism. Angiology 2002; 53(5):583–5.

68. Giannitsis E, Müller-Bardorff M, Kurowski V, et al. Independent prognostic value of cardiac troponin T in patients with confirmed pulmonary embolism. Circulation 2000;102(2):211–7.

69. Konstantinides S, Geibel A, Olschewski M, et al. Importance of cardiac troponins I and T in risk stratification of patients with acute pulmonary embolism. Circulation 2002;106(10):1263–8.

70. Tulevski II, Mulder BJM, van Veldhuisen DJ. Utility of a BNP as a marker for RV dysfunction in acute

pulmonary embolism. J Am Coll Cardiol 2002; 39(12):2080.

71. Reza N, Dudzinski DM. Pulmonary embolism response teams. Curr Treat Options Cardiovasc Med 2015;17(6):387.

72. Rodger M, Makropoulos D, Turek M, et al. Diagnostic value of the electrocardiogram in suspected pulmonary embolism. Am J Cardiol 2000;86(7): 807–9.

73. Hariharan P, Dudzinski DM, Okechukwu I, Takayesu JK, Chang Y, Kabrhel C. Association between electrocardiographic findings, right heart strain, and short-term adverse clinical events in patients with acute pulmonary embolism. Clin Cardiol 2015;38(4):236–42.

74. Co I, Eilbert W, Chiganos T. New electrocardiographic changes in patients diagnosed with pulmonary embolism. J Emerg Med 2017;52(3):280–5.

75. McGINN S, WHITE PD. Acute cor pulmonale resulting from pulmonary embolism: its clinical recognition. Journal of the American Medical Association 1935;104(17):1473–80.

76. Nallamala H, Mathis E, Sethi I. Recognizing S1q3t3 for what it is: a nonspecific pattern of right heart strain. J Hosp Med. https://shmabstracts.org/abstract/recognizing-s1q3t3-for-what-it-is-a-nonspecific-pattern-of-right-heart-strain/. [Accessed 21 June 2023].

77. Ullman E, Brady WJ, Perron AD, Chan T. Electrocardiographic manifestations of pulmonary embolism. Am J Emerg Med 2001;19(6):514–9.

78. Shopp JD, Stewart LK, Emmett TW, Kline JA. Findings from 12-lead electrocardiography that predict circulatory shock from pulmonary embolism: systematic review and meta-analysis. Acad Emerg Med 2015;22(10):1127–37.

79. Daniel KR, Courtney DM, Kline JA. Assessment of cardiac stress from massive pulmonary embolism with 12-lead ECG. Chest 2001;120(2):474–81.

80. Digby GC, Kukla P, Zhan Z, et al. The value of electrocardiographic Abnormalities in the prognosis of pulmonary embolism: a consensus Paper. Ann Noninvasive Electrocardiol 2015;20(3):207–23.

81. Golpe R, Castro-Añón O, Pérez-de-Llano LA, et al. Electrocardiogram score predicts severity of pulmonary embolism in hemodynamically stable patients. J Hosp Med 2011;6(5):285–9.

82. Kostrubiec M, Hrynkiewicz A, Pedowska-Włoszek J, et al. Is it possible to use standard electrocardiography for risk assessment of patients with pulmonary embolism? Kardiol Pol 2009;67(7):744–50.

83. Subramaniam RM, Mandrekar J, Chang C, et al. Pulmonary embolism outcome: a prospective evaluation of CT pulmonary angiographic clot burden score and ECG score. AJR Am J Roentgenol 2008;190(6):1599–604.

84. Toosi MS, Merlino JD, Leeper KV. Electrocardiographic score and short-term outcomes of acute pulmonary embolism. Am J Cardiol 2007;100(7): 1172–6.

85. Bircan A, Karadeniz N, Ozden A, et al. A simple clinical model composed of ECG, shock index, and arterial blood gas analysis for predicting severe pulmonary embolism. Clin Appl Thromb Hemost 2011;17(2):188–96.

86. Kline JA, Hernandez-Nino J, Rose GA, Norton HJ, Camargo CA. Surrogate markers for adverse outcomes in normotensive patients with pulmonary embolism. Crit Care Med 2006;34(11):2773–80.

87. Osho AA, Dudzinski DM. Interventional therapies for acute pulmonary embolism. Surg Clin North Am 2022;102(3):429–47.

88. Lyhne MD, Dudzinski DM, Andersen A, et al. Right-to-left ventricular ratio is higher in systole than diastole in patients with acute pulmonary embolism. Echocardiography 2023 09;40(9):925–31. PMID: 37477341.

89. Alerhand S, Sundaram T, Gottlieb M. What are the echocardiographic findings of acute right ventricular strain that suggest pulmonary embolism? Anaesth Crit Care Pain Med 2021;40(2):100852.

90. Bernard S, Namasivayam M, Dudzinski DM. Reflections on echocardiography in pulmonary embolism: Literally and figuratively. J Am Soc Echocardiogr 2019;32(7):807–10.

91. Fields JM, Davis J, Girson L, et al. Transthoracic echocardiography for diagnosing pulmonary embolism: a systematic review and meta-analysis. J Am Soc Echocardiogr 2017;30(7):714–23.e4.

92. Garvey S, Dudzinski DM, Giordano N, et al. Pulmonary embolism with clot in transit: an analysis of risk factors and outcomes. Thromb Res 2020;187: 139–47.

93. Torbicki A, Galié N, Covezzoli A, et al. Right heart thrombi in pulmonary embolism. J Am Coll Cardiol 2003;41(12):2245–51.

94. Darrios D, Rosa Salazar V, Morillo R, et al. Prognostic significance of right heart thrombi in patients with acute symptomatic pulmonary embolism: systematic review and meta-analysis. Chest 2017; 151(2):409–16.

95. Kinney EL, Wright RJ. Efficacy of treatment of patients with echocardiographically detected right-sided heart thrombi: a meta-analysis. Am Heart J 1989;118(3):569–73.

96. Athappan G, Sengodan P, Chacko P, Gandhi S. Comparative efficacy of different modalities for treatment of right heart thrombi in transit: a pooled analysis. Vasc Med 2015;20(2):131–8.

97. Rose PS, Punjabi NM, Pearse DB. Treatment of right heart thromboemboli. Chest 2002;121(3): 806–14.

98. Dahhan T, Siddiqui I, Tapson VF, et al. Clinical and echocardiographic predictors of mortality in acute pulmonary embolism. Cardiovasc Ultrasound 2016;14(1):44.

99. Sanchez O, Trinquart L, Caille V, et al. Prognostic factors for pulmonary embolism: the prep study, a prospective multicenter cohort study. Am J Respir Crit Care Med 2010;181(2):168–73.

100. Taylor RA, Davis J, Liu R, Gupta V. Point-of-care focused cardiac ultrasound for prediction of pulmonary embolism adverse outcomes. J Emerg Med 2013;45(3):392–9.

101. Lyhne MD, Kabrehl C, Giordano N, et al. The echocardiographic ratio tricuspid annular plane systolic excursion/pulmonary arterial systolic pressure predicts short-term adverse outcomes in acute pulmonary embolism. Eur Heart J Cardiovasc Imaging 2021;22(3):285–94.

102. Witkin A, Wilcox SR, Chang Y, et al. Impact of chronic right ventricular pressure overload in short-term outcomes of acute pulmonary embolism: a retrospective analysis. J Crit Care 2019; 51:1–5.

103. Dresden S, Mitchell P, Rahimi L, et al. Right ventricular dilatation on bedside echocardiography performed by emergency physicians aids in the diagnosis of pulmonary embolism. Ann Emerg Med 2014;63(1):16–24.

104. Zhu R, Ma XC. Clinical value of Ultrasonography in diagnosis of pulmonary embolism in critically ill patients. J Transl Int Med 2017;5(4):200–4.

105. Kaptein FHJ, Kroft LJM, Hammerschlag G, et al. Pulmonary infarction in acute pulmonary embolism. Thromb Res 2021;202:162–9.

106. Elliott CG, Goldhaber SZ, Visani L, DeRosa M. Chest radiographs in acute pulmonary embolism: results from the International Cooperative pulmonary embolism registry. Chest 2000; 118(1):33–8.

107. Hampton AO. Correlation of postmortem chest teleroentogenograms with autopsy findings, with special reference to pulmonary embolism and infarction. Am J Roentgenol 1940;43:305–25.

108. Worsley DF, Alavi A, Aronchick JM, Chen JT, Greenspan RH, Ravin CE. Chest radiographic findings in patients with acute pulmonary embolism: observations from the PIOPED Study. Radiology 1993;189(1):133–6.

109. Talbot S, Worthington BS, Roebuck EJ. Radiographic signs of pulmonary embolism and pulmonary infarction. Thorax 1973;28(2):198–203.

110. van der Pol LM, Tromeur C, Faber LM, et al. Chest X-ray not routinely indicated prior to the YEARS algorithm in the diagnostic management of suspected pulmonary embolism. TH Open 2019;3(1):e22–7.

111. Kruger PC, Eikelboom JW, Douketis JD, Hankey GJ. Pulmonary embolism: update on diagnosis and management. Med J Aust 2019; 211(2):82–7.

112. Carrier M, Righini M, Wells PS, et al. Subsegmental pulmonary embolism diagnosed by computed tomography: incidence and clinical implications. A systematic review and meta-analysis of the management outcome studies. J Thromb Haemost 2010;8(8):1716–22.

113. Stein PD, Fowler SE, Goodman LR, et al. Multidetector computed tomography for acute pulmonary embolism. N Engl J Med 2006;354(22): 2317–27.

114. Dudzinski DM, Hariharan P, Parry BA, Chang Y. Assessment of right ventricular strain by computed tomography versus echocardiography in acute pulmonary embolism. Acad Emerg Med 2017; 24(3):337–43.

115. Lyhne MD, Giordano N, Dudzinski D, et al. Low concordance between CTPA and echocardiography in identification of right ventricular strain in PERT patients with acute pulmonary embolism. Emerg Radiol 2023;30(3):325–31.

116. Furlan A, Aghayev A, Chang CCH, et al. Short-term mortality in acute pulmonary embolism: clot burden and signs of right heart dysfunction at CT pulmonary angiography. Radiology 2012;265(1):283–93.

117. Hariharan P, Dudzinski DM, Rosovsky R, et al. Relation among clot burden, right-sided heart strain, and adverse events after acute pulmonary embolism. Am J Cardiol 2016;118(10):1568–73.

118. Reid JH, Coche EE, Inoue T, et al. Is the lung scan alive and well? Facts and controversies in defining the role of lung scintigraphy for the diagnosis of pulmonary embolism in the era of MDCT. Eur J Nucl Med Mol Imaging 2009;36(3):505–21.

119. Lyhne MD, Witkin AS, Dasegowda G, et al. Evaluating cardiopulmonary function following acute pulmonary embolism. Expert Rev Cardiovasc Ther 2022;20(9):747–60.

120. Anderson DR, Kahn SR, Rodger MA, et al. Computed tomographic pulmonary angiography vs ventilation-perfusion lung scanning in patients with suspected pulmonary EmbolismA randomized controlled trial. JAMA 2007;298(23):2743–53.

121. Glaser JE, Chamarthy M, Haramati LB, Esses D, Freeman LM. Successful and safe implementation of a trinary interpretation and reporting strategy for V/Q lung scintigraphy. J Nucl Med 2011; 52(10):1508–12.

122. Aziz MU, Hall MK, Pressacco J, Maki JH. Magnetic resonance angiography in pulmonary embolism: a review. Curr Probl Diagn Radiol 2019;48(6): 586–91.

123. Revel MP, Sanchez O, Couchon S, et al. Diagnostic accuracy of magnetic resonance imaging for an acute pulmonary embolism: results of the "IRM-EP" study. J Thromb Haemost 2012;10(5):743–50.

124. Stein PD, Chenevert TL, Fowler SE, et al. Gadolinium-enhanced magnetic resonance angiography for pulmonary embolism: a multicenter prospective study (PIOPED III). Ann Intern Med 2010;152(7): 434–43. W142-143.

125. Schiebler ML, Nagle SK, François CJ, et al. Effectiveness of MR angiography for the primary diagnosis of acute pulmonary embolism: clinical outcomes at 3 months and 1 year. J Magn Reson Imaging 2013;38(4):914–25.

126. Murphy SP, Urbut SM, Dudzinski DM. Progress toward prognosis in patients with pulmonary embolism. J Am Soc Echocardiogr 2023.

127. Bangalore S, Horowitz JM, Beam D, et al. Prevalence and predictors of Cardiogenic shock in intermediate-risk pulmonary embolism: Insights from the FLASH registry. J Am Coll Cardiol Intv 2023;16(8):958–72.

128. Bova C, Sanchez O, Prandoni P, et al. Identification of intermediate-risk patients with acute symptomatic pulmonary embolism. Eur Respir J 2014; 44(3):694–703.

129. Aujesky D, Obrosky DS, Stone RA, et al. Derivation and validation of a prognostic model for pulmonary embolism. Am J Respir Crit Care Med 2005;172(8):1041–6.

130. Jiménez D, Aujesky D, Moores L, et al. Simplification of the pulmonary embolism severity index for prognostication in patients with acute symptomatic pulmonary embolism. Arch Intern Med 2010; 170(15):1383–9.

131. Elias A, Mallett S, Daoud-Elias M, Poggi JN, Clarke M. Prognostic models in acute pulmonary embolism: a systematic review and meta-analysis. BMJ Open 2016;6(4):e010324.

132. Donzé J, Le Gal G, Fine MJ, et al. Prospective validation of the Pulmonary Embolism Severity Index. A clinical prognostic model for pulmonary embolism. Thromb Haemost 2008;100(5):943–8.

133. Righini M, Roy PM, Meyer G, Verschuren F, Aujesky D, Le Gal G. The Simplified Pulmonary Embolism Severity Index (PESI): validation of a clinical prognostic model for pulmonary embolism. J Thromb Haemost 2011;9(10):2115–7.

134. Barnes GD, Muzikansky A, Cameron S, et al. Comparison of 4 acute pulmonary embolism mortality risk scores in patients evaluated by pulmonary embolism response teams. JAMA Netw Open 2020; 3(8):e2010779.

135. Dudzinski DM, Piazza G. Multidisciplinary pulmonary embolism response teams. Circulation 2016; 133(1):98–103.

136. Provias T, Dudzinski DM, Jaff MR, et al. The Massachusetts General Hospital Pulmonary Embolism Response Team (MGH PERT): creation of a multidisciplinary program to improve care of patients with massive and submassive pulmonary embolism. Hosp Pract 2014;42(1):31–7.

137. Root CW, Dudzinski MD, Zakhary B, et al. Multidisciplinary approach to the management of pulmonary embolism patients: the pulmonary embolism response team (PERT). J Multidiscip Healthc 2018;11:187–95.

138. Kabrhel C, Rosovsky R, Channick R, et al. A multidisciplinary pulmonary embolism response team: initial 30-month experience with a Novel approach to Delivery of care to patients with submassive and massive pulmonary embolism. Chest 2016;150(2):384–93.

139. Dudzinski DM, Horowitz JM. Start-up, Organization and Performance of a multidisciplinary pulmonary embolism response team for the diagnosis and treatment of acute pulmonary embolism. Rev Esp Cardiol 2017;70(1):9–13.

140. Mahar JH, Haddadin I, Sadana D, et al. A pulmonary embolism response team (PERT) approach: initial experience from the Cleveland Clinic. J Thromb Thrombolysis 2018;46(2):186–92.

141. Fleitas Sosa D, Lehr AL, Zhao H, et al. Impact of pulmonary embolism response teams on acute pulmonary embolism: a systematic review and meta-analysis. Eur Respir Rev 2022;31(165):220023.

142. Wright C, Goldenberg I, Schleede S, et al. Effect of a multidisciplinary pulmonary embolism response team on patient mortality. Am J Cardiol 2021;161: 102–7.

143. Xenos ES, Davis GA, He Q, Green A, Smyth SS. The implementation of a pulmonary embolism response team in the management of intermediate- or high-risk pulmonary embolism. J Vasc Surg Venous Lymphat Disord 2019;7(4):493–500.

144. Hobohm L, Farmakis IT, Keller K, et al. Pulmonary embolism response team (PERT) implementation and its clinical value across countries: a scoping review and meta-analysis. Clin Res Cardiol 2022; 1–11. https://doi.org/10.1007/s00392-022-02077-0.

145. Rali P, Sacher D, Rivera-Lebron B, et al. Interhospital transfer of patients with acute pulmonary embolism: challenges and Opportunities. Chest 2021;160(5): 1844–52.

146. Perez-Nieto OR, Gomez-Oropeza I, Quintero-Leyra A, et al. Hemodynamic and respiratory support in pulmonary embolism: a narrative review. Front Med 2023;10:1123793.

147. Available at: https://pubmed.ncbi.nlm.nih.gov/ 32551849/. Accessed March 23, 2024. DOI: 10. 1177/1076029620933944

148. Bělohlávek J, Dytrych V, Linhart A. Pulmonary embolism, part II: management. Exp Clin Cardiol 2013;18(2):139–47.

149. Manier G, Castaing Y. Influence of cardiac output on oxygen exchange in acute pulmonary embolism. Am Rev Respir Dis 1992;145(1):130–6.

150. Yamamoto T. Management of patients with high-risk pulmonary embolism: a narrative review. Journal of Intensive Care 2018;6(1):16.

151. Duran D, Barrios D, Moises J, et al. The rationale, design, and methods of a trial to evaluate the efficacy and safety of oxygen therapy in patients with intermediate-risk acute pulmonary embolism. Am Heart J 2023;257:62–8.

152. Layish DT, Tapson VF. Pharmacologic hemodynamic support in massive pulmonary embolism. Chest 1997;111(1):218–24.

153. Piazza G. Advanced management of intermediate- and high-risk pulmonary embolism. J Am Coll Cardiol 2020;76(18):2117–27.

154. Mercat A, Diehl JL, Meyer G, Teboul JL, Sors H. Hemodynamic effects of fluid loading in acute massive pulmonary embolism. Crit Care Med 1999;27(3):540–4.

155. Ghignone M, Girling L, Prewitt RM. Volume Expansion versus norepinephrine in treatment of a low cardiac output complicating an acute increase in right ventricular afterload in Dogs. Anesthesiology 1984;60(2):132–5.

156. Ventetuolo CE, Klinger JR. Management of acute right ventricular failure in the intensive care Unit. Annals ATS 2014;11(5):811–22.

157. Kline JS, Puskarich MA, Jones AE, et al. Inhaled nitric oxide to treat intermediate risk pulmonary embolism: a multicenter randomized controlled trial. Nitric Oxide 2019;84:60–8.

158. Summerfield DT, Desai H, Levitov A, Grooms DA, Marik PE. Inhaled nitric oxide as salvage therapy in massive pulmonary embolism: a case series. Respir Care 2012;57(3):444–8.

159. Andersen A, Waziri F, Schultz JG, et al. Pulmonary vasodilation by sildenafil in acute intermediate-high risk pulmonary embolism: a randomized explorative trial. BMC Pulm Med 2021;21(1):72.

160. O'Malley TJ, Choi JH, Maynes EJ, et al. Outcomes of extracorporeal life support for the treatment of acute massive pulmonary embolism: a systematic review. Resuscitation 2020;146:132–7.

161. Yusuff HO, Zochios V, Vuylsteke A. Extracorporeal membrane oxygenation in acute massive pulmonary embolism: a systematic review. Perfusion 2015;30(8):611–6.

162. Weinberg A, Tapson VF, Ramzy D. Massive pulmonary embolism: extracorporeal membrane oxygenation and surgical pulmonary embolectomy. Semin Respir Crit Care Med 2017;38(1):66–72.

163. Scott JH, Gordon M, Vender R, et al. Venoarterial extracorporeal membrane oxygenation in massive pulmonary embolism-related cardiac arrest: a systematic review. Crit Care Med 2021;49(5):760–9.

164. Smith SB, Geske JB, Maguire JM, Zane NA, Carter RE, Morgenthaler TI. Early anticoagulation is associated with reduced mortality for acute pulmonary embolism. Chest 2010;137(6):1382–90.

165. Cossette B, Pelletier ME, Carrier N, et al. Evaluation of bleeding risk in patients exposed to therapeutic unfractionated or low-molecular-weight heparin: a cohort study in the context of a quality improvement initiative. Ann Pharmacother 2010;44(6): 994–1002.

166. Stein PD, Hull RD, Matta F, Yaekoub AY, Liang J. Incidence of thrombocytopenia in hospitalized patients with venous thromboembolism. Am J Med 2009;122(10):919–30.

167. Leentjens J, Peters M, Esselink AC, Smulders Y, Kramers C. Initial anticoagulation in patients with pulmonary embolism: thrombolysis, unfractionated heparin, LMWH, fondaparinux, or DOACs? Br J Clin Pharmacol 2017;83(11):2356–66.

168. Kearon C, Akl EA, Ornelas J, et al. Antithrombotic therapy for VTE disease: CHEST guideline and expert Panel Report. Chest 2016;149(2):315–52.

169. Meyer G, Vicaut E, Danays T, et al. Fibrinolysis for patients with intermediate-risk pulmonary embolism. N Engl J Med 2014;370(15):1402–11.

170. Marti C, John G, Konstantinides S, et al. Systemic thrombolytic therapy for acute pulmonary embolism: a systematic review and meta-analysis. Eur Heart J 2015;36(10):605–14.

171. Chatterjee S, Chakraborty A, Weinberg I, et al. Thrombolysis for pulmonary embolism and risk of all-cause mortality, major bleeding, and intracranial hemorrhage: a meta-analysis. JAMA 2014;311(23): 2414–21.

172. Grant PJ, Courey AJ, Hanigan S, et al. Table 6, [Indications and contraindications for systemic...]. Published February 2019.. Available at: https://www.ncbi.nlm.nih.gov/books/NBK544377/table/T6/. [Accessed 27 July 2023].

173. Konstantinides SV, Torbicki A, Agnelli G, et al. 2014 ESC guidelines on the diagnosis and management of acute pulmonary embolism. Eur Heart J 2014; 35(43):3033–69.

174. Forry J, Chappell A. Tenecteplase: a review of its Pharmacology and Uses. AACN Adv Crit Care 2023;34(2):77–83.

175. Shukla AN, Thakkar B, Jayaram AA, Madan TH, Gandhi GD. Efficacy and safety of tenecteplase in pulmonary embolism. J Thromb Thrombolysis 2014;38(1):24–9.

176. Zhang L, Yang X, Li S, Liao T, Pan G. Answering medical questions in Chinese using automatically mined knowledge and deep neural networks: an end-to-end solution. BMC Bioinf 2022;23(1):136.

177. Meneveau N, Séronde MF, Blonde MC, et al. Management of unsuccessful thrombolysis in acute massive pulmonary embolism. Chest 2006;129(4): 1043–50.

178. Singh M, Shafi I, Rali P, Panaro J, Lakhter V, Bashir R. Contemporary catheter-based treatment options for management of acute pulmonary embolism. Curr Treat Options Cardio Med 2021; 23(7):44.

179. Mostafa A, Briasoulis A, Telila T, Belgrave K, Grines C. Treatment of massive or submassive acute pulmonary embolism with catheter-directed thrombolysis. Am J Cardiol 2016;117(6):1014–20.

180. Furfaro D, Stephens RS, Streiff MB, Brower R. Catheter-directed thrombolysis for intermediate-risk pulmonary embolism. Ann Am Thorac Soc 2018;15(2):134–44.

181. Piazza G, Hohlfelder B, Jaff MR, et al. A prospective, single-arm, multicenter trial of ultrasound-facilitated, catheter-directed, low-Dose fibrinolysis for acute massive and submassive pulmonary embolism: the SEATTLE II study. JACC Cardiovasc Interv 2015;8(10):1382–92.

182. Kucher N, Boekstegers P, Müller OJ, et al. Randomized, controlled trial of ultrasound-assisted catheter-directed thrombolysis for acute intermediate-risk pulmonary embolism. Circulation 2014;129(4):479–86.

183. Bruno ES, Mujer MTP, Desai V, Brailovsky Y. A meta-analysis of standard versus ultrasound-assisted catheter-directed thrombolysis in the management of acute pulmonary embolism. JSCAI 2023;2(1):100514.

184. Tapson VF, Sterling K, Jones N, et al. A randomized trial of the Optimum duration of Acoustic Pulse thrombolysis procedure in acute intermediate-risk pulmonary embolism: the OPTALYSE PE trial. J Am Coll Cardiol Intv 2018;11(14):1401–10.

185. Klok FA, Piazza G, Sharp ASP, et al. Ultrasound-facilitated, catheter-directed thrombolysis vs anticoagulation alone for acute intermediate-high-risk pulmonary embolism: rationale and design of the HI-PEITHO study. Am Heart J 2022;251:43–53.

186. Tu T, Toma C, Tapson VF, et al. A prospective, single-arm, multicenter trial of catheter-directed mechanical thrombectomy for intermediate-risk acute pulmonary embolism: the FLARE study. JACC Cardiovasc Interv 2019;12(9):859–69.

187. Toma C, Jaber WA, Weinberg MD, et al. Acute outcomes for the full US cohort of the FLASH mechanical thrombectomy registry in pulmonary embolism. Eurointervention 2023;18:1201–12.

188. Sista AK, Horowitz JM, Tapson VF, et al. Indigo aspiration system for treatment of pulmonary embolism: results of the EXTRACT-PE trial. JACC Cardiovasc Interv 2021;14(3):319–29.

189. Sedhom R, Elbadawi, Megaly M, et al. Outcomes with catheter-directed thrombolysis vs. catheter-directed embolectomy among patients with high-risk pulmonary embolism: a nationwide analysis. European Heart Journal. Acute Cardiovascular Care 2023;12(Issue 4):224–31.

190. Choi JH, O'Malley TJ, Maynes EJ, et al. Surgical pulmonary embolectomy outcomes for acute pulmonary embolism. Ann Thorac Surg 2020;110(3):1072–80.

191. Dudzinski DM, Giri J, Rosenfield K. Interventional treatment of pulmonary embolism. Circ Cardiovasc Interv 2017;10(2):e004345.

192. Nakamura K, Alba GA, Scheske JA, et al. A 57-year-old man with Insidious dyspnea and Non-pleuritic chest and back pain. Chest 2016;150(2): e41–7.

193. Kabrhel C, Rempell JS, Avery LL, Dudzinski DM, Weinberg I. Case records of the Massachusetts General Hospital. Case 29-2014. A 60-year-old woman with syncope. N Engl J Med 2014; 371(12):1143–50.

194. Keeling WB, Sundt T, Leacche M, et al. Outcomes after surgical pulmonary embolectomy for acute pulmonary Embolus: a multi-Institutional study. Ann Thorac Surg 2016; 102(5):1498–502.

195. Zarrabi K, Zolghadrasli A, Ostovan MA, Azimifar A. Short-term results of retrograde pulmonary embolectomy in massive and submassive pulmonary embolism: a single-center study of 30 patients. Eur J Cardio Thorac Surg 2011;40(4):890–3.

196. Pasrija C, Kronfli A, Rouse M, et al. Outcomes after surgical pulmonary embolectomy for acute submassive and massive pulmonary embolism: a single-center experience. J Thorac Cardiovasc Surg 2018;155(3):1095–106.e2.

Acute Heart Valve Emergencies

Ryan R. Keane, MD, Venu Menon, MD, Paul C. Cremer, MD, MS*

KEYWORDS

- Acute aortic regurgitation • Acute mitral regurgitation • CICU • Severe aortic stenosis
- Severe mitral stenosis • Tricuspid regurgitation • Tricuspid stenosis • Valvular emergency

KEY POINTS

- Acute aortic regurgitation results in rapid equilibration of aortic and left ventricular diastolic pressures, which increases left ventricular wall stress and decreases coronary perfusion. Goals of therapy include decreasing the diastolic filling period with reduction in regurgitant volume.
- Severe aortic stenosis resulting in decompensated heart failure or cardiogenic shock is due to a fixed obstruction, which increases left ventricular wall stress and decreases stroke volume. Management includes decreasing the left ventricular to aortic gradient.
- Acute mitral regurgitation results in a precipitous increase in pressure within an unprepared left atrium, and left ventricular ejection fraction may appear seemingly preserved despite cardiogenic shock. Treatment includes optimizing forward flow and decreasing pulmonary edema.
- Severe mitral stenosis results in an elevated left atrial pressure with a normal or low left ventricular end-diastolic pressure. Cardiogenic shock can occur from right ventricular failure with enhanced interventricular interaction.
- For all severe valvular lesions that result in decompensated heart failure or cardiogenic shock, appropriate medical therapy is essential for stabilization, but expeditious correction of the underlying anatomic problem should not be delayed.

 Video content accompanies this article at http://www.cardiology.theclinics.com.

INTRODUCTION

Although many patients in the cardiac intensive care unit (CICU) have chronic valvular heart disease, a primary valvular problem accounts for approximately 8% of all admissions.[1] In this setting, valvular emergencies can encompass both acute dysfunction and decompensation due to a progressive valvular lesion. For both scenarios, but especially for acute lesions where compensatory cardiac remodeling has not occurred, prompt recognition, stabilization, and definitive treatment are essential for optimal patient outcomes. Accordingly, the aim of the current article is to highlight commonly encountered acute valvular emergencies with a focus on pertinent clinical and hemodynamic findings, essential echocardiographic features, medical and temporary mechanical circulatory support management, and finally, definitive repair with transcatheter based intervention or surgery.

AORTIC REGURGITATION

Acute, severe aortic regurgitation (AR) must be promptly recognized to prevent multi-organ failure and hemodynamic collapse. Once cardiogenic shock has occurred, medical options are limited, and emergency intervention is often required.

Department of Cardiovascular Medicine, Cleveland Clinic Coordinating Center for Clinical Research, Heart Vascular and Thoracic Institute, 9500 Euclid Ave: Desk J1-5, Cleveland, OH 44195, USA
* Corresponding author. Heart, Vascular and Thoracic Institute, Cleveland Clinic, 9500 Euclid Avenue, Desk J1-5, Cleveland, OH 44195.
E-mail address: cremerp@ccf.org
Twitter: @PaulCremerMD (P.C.C.)

Cardiol Clin 42 (2024) 237–252
https://doi.org/10.1016/j.ccl.2024.02.009
0733-8651/24/© 2024 Elsevier Inc. All rights reserved.

Causes

Acute AR can result from infective endocarditis, aortic dissection, prosthetic or allograft valve dysfunction, and trauma/iatrogenic injury.[2] In categorizing the mechanism of AR, the Carpentier classification is often employed: type I (normal leaflet excursion, ie, annular dilation or leaflet perforation), type II (cusp prolapse or flail), and type III (cusp restriction).[3] Infective endocarditis can cause leaflet perforation and/or leaflet flail. In particular with prosthetic valves, perivalvular extension of infection (ie, aortic root abscess) can result in complete or partial valve dehiscence and paravalvular leak. Aortic dissections can result in acute AR through annular dilation leading to incomplete coaptation of the aortic valve leaflets, direct extension of the dissection resulting in a flail leaflet or commissural disruption, and prolapse of the dissection flap into the left ventricular outflow tract (LVOT). Iatrogenic acute AR can result from leaflet perforation or impingement during left heart catheterization, and during balloon valvuloplasty of a stenotic aortic valve. Blunt trauma to the chest is a rare but reported etiology of acute AR.[4] Patients with a bicuspid aortic valve are also at increased risk of developing acute AR due to either infection, dissection, or trauma.

Clinical and Hemodynamic Presentation

In acute AR, there is a rapid influx of blood into the left ventricle (LV) during diastole, leading to an equalization of LV and aortic pressures and a precipitous rise in left ventricular end-diastolic pressure (LVEDP). This initially leads to premature closing of the mitral valve in diastole and incomplete left atrial emptying with resultant pulmonary edema. If the LVEDP continues to increase and exceeds left atrial pressure, diastolic mitral regurgitation (MR) can occur. In addition, effective forward stroke volume is reduced, and in a chronotropically competent patient, heart rate increases in an attempt to maintain cardiac output. An invasive hemodynamic assessment often reveals elevated filling pressures and a low cardiac index. In acute AR, when there has not been time for compensatory LV enlargement, the pulse pressure may be normal or even reduced if the stroke volume is low.

Echocardiographic Diagnosis

AR is initially assessed with transthoracic echocardiography (TTE), although transesophageal echocardiography (TEE) is often required to better delineate the anatomic mechanism of AR and to aid in surgical/procedural planning.[3,5–7] On TTE, color flow Doppler can be used to identify the presence or absence of AR, particularly in a parasternal long or apical 5-chamber view. The ratio of the AR jet width to LVOT diameter is a simple, relatively sensitive screen for AR. However, this methodology can underestimate eccentric jets of AR and is affected by the diameter of the LVOT. A vena contracta can also be measured while in a parasternal long axis view and can help delineate mild (VC < 0.3 cm) from severe AR (>0.7 cm). This method is also prone to measurement error and is less reliable with bicuspid aortic valves.

Continuous wave Doppler can be used to evaluate the severity of acute AR. The pressure half-time (PHT) is a measure of equalization of pressures between the LV and aorta, and a PHT less than 200 m sec is compatible with severe AR.[3,5] However, this parameter reflects the time course of AR development more than the severity. Specifically, in acute severe AR, when the LV has not had time to remodel to accommodate the increased LVEDP, the PHT will be short. Conversely, in chronic severe AR with LV remodeling, the PHT is not a reliable measure of AR severity.

The presence of flow reversal in the thoracic and abdominal aorta is another useful semiquantitative parameter to assess the severity of AR. Any degree of diastolic flow reversal in the abdominal aorta is compatible with severe AR. Of note, in acute severe AR, due to the rapid equalization of pressures between the LV and aorta, flow reversal may not be holo-diastolic. Finally, assessment of the LV response is crucial. In acute AR, left ventricular size is normal, and LV ejection fraction may be reduced because of increased wall stress and decreased coronary perfusion pressure.

Medical Management and Mechanical Support Options

In acute severe AR, urgent medical stabilization is critical to prevent further deterioration. A cornerstone of medical management in AR is reducing diastolic filling time to maintain cardiac output and reduce LVEDP. The avoidance of bradycardia is essential, and even a normal sinus rhythm (ie, 70 beats/min) may be inadequate. Temporary transvenous pacing or inotropes should be considered in patients with acute AR with bradycardia or normal sinus rhythm who have acute decompensated heart failure or cardiogenic shock. In patients with AR in the setting of an aortic root abscess who are at high risk of progression to complete heart block, which can precipitate rapid hemodynamic collapse, temporary pacing can also be considered. Atrioventricular nodal blockade should be avoided in patients with acute severe AR, including patients with an acute ascending aortic dissection.[7]

Afterload reduction with intravenous (IV) vasodilators can reduce the regurgitant flow and help stabilize patients.[7] Preload reduction with diuretics can also aid in reducing pulmonary edema. Mechanical circulatory support (MCS) in acute or severe AR is relatively contraindicated as currently available MCS options require a competent aortic valve. An intra-aortic balloon pump will worsen AR regurgitant volume. An Impella device (AbioMed, Danvers, MA), which must cross the aortic valve and rests in the LV, will also worsen AR due impaired leaflet coaptation (and possible leaflet damage). Veno-arterial extracorporeal membrane oxygenation (ECMO) increases LV afterload, LV wall stress, and results in pulmonary edema. An additional venous cannula can be placed in the left atrium to attenuate pulmonary edema (LAVA ECMO). However, this approach is reserved for the rare patients in extremis who are not currently candidates for emergency intervention, but definitive repair is planned in the near-term.

Definitive Repair

Surgical repair or aortic valve replacement (SAVR) carries a class I indication in acute, severe AR (**Fig. 1**, Videos 1–3).[7] In patients with decompensated heart failure or cardiogenic shock, surgical replacement should not be delayed unless the intraoperative risk is prohibitive. Transcatheter aortic valve replacement (TAVR) for severe AR has traditionally been considered a contraindication in native valves, as earlier generation TAVR valves were associated with valve embolization and paravalvular leak (due to a dilated aortic annulus). However, newer generation TAVR valves have shown an improvement in clinical outcomes (**Fig. 2**, Videos 4–6).[7–9] Moreover, transcatheter

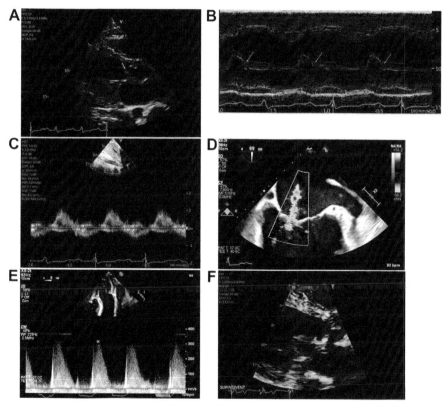

Fig. 1. 40-year-old intravenous drug user with group B streptococcus bacteremia presenting with hypotension. (A) Parasternal long-axis view shows a flail non-coronary cusp, and pre-mature closure of the mitral valve in keeping with elevated left ventricular diastolic pressure. (B) M-mode through the mitral valve from a parasternal long-axis view confirms premature closure (*arrows*). (C) Diastolic flow reversal in the abdominal aorta compatible with severe aortic regurgitation. (D) Transesophageal echo shows diastolic mitral regurgitation in the setting of acute severe aortic regurgitation, reflective of increased left ventricular diastolic pressure. (E) Short pressure half-time consistent with rapid equilibration of aortic and left ventricular diastolic pressures. (F) Patient underwent successful aortic valve replacement with a bioprosthesis as well as mitral valve repair including repair of aortic-mitral continuity.

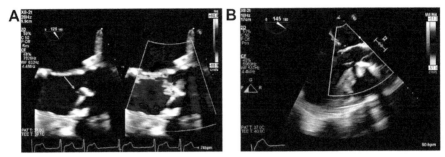

Fig. 2. 60-year-old with multiple prior cardiac surgeries, most recently with aortic valve replacement with a homograft as well as mitral valve repair with an annuloplasty band and reconstruction of the aortic-mitral continuity presents with (A) flail of the anterior cusp (arrow) and eccentric posteriorly directed aortic regurgitation, noted on long-axis view of the aortic valve with TEE. (B) Status post 29 mm Edwards S3 valve within the aortic homograft with no residual aortic regurgitation.

aortic valves designed specifically for AR are currently being investigated in clinical trials.

AORTIC STENOSIS

In the elderly population, aortic stenosis (AS) is the most prevalent valvular heart disease.[10,11] The most common causes are calcific and congenital AS (ie, due to a bicuspid aortic valve). When severe AS results in decompensated heart failure or cardiogenic shock, urgent or emergency intervention is required.

Clinical and Hemodynamic Presentation

On exam, patients with severe AS have a late-peaking crescendo-decrescendo systolic murmur

with a diminished or absent A2 and pulsus parvus et tardus. In the setting of decompensated heart failure, patients with severe AS will have elevated biventricular filling pressures and may have a reduced cardiac index. In a tenuous patient, invasive hemodynamic monitoring is essential because the fixed obstruction from AS renders the patient sensitive to shifts in preload and afterload.

Echocardiography

The initial assessment of AS severity is based on peak jet velocity, mean transvalvular gradient, aortic valve area, and the dimensionless index (DI).[12] Peak jet velocity and mean gradient are measured using continuous wave Doppler in

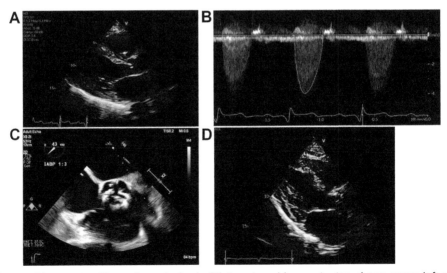

Fig. 3. 70-year-old presents with cardiogenic shock. (A) Parasternal long axis view shows severe left ventricular systolic dysfunction with thickened aortic valve leaflets. (B) Continuous wave Doppler shows a peak gradient of 63 mm Hg and a mean gradient of 37 mm Hg compatible with severe aortic stenosis. (C) Short axis transesophageal echo shows a trileaflet aortic valve with limited leaflet excursion. The patient was supported with an intra-aortic balloon pump (IABP) for cardiogenic shock. (D) The patient underwent transcatheter aortic valve replacement with a 26 mm Edwards S3 valve with improvement in left ventricular systolic function.

multiple acoustic windows to obtain the highest velocity. A peak velocity of greater than 4.0 metre per second and a mean gradient of greater than 40 millimetre Hg is consistent with severe AS, whereas a velocity of greater than 5.0 metre per second indicates very severe AS. AS severity is also assessed with aortic valve area (AVA), and an AVA of less than 1.0 square centimetre (<0.6 cm^2/m^2) is compatible with severe AS. Finally, the ratio of the LVOT and AV velocity time integrals (DI or velocity ratio) is standard in the assessment of AS, and a ratio of less than 0.25 is in keeping with severe AS.

In patients with a reduced stroke volume, transvalvular gradients may not reach classic severe thresholds despite severe AS (low-flow, low-gradient (LFLG)). In this setting, the AVA and DI may be more informative, and further imaging with TEE or computed tomography can aid in confirming severe AS. Moreover, as AS progresses, the time to peak velocity (acceleration time [AT]) increases, analogous to the physical exam finding of *pulsus tardus*. Therefore, an increased AT, or an elevated AT to ejection time ratio, is associated with AS severity. Similarly, in patients with prosthetic valves, severe stenosis is suspected when

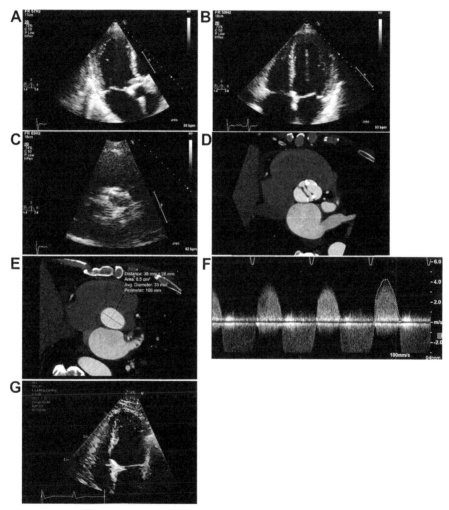

Fig. 4. 65-year-old presents with decompensated heart failure in setting of aortic stenosis. (*A*) Apical long axis view shows severely reduced left ventricular systolic function with hyperechoic and thickened aortic valve leaflets with decreased excursion. (*B*) Apical 4 chamber view show reduced left and right ventricular systolic function. (*C*) Aortic valve morphology is difficult to delineate on this short-axis view. (*D*) 4D CTA showed a bicuspid aortic valve with asymmetric calcification of the sinuses. (*E*) On CTA, the aortic annulus was enlarged, which favored surgical versus transcatheter aortic valve replacement. (*F*) Continuous wave Doppler from the right upper sternal border is compatible with severe aortic stenosis with a prolonged acceleration time and increased acceleration time (AT) to ejection time (ET) ratio. (*G*) Left and right ventricular systolic function is improved after surgical aortic valve replacement.

the DI is less than 0.25 and the AT is greater than 100 metre per sec.[13]

Medical Stabilization and Mechanical Support Options

Medical stabilization focuses on optimizing afterload and preload. Nitroprusside can be useful in reducing the LV to aorta gradient and improving cardiac output,[14] though invasive hemodynamic monitoring is essential because overly zealous treatment can result in hypotension and reduced coronary perfusion. With preload, an adequate LV end-diastolic volume is necessary to maintain an acceptable stroke volume. However, compensatory remodeling from AS reduces LV compliance and excess preload will result in pulmonary edema and pulmonary hypertension. Reducing preload with IV diuresis can ameliorate pulmonary edema, but over-diuresis can lead to a reduction in stroke volume and hypotension.

Regarding MCS options in a patient with cardiogenic shock despite medical therapy, an IABP will reduce afterload and improve coronary perfusion. Few data are available regarding percutaneous left ventricular assist devices, such as the Impella, and there is a manufacturer recommendation against its use with an AVA of less than 0.6 square centimetre. Finally,

venoarterial extracorporeal membrane oxygenation (VA-ECMO) may be considered to support end-organ perfusion in refractory shock. However, the fixed obstruction increases LV afterload as well as the risk for aortic valve and LV thrombus, and expeditiously correcting the valvular stenosis is indicated.[15]

Definitive Repair

With decompensated heart failure or cardiogenic shock due to AS, aortic valve replacement (AVR) carries a class 1A indication.[7] Given the limitations of medical therapy, unless AVR is prohibitive-risk, definitive treatment should not be delayed. If the anatomy is amenable to TAVR, this approach has emerged as a good treatment option for the extreme-risk patient (**Fig. 3**, Videos 7–9).[16] Importantly, for patients with embarrassed left ventricular systolic function due to high gradient AS, rapid improvement in left ventricular ejection fraction (LVEF) is expected after AVR with relief of the afterload mismatch. In a situation, where there is uncertainty regarding the contribution of AS to the clinical deterioration, percutaneous balloon aortic valvuloplasty (PBAV) can be a diagnostic as well as a therapeutic measure.[7,17–19] However, PBAV is contraindicated in patients with moderate or greater AR.

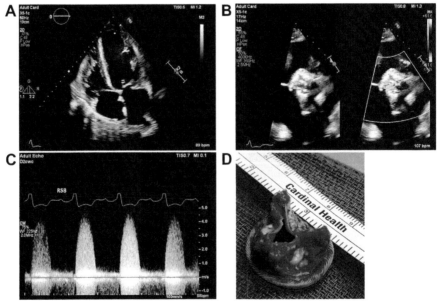

Fig. 5. 38-year-old with a history of congenital aortic stenosis and two prior cardiac surgeries, most recently with bioprosthetic aortic valve replacement, presented in cardiogenic shock. (A) Apical 4 chamber view shows severe left and right ventricular systolic dysfunction. Given progressive cardiogenic shock, she was placed on VA ECMO as a bridge to cardiac surgery. (B) Short axis view of the bioprosthetic aortic valve with color compare shows hyperechoic immobile leaflets. (C) Continuous wave Doppler from the right upper sternal border (RSB) shows peak and mean gradients of 76 and 44 mm Hg, respectively. (D) Given the small annulus and valve, she underwent surgery. The bioprosthetic leaflets were severely calcified and immobile with no signs of infection.

Patients with bicuspid aortic valves present a unique challenge.[20] Specifically, anatomic considerations such as an enlarged annulus, asymmetric sinuses, or raphae calcifications may make TAVR less favorable (**Fig. 4**, Videos 10–14). In addition, these patients may have an associated aortopathy that warrants surgical correction. Therefore, many of these patients should undergo surgery unless the risk is prohibitive. Anatomic considerations are also paramount for decision-making in patients with prosthetic AS. For example, patients with decompensated heart failure or cardiogenic shock may preferentially undergo TAVR unless there are concerns such as a small annulus, potential coronary artery obstruction, or active infective endocarditis (**Figs. 5** and **6**, Videos 15–17).

ACUTE MITRAL REGURGITATION

Similar to acute AR, when an acute onset has precluded gradual compensatory remodeling of the left-sided chambers, severe MR can result in florid pulmonary edema and cardiogenic shock, which requires emergency intervention.

Causes

In general, MR is classified according to whether the valvular pathology is primary or secondary, and the Carpentier methodology is also employed: type I (normal leaflet excursion), type II (leaflet prolapse or flail), and type III (restricted leaflet motion). With myocardial ischemia, acute MR can occur through 2 mechanisms. First one is posterior papillary muscle rupture (either partial or complete) and is generally seen with an inferior myocardial infarction because the posterior papillary muscle has a single arterial supple, unlike the anterior papillary muscle.[21,22] The second mechanism is restricted posterior leaflet motion due to regional wall motion abnormalities, again most commonly encountered with an inferior myocardial infarction. Non-ischemic acute MR can result from chordal rupture with leaflet prolapse and flail in the setting of degenerative mitral valve disease and may also occur due to infective endocarditis.

Clinical and Hemodynamic Presentation

In acute severe MR, the left atrial pressure increases precipitously, and forward stroke volume dramatically decreases. The result is a decreased transmitral gradient and potential underestimated of MR on both echo and auscultation (ie, "silent MR"). With invasive hemodynamic monitoring, although no feature is pathognomonic for acute severe MR, pulmonary hypertension, and an

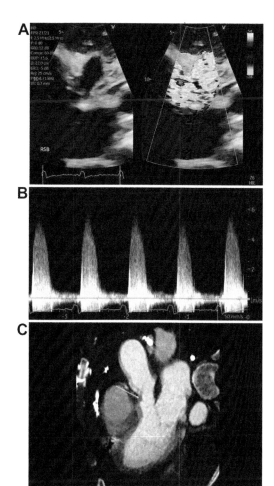

Fig. 6. 55-year-old presented in cardiogenic shock after recent aortic homograft placement at an outside institution for infective endocarditis. (*A*) Echocardiography at the right upper sternal border shows turbulent flow across the homograft. (*B*) Continuous wave Doppler at the right upper sternal border shows peak and mean gradients of 138 and 76 mm Hg, respectively. (*C*) On CTA, there was suggestion of kinking of the proximal aspect of the aortic homograft, which was confirmed at the time of repeat cardiac surgery.

increased pulmonary capillary wedge pressure with tall v waves are observed.

Echocardiography

When acute MR is suspected, echocardiography should be performed at the bedside with the goals of classifying severity, assessing LV response, and delineating MR mechanism.[23] Oftentimes, TEE is necessary to expeditiously achieve these objectives.[3] Color flow imaging can be useful for an initial assessment of the size, geometry, and direction of the MR jet. In acute severe MR, continuous Doppler demonstrates a dense triangular profile

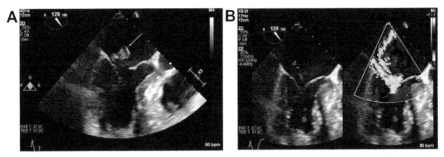

Fig. 7. 78-year-old presented with inferior STEMI, distal RCA occlusion, and cardiogenic shock. Given hemodynamic instability, emergency transesophageal echocardiogram was performed (*A*) which showed rupture of the posteromedial papillary muscle (*arrow*). (*B*) Left ventricular ejection fraction was preserved, which is often the case with acute papillary muscle rupture, and there was severe mitral regurgitation.

indicating rapid equilibration of left ventricular and atrial pressures. Importantly, if the left atrial pressure is markedly elevated and/or systolic blood pressure is low, the MR jet will have a low velocity reflective of a decreased gradient between left ventricular and atrial pressures. On mitral inflow, the E velocity is generally elevated (>1.2 m/sec) indicating increased flow.[3]

Additional measures of MR focus on calculating the regurgitant volume and effective orifice area, although these methods may be technically challenging. The proximal isovelocity surface area (PISA) method is most commonly employed, and in general, an effective regurgitant orifice area (EROA) of greater than 0.4 square centimetre is consistent with severe MR. However, this method is not reliable with multiple or eccentric jets. Moreover, the simplified PISA equation ($r^2/2$) assumes an LV to left atrial pressure gradient of 100 millimetre Hg and should be avoided in the acute setting, where this may not be accurate.

Medical Stabilization and Mechanical Circulatory Support Options

Prompt medical stabilization focuses on reducing pulmonary edema and increasing forward stroke volume. Intravenous vasodilator therapy, such as with nitroprusside, which is rapidly titratable and has a short half-life, and fluid removal are mainstays of acute management. Unfortunately, acute MR can present with hypotension and MCS may be needed for stabilization. Intra-aortic balloon counter pulsation can be utilized to reduce afterload and improve coronary perfusion.[15] Similarly, a percutaneous temporary LVAD such as the Impella (Abiomed, Danvers, and MA) can be used to offload the LV and reduce left atrial pressure.[24] Venoarterial extracorporeal membrane oxygenation may be indicated with profound cardiogenic shock or when biventricular support is necessary. In this setting, given the increase in LV wall stress and potential worsening of pulmonary edema, an LV vent (such as with an Impella or IABP) is often employed.[25]

Definitive Repair

Acute MR with decompensated heart failure and/or cardiogenic shock requires immediate surgical intervention (**Figs. 7–9**, Videos 18–25). With papillary muscle rupture, mitral valve replacement is more common that mitral valve repair (see **Fig. 7**).[26] For ischemic MR, although replacement may be generally preferred, the decision is more nuanced and should account for the patient's age and expected prognosis, as well as the potential

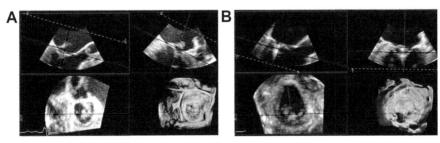

Fig. 8. 50-year-old with a history of coronary artery disease presented with decompensated heart failure and cardiogenic shock. (*A*) 3D multiplanar reconstruction shows rupture of the posteromedial papillary muscle. (*B*) Due to medical comorbidities including cirrhosis, the patient underwent successful transcatheter edge-to-edge mitral valve repair.

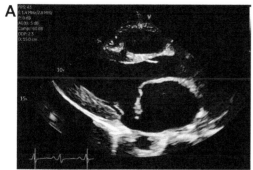

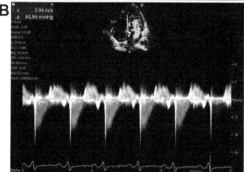

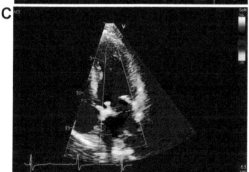

Fig. 9. 39-year-old with oral streptococcal bacteremia presented with cardiogenic shock, acute kidney injury, ischemic hepatitis, and disseminated intravascular coagulation. (*A*) Echocardiogram shows an echodensity associate with the mitral valve, compatible with a vegetation, and a large coaptation defect consistent with severe mitral regurgitation. (*B*) On continuous wave Doppler assessment of the mitral regurgitation, the jet has an early peak and is low velocity. These findings are reflective of a rapid equalization of systolic pressures between the left ventricle and left atrium, as well as markedly increased left atrial pressure with systemic hypotension. (*C*) Given the degree of multiorgan failure, he was initially supported with VA ECMO, and then underwent bioprosthetic mitral valve replacement with good result.

for LV remodeling with surgery. For both ischemia MR and papillary muscle rupture, transcatheter edge-to-edge repair (TEER) has been reported, and should be considered when operative risk is extremely high or prohibitive (see **Fig. 8**).[27]

SEVERE MITRAL STENOSIS

In the developing world, mitral stenosis (MS) is most commonly due to rheumatic heart disease.[28] The most common cause of non-rheumatic MS is mitral annular calcification (MAC) which encroaches on the leaflets and restricts motion.[29–31] In patients with prosthetic mitral valves, stenosis can result from structural valve degeneration, thrombosis, or endocarditis. With the exception of prosthetic valve thrombosis and endocarditis, MS does not generally occur acutely, and presentation to theCICU with MS as the primary problem may reflect a lack of appropriate follow-up or a missed diagnosis.

Clinical and Hemodynamic Presentation

Patients with severe MS will have elevated left atrial pressures with a low or normal LVEDP. With this fixed obstruction, a prolonged diastolic filling period will decrease the gradient between the left atrium and ventricle and reduce pulmonary edema. However, when a patient develops cardiogenic shock due to severe MS, this presentation is often the result of a right ventricle that is failing because of pulmonary hypertension.

Echocardiographic Assessment

Measurement of the mitral valve area (MVA) is an essential step in the assessment of MS. MVA can be measured directly with planimetry, though accurate assessment at the leaflet tips is necessary.[32] The MVA can also be calculated via the PHT, and even though there are limitations of this approach, a prolonged PHT is associated with more significant MS. The mean gradient is also correlated with MS severity, and a mean gradient of greater than 10 millimetre Hg is compatible with severe MS. However, the mean gradient is dependent on flow (ie, stroke volume) and heart rate, and both of these parameters may be perturbed for a patient in the CICU.

The downstream consequences of MS should also be well interrogated. The left atrium is invariably enlarged, and estimated pulmonary pressures are elevated. Right ventricular systolic function may also be impaired. In the setting of right ventricular pressure overload, the interventricular septum may shift to the left during systole, and this interventricular interaction can also negatively impact stroke volume.

Medical Stabilization and Mechanical Support Options

MS is a fixed obstruction that results in reduced LV diastolic filling. Medical stabilization balances optimizing left ventricular diastolic volume and

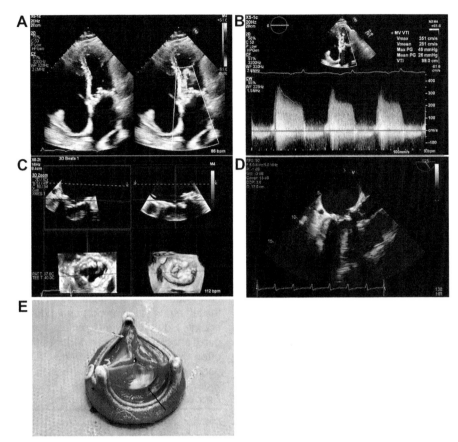

Fig. 10. 50-year-old with a history of an inferior myocardial infarction complicated by papillary muscle rupture status post bioprosthetic mitral valve replacement 10 years prior is admitted with cardiogenic shock. (*A*) Apical 4 chamber view shows thickened, hyperechoic mitral valve leaflets with aliasing on color flow map across the mitral inflow, as well as a dilated and dysfunction right ventricle. (*B*) Continuous wave Doppler of the mitral inflow shows markedly elevated peak and mean gradients at 49 and 26 mm Hg, respectively, with a prolonged pressure half-time (~320 msec) compatible with severe mitral stenosis. (*C*) 3D multiplanar reconstruction shows severely thickened mitral valve leaflet with limited opening during diastole. (*D*) Marked shift of the interventricular septum was noted which contributed to an underfilled left ventricle and raised concern about left ventricular outflow tract obstruction if valve in valve transcatheter therapy was pursued. (*E*) Patient underwent repeat mitral valve replacement. The explanted bioprosthesis showed severe calcification (*orange arrow*) and pannus (*black arrow*) restricting leaflet motion.

reducing pulmonary edema. Decreasing heart rate is often essential in achieving this balance by increasing diastolic filling time. For this reason, beta-blockers are often used, though may be contraindicated in a patient with cardiogenic shock with a prominent component of right ventricular failure. When atrial fibrillation develops, hemodynamic decompensation may occur due to the loss of atrial contraction, and restoration of sinus rhythm should be pursued if feasible. In severe MS, the LV is typically underfilled and vasodilators should be avoided as they may further decrease preload and result in hypotension.

Mechanical circulatory support options are limited in MS. An IABP would provide minimal benefit in augmenting cardiac output, and successful placement of a percutaneous LVAD such as an Impella

wound not benefit an underfilled LV. Venoarterial extracorporeal membrane oxygenation with an left artrial (LA) vent (LAVA-ECMO) or a TandemHeart would be feasible MCS options in offloading LA pressure and providing adequate end-organ perfusion, but should only be considered when needed as a short-term bridge to definitive repair.

Definitive Repair

For rheumatic MS, percutaneous mitral balloon valvuloplasty or surgery are considered standard of care.[33,34] With stenosis due to MAC, surgery is first-line, though transcatheter based procedures are promising. If the anatomy is favorable, transcatheter valve-in-valve therapy is a good treatment option for the critically ill patient with

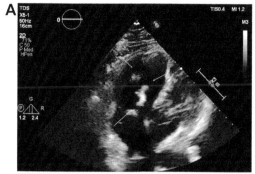

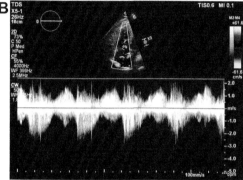

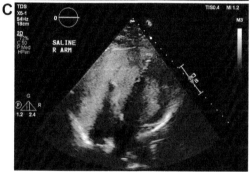

Fig. 11. 38-year-old admitted with refractory hypoxemia. (*A*) Apical 4 chamber view with a focus on the right ventricle shows multiple hypodensities (*arrows*) associated with an intracardiac device lead, which was known to be fractured. The right ventricle is dilated and dysfunctional. (*B*) On continuous wave Doppler assessment, there is a dense and triangular profile compatible with severe, laminar TR. (*C*) On agitated saline study, there is a large right to left shunt across a patent foramen ovale in the setting of elevated right sided pressures and severe TR.

MS due to small vessel disease (SVD. Otherwise, surgery is preferred (**Fig. 10**, Videos 26–28) and is also indicated in patient with prosthetic valve thrombosis or endocarditis.

SEVERE TRICUSPID AND PULMONIC LESIONS
Causes

Severe tricuspid regurgitation (TR) is often a result of other cardiac conditions and can occur from secondary to annular dilation. Primary TR can result from trauma (such as impingement by pacemaker lead placement, or flail leaflet from an endomyocardial biopsy), myxomatous degeneration or from carcinoid syndrome causing leaflet fixation, and lack of coaptation. Native tricuspid stenosis (TS) is rare and is usually caused by mechanical obstruction from an intracardiac mass, such as a tumor or a vegetation. Tricuspid stenosis can also occur with prosthetic valves due to endocarditis, thrombus, or SVD. Pulmonic stenosis (PS) is most commonly congenitally acquired as an isolated lesion or as part of a syndrome such as Tetralogy of Fallot.

Clinical Presentation and Hemodynamics

Severe tricuspid or pulmonic valve disease can present with signs and symptoms of right heart failure including lower extremity edema, ascites, congestive hepatopathy, and cardiorenal syndrome. In severe TR, measurement of right atrial (RA) pressure will demonstrate elevated mean pressures, a steep y descent, and potential ventricularization of RA pressures.[35,36] Patients with severe TS will have an elevated RA:RV gradient. In severe PR, elevated RV and RA pressures are noted with a widened pulmonary artery pulse pressure.

Echocardiographic Assessment

Assessment of the tricuspid valve (TV) anatomy on transthoracic echocardiogram (TTE) can be challenging, though the anterior leaflet can be readily evaluated on parasternal long RV inflow and apical 4 chamber views.[3] Assessment of severe TR with continuous wave Doppler demonstrates a dense triangular shape. With severe secondary TR, annular dilation and a large central jet are present. In primary severe TR due to leaflet perforation, an eccentric jet may be noted. Systolic flow reversal in the hepatic veins and a plethoric inferior vena cava (IVC) are also characteristic of severe TR. Tricuspid stenosis can be evaluated in a similar manner to MS and is considered severe if the mean gradient is greater than 5 millimetre Hg.[36–38] Pulmonic stenosis is severe when peak and mean gradients are greater than 64 millimetre Hg and 35 millimetre Hg, respectively.[34]

Medical Stabilization and Mechanical Support Options

Medical management of severe right sided regurgitant lesions involves diuresis for right heart failure, and the approach is similar for stenotic lesions, though with more caution given preload dependence. When cardiogenic shock occurs

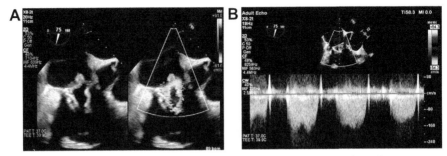

Fig. 12. 37-year-old with a history of tricuspid valve replacement for infective endocarditis presents with fevers and right-sided heart failure. (*A*) Transesophageal echo with a focus on the bioprosthetic tricuspid valves shows associated echodensities in keeping with vegetations. Color Doppler shows aliasing of flow across the tricuspid bioprosthesis and no significant TR. (*B*) Continuous wave Doppler across the bioprosthetic tricuspid valve shows severe TS with peak and mean gradients of 16 and 10 mm Hg, respectively.

from RV failure, inotropes can be used. MCS options are limited, though VA-ECMO will support end-organ perfusion. Percutaneous right ventricular assist devices are also available even though severe stenotic right-sided lesions are a contraindication to their use.

Definitive Repair

For severe TR, TV repair is preferred to replacement when feasible (**Figs. 11** and **12**, Videos 29–31), especially in the setting of endocarditis, where the risk of re-infection is high.[38,39] In general, isolated TV surgery is higher risk compared to surgery for another primary indication with concomitant TV repair. Hemodynamic factors that increase surgical risk include pulmonary hypertension and a decreased cardiac index. When surgical risk is prohibitive, transcatheter approaches can be considered.[40]

Isolated pulmonary stenosis (PS) can be treated with balloon valvuloplasty with reasonable long term outcomes.[41,42] In patients with prior surgery, a transcatheter pulmonic valve can be used within

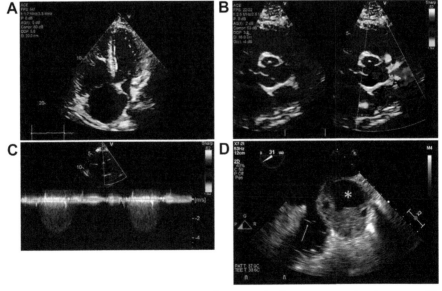

Fig. 13. 57-year-old with a history of coronary artery disease and prior coronary artery bypass grafting presents with cardiogenic shock. (*A*) Apical four chamber shows a dilated and dysfunctional right ventricle. The interatrial septum is also fixed in the left atrium suggesting elevated right atrial pressures. (*B*) Short axis view at the level of the aortic valve shows turbulent flow on color Doppler in the right ventricular outflow tract. (*C*) Continuous wave Doppler across the right ventricular outflow tract demonstrates a late peaking systolic velocity with a peak gradient of 51 mm Hg consistent with significant stenosis. (*D*) On transesophageal echocardiogram, there is a partially thrombosed saphenous vein graft aneurysm (***) extrinsically compressing the proximal pulmonary artery immediately distal to the pulmonic valve (*arrow*).

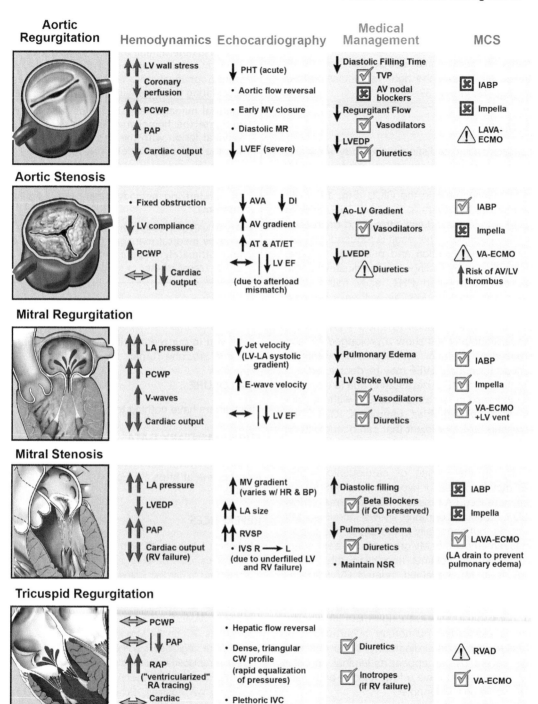

Fig. 14. Central illustration describing the main echo and hemodynamic findings in each valvular lesion, as well as the guiding principles in medical and device management. Green check mark means "clearly beneficial," yellow sign means "use with caution", and red circle indicates "contraindicated". AT, acceleration time; AVA, aortic valve area; CW, continuous wave; ET, ejection time; IABP, intra-aortic balloon pump; IVC, inferior vena cava; LAVA-ECMO, left atrial venoarterial extracorpeal membranous oxygenation; LVEDP, left ventricular end diastolic pressure; LVEF, left ventricular ejection fraction; MR, mitral regurgitation; MV, mitral valve; NSR, normal sinus rhythm; PAP, pulmonary artery pressure; PCWP, pulmonary capillary wedge pressure; PHT, pressure half time; RAP, right atrial pressure; RVAD, right ventricular assist device; RVSP, right ventricular systolic pressure; TVP, temporary venous pacing. (Reprinted with permission, Cleveland Clinic, Cardiology Graphics and Design © 2023. All Rights Reserved.)

a bioprosthetic valve.[43] However, little data are available regarding the optimal management of patients in cardiogenic shock due to PS or extrinsic stenosis of the right ventricular outflow tract (**Fig. 13**, Videos 32–34).

SUMMARY

An understanding of distinctive hemodynamic and echocardiographic features of acute valvular emergencies is essential to guiding medical and device management in the CICU (**Fig. 14**). With acute severe AR, there is a dramatic increase in LVEDP with increased wall stress and decreased coronary perfusion. The result is reduced left ventricular systolic function and pulmonary edema. Echocardiography findings include diastolic aortic flow reversal, a short PHT, early mitral valve closure and diastolic MR, as well as a reduced LVEF. In AS, a fixed obstruction leads to a noncompliant LV. In addition to a low AVA and DI, echocardiography will show a prolonged AT and increased AT/ET ratio. With severe or prolonged afterload mismatch, LVEF may be decreased.

Acute severe MR is devastating due to a precipitous increase in left atrial pressure without prior remodeling of left-sided chambers. Given the decreased LV-LA gradient that can occur with an increased LA pressure and low systolic blood pressure, the MR jet on CW Doppler may be low velocity. In the setting of cardiogenic shock, LVEF may be normal or hyperdynamic. MS results in an increased LA pressure with a normal or low LVEDP. Echocardiography shows increased MV gradients, but especially in the CICU, it is important to remember that MV gradients are dependent on flow (stroke volume) and heart rate. When shock from MS develops, related RV failure is often present with associated accentuated interventricular interaction. Severe TR rarely presents with cardiogenic shock, though this can occur if there is associated pulmonary hypertension or RV failure. On echocardiography, if the orifice is large, severe TR can appear as laminar on color flow mapping and have a low velocity and triangular profile on CW Doppler.

CLINICS CARE POINTS

- Comprehensive assessment of acute valvular emergencies involves a focused physical and echocardiographic examination, with the supplementation of invasive hemodynamics in select cases to guide both diagnosis and management.

- The underlying etiology of the valvular lesion is crucial in determining the appropriate temporizing medical therapy and definitive repair. A transesophageal can often be useful in better elucidating the underlying mechanism.
- Medical management should be tailored to mitigate the hemodynamic insult from the valvular lesion with the end goal of stabilizing the patient for a definitive repair.
- Decision making regarding MCS should be approached with careful consideration of the underlying hemodynamics and valvular anatomy.
- Acute valvular emergencies cannot be remedied by medical management or MCS alone and ultimately require a definitive repair, either transcatheter or surgical.

ACKNOWLEDGMENTS

Thank you to our medical illustrators Dave Schumick and Suzzane Turner.

DISCLOSURE

The authors have nothing to disclosures.

SUPPLEMENTARY DATA

Supplementary data related to this article can be found online at https://doi.org/10.1016/j.ccl.2024.02.009.

REFERENCES

1. Bohula EA, Katz JN, van Diepen S, et al. Demographics, care patterns, and outcomes of patients admitted to cardiac intensive care units: the critical care cardiology trials network prospective north american multicenter registry of cardiac critical illness. JAMA Cardiol 2019;4(9):928–35.
2. Roberts WC, Ko JM, Moore TR, et al. Causes of pure aortic regurgitation in patients having isolated aortic valve replacement at a single US tertiary hospital (1993 to 2005). Circulation 2006;114(5):422–9.
3. Zoghbi WA, Adams D, Bonow RO, et al. Recommendations for noninvasive evaluation of native valvular regurgitation. J Am Soc Echocardiogr 2017;30(4):303–71.
4. Prêtre R, Chilcott M. Blunt trauma to the heart and great vessels. N Engl J Med 1997;336(9):626–32.
5. Teague SM, Heinsimer JA, Anderson JL, et al. Quantification of aortic regurgitation utilizing continuous wave Doppler ultrasound. J Am Coll Cardiol 1986;8(3):592–9.
6. Effron MK, Popp RL. Two-dimensional echocardiographic assessment of bioprosthetic valve dysfunction

and infective endocarditis. J Am Coll Cardiol 1983; 2(4):597–606.

7. Otto CM, Nishimura RA, Bonow RO, et al. 2020 ACC/AHA guideline for the management of patients with valvular heart disease: a report of the American college of cardiology/American heart association joint committee on clinical practice guidelines. Circulation 2021;143(5). https://doi.org/10.1161/CIR.0000000000000923.

8. Sawaya FJ, Deutsch MA, Seiffert M, et al. Safety and efficacy of transcatheter aortic valve replacement in the treatment of pure aortic regurgitation in native valves and failing surgical bioprostheses: results from an international registry study. JACC Cardiovasc Interv 2017;10(10):1048–56.

9. Jiang J, Liu X, He Y, et al. Transcatheter aortic valve replacement for pure native aortic valve regurgitation: a systematic review. Cardiology 2018;141(3):132–40.

10. Iung B, Baron G, Butchart EG, et al. A prospective survey of patients with valvular heart disease in europe: the euro heart survey on valvular heart disease. Eur Heart J 2003;24(13):1231–43.

11. Osnabrugge RLJ, Mylotte D, Head SJ, et al. Aortic stenosis in the elderly: disease prevalence and number of candidates for transcatheter aortic valve replacement: a meta-analysis and modeling study. J Am Coll Cardiol 2013;62(11):1002–12.

12. Echocardiographic assessment of aortic valve stenosis: a focused update from the european association of cardiovascular imaging and the american society of echocardiography. https://www.asecho.org/guideline/echocardiographic-assessment-of-aortic-valve-stenosis-a-focused-update/. [Accessed 28 June 2023].

13. Zoghbi WA, Chambers JB, Dumesnil JG, et al. Recommendations for evaluation of prosthetic valves with echocardiography and Doppler ultrasound. J Am Soc Echocardiogr 2009;22(9):975–1014.

14. Khot UN, Novaro GM, Popović ZB, et al. Nitroprusside in critically ill patients with left ventricular dysfunction and aortic stenosis. N Engl J Med 2003;348(18):1756–63.

15. Santana JM, Dalia AA, Newton M, et al. Mechanical circulatory support options in patients with aortic valve pathology. J Cardiothorac Vasc Anesth 2022; 36(8):3318–26.

16. Steffen J, Stocker A, Scherer C, et al. Emergency transcatheter aortic valve implantation for acute heart failure due to severe aortic stenosis in critically ill patients with or without cardiogenic shock. Eur Heart J Acute Cardiovasc Care 2022;11(12):877–86.

17. Dall'Ara G, Saia F, Moretti C, et al. Incidence, treatment, and outcome of acute aortic valve regurgitation complicating percutaneous balloon aortic valvuloplasty. Catheter Cardiovasc Interv 2017; 89(4):E145–52.

18. Arsalan M, Khan S, Golman J, et al. Balloon aortic valvuloplasty to improve candidacy of patients evaluated for transcatheter aortic valve replacement. J Intervent Cardiol 2018;31(1):68–73.

19. Kawsara A, Alqahtani F, Eleid MF, et al. Balloon aortic valvuloplasty as a bridge to aortic valve replacement: a contemporary nationwide perspective. JACC Cardiovasc Interv 2020;13(5):583–91.

20. Takagi H, Hari Y, Kawai N, et al, ALICE All-Literature Investigation of Cardiovascular Evidence Group. ALICE (All-Literature Investigation of Cardiovascular Evidence) Group. Meta-analysis of transcatheter aortic valve implantation for bicuspid versus tricuspid aortic valves. J Cardiol 2019;74(1):40–8.

21. Voci P, Bilotta F, Caretta Q, et al. Papillary muscle perfusion pattern. A hypothesis for ischemic papillary muscle dysfunction. Circulation 1995;91(6):1714–8.

22. Birnbaum Y, Chamoun AJ, Conti VR, et al. Mitral regurgitation following acute myocardial infarction. Coron Artery Dis 2002;13(6):337–44.

23. El Sabbagh A, Reddy YNV, Nishimura RA. Mitral valve regurgitation in the contemporary era. JACC Cardiovasc Imaging 2018;11(4):628–43.

24. Nakata J, Saku K, Nishikawa T, et al. Substantial reduction of acute ischemic mitral regurgitation using impella in AMI complicated with cardiogenic shock. Int Heart J 2023;64(2):294–8.

25. Ekanem E, Gattani R, Bakhshi H, et al. Combined venoarterial ECMO and impella-CP circulatory support for cardiogenic shock due to papillary muscle rupture. JACC Case Rep 2020;2(14):2169–72.

26. Russo A, Suri RM, Grigioni F, et al. Clinical outcome after surgical correction of mitral regurgitation due to papillary muscle rupture. Circulation 2008;118(15):1528–34.

27. Adamo M, Curello S, Chiari E, et al. Percutaneous edge-to-edge mitral valve repair for the treatment of acute mitral regurgitation complicating myocardial infarction: a single centre experience. Int J Cardiol 2017;234.53–7.

28. Watkins DA, Johnson CO, Colquhoun SM, et al. Global, regional, and national burden of rheumatic heart disease, 1990-2015. N Engl J Med 2017; 377(8):713–22.

29. Abramowitz Y, Jilaihawi H, Chakravarty T, et al. Mitral annulus calcification. J Am Coll Cardiol 2015;66(17):1934–41.

30. Churchill TW, Yucel E, Deferm S, et al. Mitral valve dysfunction in patients with annular calcification. J Am Coll Cardiol 2022;80(7):739–51.

31. Labovitz AJ, Nelson JG, Windhorst DM, et al. Frequency of mitral valve dysfunction from mitral anular calcium as detected by Doppler echocardiography. Am J Cardiol 1985;55(1):133–7.

32. Wunderlich NC, Beigel R, Siegel RJ. Management of mitral stenosis using 2D and 3D echo-Doppler

imaging. JACC Cardiovasc Imaging 2013;6(11): 1191–205.

33. Song JK, Kim MJ, Yun SC, et al. Long-term outcomes of percutaneous mitral balloon valvuloplasty versus open cardiac surgery. J Thorac Cardiovasc Surg 2010;139(1):103–10.

34. 2018 AHA/ACC guideline for the management of adults with congenital heart disease: a report of the american college of cardiology/american heart association task force on clinical practice guidelines | Circulation. https://www.ahajournals.org/doi/10.1161/CIR.0000000000000603. [Accessed 4 July 2023].

35. Rao S, Tate DA, Stouffer GA. Hemodynamic findings in severe tricuspid regurgitation. Catheter Cardiovasc Interv 2013;81(1):162–9.

36. Fawzy ME, Mercer EN, Dunn B, et al. Doppler echocardiography in the evaluation of tricuspid stenosis. Eur Heart J 1989;10(11):985–90.

37. Baumgartner H, Hung J, Bermejo J, et al. Echocardiographic assessment of valve stenosis: EAE/ASE recommendations for clinical practice. J Am Soc Echocardiogr 2009;22(1):1–23.

38. Axtell AL, Bhambhani V, Moonsamy P, et al. Surgery does not improve survival in patients with isolated severe tricuspid regurgitation. J Am Coll Cardiol 2019;74(6):715–25.

39. Zack CJ, Fender EA, Chandrashekar P, et al. National trends and outcomes in isolated tricuspid valve surgery. J Am Coll Cardiol 2017;70(24):2953–60.

40. Sorajja P, Whisenant B, Hamid N, et al. Transcatheter repair for patients with tricuspid regurgitation. N Engl J Med 2023;388(20):1833–42.

41. Taggart NW, Cetta F, Cabalka AK, et al. Outcomes for balloon pulmonary valvuloplasty in adults: comparison with a concurrent pediatric cohort. Catheter Cardiovasc Interv 2013;82(5):811–5.

42. Kaul UA, Singh B, Tyagi S, et al. Long-term results after balloon pulmonary valvuloplasty in adults. Am Heart J 1993;126(5):1152–5.

43. Jones TK, McElhinney DB, Vincent JA, et al. Long-term outcomes after melody transcatheter pulmonary valve replacement in the us investigational device exemption trial. Circ Cardiovasc Interv 2022;15(1):e010852.

Complex Heart–Lung Ventilator Emergencies in the CICU

Mireia Padilla Lopez, MD[a], Willard Applefeld, MD[b], Elliott Miller, MD, MHS[c], Andrea Elliott, MD[d], Courtney Bennett, DO[e], Burton Lee, MD[f], Christopher Barnett, MD, MPH[g], Michael A. Solomon, MD, MBA[h], Francesco Corradi, MD, PhD[i], Alessandro Sionis, MD[a], Eduardo Mireles-Cabodevila, MD[j], Guido Tavazzi, MD, PhD[k], Carlos L. Alviar, MD[l],*

KEYWORDS

- Cardiopulmonary interactions • Mechanical ventilation • Hemodynamics • Cardiogenic shock

KEY POINTS

- Understanding the complex interplay between the cardiovascular and respiratory systems is essential for clinicians to provide optimal management and improve patient outcomes across diverse scenarios in the critically ill cardiac patient.
- Mechanical ventilation effects can be beneficial or detrimental, depending on the specific patient's physiology, cardiopulmonary reserve, hemodynamics, right and left ventricular function, and loading conditions.
- Monitoring and management of cardiopulmonary function during mechanical ventilation is critical in optimizing gas exchange and hemodynamics in the critically ill cardiac patient.

INTRODUCTION

The complexity and morbidity of patients admitted to the cardiac intensive care unit (CICU) has increased over the last few decades,[1,2] with respiratory failure complicating CICU admissions in 23% to 37% of the cases and representing one of the most common indications for admission to the CICU.[3–5] The presence of respiratory failure in the CICU patients represents a higher risk of adverse effects and mortality, particularly when requiring respiratory support with invasive mechanical ventilation,[4] underscoring the importance of proper coordination between cardiovascular and pulmonary systems.

This review summarizes the cardiopulmonary interactions during the use of invasive mechanical ventilation (IMV) in different clinical scenarios and provides insights for practical management of patients in these situations.

[a] Department of Cardiology, Hospital de la Santa Creu i Sant Pau, Biomedical Research Institute IIB Sant Pau, Universitat Autònoma de Barcelona, Barcelona, Spain; [b] Division of Cardiology, Duke University Medical Center, Durham, NC, USA; [c] Division of Cardiovascular Medicine, Yale University School of Medicine, New Haven, CT, USA; [d] Division of Cardiology, University of Minnesota, Minneapolis, MN, USA; [e] Heart and Vascular Institute, Leigh Valley Health Network, Allentown, PA, USA; [f] Department of Critical Care Medicine, National Institutes of Health Clinical Center, Bethesda, MA, USA; [g] Division of Cardiology, Department of Medicine, University of California San Francisco, San Francisco, CA, USA; [h] Clinical Center and Cardiology Branch, Critical Care Medicine Department, National Heart, Lung, and Blood Institute, National Institutes of Health, Bethesda, MA, USA; [i] Department of Surgical, Medical, Molecular Pathology and Critical Care Medicine, University of Pisa, Pisa, Italy; [j] Respiratory Institute, Cleveland Clinic, Ohio and the Lerner College of Medicine of Case Western Reserve University, Cleveland, OH, USA; [k] Department of Critical Care Medicine, Intensive Care Fondazione IRCCS Policlinico San Matteo, Pavia, Italy; [l] The Leon H. Charney Division of Cardiovascular Medicine, New York University School of Medicine, USA
* Corresponding author. 462 First Avenue, Suite 10W17, New York, NY 10016.
E-mail address: carlosalviar@gmail.com

Cardiol Clin 42 (2024) 253–271
https://doi.org/10.1016/j.ccl.2024.02.010
0733-8651/24/© 2024 Elsevier Inc. All rights reserved.

PATHOPHYSIOLOGY IN HEART–LUNG INTERACTIONS
Effect of Spontaneous Respiration on Cardiac Function

The heart and lungs have a complex, tightly coupled relationship such that intrathoracic pressures modulate cardiac hemodynamics while cardiac pathology can adversely impact respiratory function. Breathing involves pressure–volume work, consuming oxygen and producing carbon dioxide.[6,7] The elastic and resistive components of work of breathing (WOB) can increase with states of decreased respiratory compliance, increased airway resistance, and increased gas flow demands. During spontaneous respiration, inspiration is an active process, and expiration is typically passive. However, a patient in respiratory distress will not only have increased inspiratory WOB but may also involve active inspiratory or expiratory efforts, increasing overall metabolic demand, resulting in profound pleural pressure swings as well as increased oxygen consumption, carbon dioxide production, and alterations in acid–base balance. Thus, states of respiratory distress can strain the myocardium, with specific detrimental effects to the right ventricle (RV) and left ventricle (LV), which is poorly tolerant of hypoxia, hypercarbia, and acidosis.

Flow through the pulmonary circuit is determined by the gradient between the RV intracavitary and left atrial pressures as well as by the pulmonary vasculature resistance (PVR), which in turn is affected by both lung volume and fluctuation in pleural pressure.[8] At low lung volumes, extra-alveolar vessels collapse, while alveolar vessels dilate; however, at high lung volumes, alveolar vessels compress, while extra-alveolar vasculature is tethered open.[9] Therefore, the relationship between lung volume and PVR is U-shaped, with PVR being minimized at functional residual lung capacity. For patients in respiratory distress, profoundly negative pleural pressures are transmitted to the heart so that the left atrial pressure may drop below alveolar pressure and the pulmonary vessels collapse. If so, the flow through the pulmonary circuit is now driven by the gradient between RV intracavitary and alveolar pressures, rather than the left atrial pressures, establishing a Starling Resistor effect.[5] Furthermore, as pericardial pressure drops and is transmitted to the RV, the RV intracavitary pressure becomes closer to alveolar pressure and there is less of a pressure gradient driving blood forward.

During inspiration, inferior diaphragmatic displacement decreases the pleural pressure which is transmitted to the pericardium and subsequently the right atrium while increasing the intra-abdominal pressure which is transmitted to the inferior vena cava (IVC). This pressure gradient established between the more negative atrial pressure and more positive pressures in the IVC favors blood return to the right heart. However, this augmentation of venous return to the right heart only occurs up to a point. For example, during states of respiratory distress, wide excursions of the diaphragm inferiorly can create intensely negative inspiratory pleural pressures which keeps the intrathoracic venous channels patent while raising the intra-abdominal pressure and collapsing the extrathoracic IVC, impairing right heart preload, and increasing left ventricular afterload.[10]

As estimated by Laplace's law, the wall stress of the left ventricle (LV) increases with increasing transmural pressure difference (LV end-diastolic pressure—pericardial pressure) and the chamber size (radius^2) and decreases with the wall thickness (h). Pleural pressure changes that occur with spontaneous inspiration also increase LV afterload by increasing the transmural pressure gradient between the intracavitary pressure and pericardial pressure, which mirrors the pleural pressure. Thus, wide swings in pleural pressure increase the pressure gradient between intracavitary and pericardial pressure, increasing wall stress and LV afterload.[11]

Basics of Ventilator Modes

Mechanical ventilation can profoundly alter cardiopulmonary relationships that characterize normal physiologic breathing. Of the numerous modes of mechanical ventilation available (**Box 1**), we will focus on common types. Depending on the chosen mode, clinicians are generally able to prescribe the fraction of inspired oxygen (Fio_2), the positive end-expiratory pressure (PEEP), the minimum respiratory rate, and either a set volume (volume control) or inspiratory pressure (pressure control). In all modes, expiration is normally a passive process dictated by resistance and compliance of the respiratory system.[12] A variant of pressure control ventilation allows clinician to set a targeted volume (volume target) where the ventilator uses the minimal pressure above PEEP necessary to achieve the prescribed tidal volume. This breath type is known by various names such as pressure regulated volume control or volume control plus depending on the ventilator manufacturer. With this breath type, if the resulting tidal volume exceeds the volume targeted by the clinician, the ventilator will automatically deliver a lower pressure for subsequent breaths and vice versa. While this self-adjusting pressure mechanism

---

Box 1
Modes of mechanical ventilation

Ventilator Modes by Taxonomy

  Control Variable

    Pressure control ventilation

    Volume control ventilation

  Breath Sequence

    Continuous spontaneous ventilation

    Continuous mandatory ventilation (CMV)

    Intermittent mandatory ventilation

  Targeting Scheme

    Set point

    Adaptive

    Dual

    Optimal

    Bio-variable

    Intelligent

    Servo

Examples of Conventional Ventilator Modes

- CMV or assist/control
  - Volume control CMV
  - Pressure control CMV
- Synchronous intermittent mandatory ventilation
- Spontaneous ventilatory modes
  - Continuous positive airway pressure
  - Pressure support ventilation
  - Volume support

Examples of Other Ventilatory Modes

- CMV
- Airway pressure release ventilation
- Mandatory minute ventilation
- Inverse ratio ventilation
- Pressure-regulated volume control
- Proportional assist ventilation
- Adaptive support ventilation
- Adaptive pressure control
- Volume-assured pressure support
- Neurally adjusted ventilatory assist
- Automatic tube compensation
- High-frequency oscillatory ventilation

---

clearly has advantages, an important caution is warranted for patients with strong spontaneous inspiratory efforts, as the ventilator may gradually withdraw inspiratory pressure until the patient assumes the entire WOB, potentially leading to fatigue, despite ventilation support.

In assist control (AC) mode, patients trigger breaths if they meet the trigger threshold. If no trigger attempts are detected, the ventilator will deliver controlled breaths at the set rate with the prescribed volume or pressure. Further successful triggers above the set rate result in assisted breaths identical to the controlled ones. Synchronized IMV (SIMV) allows patient-triggered breaths, delivering controlled breaths if no triggers are detected.[13] Spontaneous inspiratory efforts beyond the set rate are managed similarly to pressure support or continuous positive airway pressure (CPAP): the patient must use their respiratory muscles to entrain gas and is allowed to determine their own inspiratory time and flow. Frequently, this mode is modified to provide pressure support above PEEP during these spontaneous breaths, potentially increasing WOB compared to assist-controlled ventilation and the unsupported breaths can lead intrathoracic pressure swings resulting in adverse hemodynamic consequences, such as increasing LV afterload.[14] For AC or SIMV modes, ventilators allow manipulation of inspiratory time or gas flow rate and pattern. During spontaneous ventilation, the patient must initiate all breaths as respiratory rate or inspiratory time is not prescribed by the clinician. The most common spontaneous mode is pressure support ventilation, where a clinician sets the Fio_2, PEEP, and an inspiratory pressure above PEEP. CPAP represents a variant of pressure support where clinicians do not prescribe any pressure above PEEP and instead rely entirely on patient muscular effort to assume the totality of the WOB.

According to the equation of motion (P_{aw} − P_{mus} = $F*R$ + V/C + $PEEP_{total}$; **Fig. 1**), alveolar pressure (P_{alv}) measured at the end-inspiration represents plateau pressure (P_{plat}) and is equivalent to the highest P_{alv} in the respiratory cycle, reflecting the total volume and the static compliance of the lung and the chest wall. This parameter (P_{plat}) should be routinely monitored to minimize ventilator-associated lung injury. The set PEEP ($PEEP_{set}$), also known as extrinsic PEEP, is provided throughout the respiratory cycle. The sum of $PEEP_{set}$ and autoPEEP ($PEEP_i$) is the total PEEP ($PEEP_{total}$). For a sedated passive patient on pressure control ventilation, P_{mus} which refers to the pressure caused by respiratory muscles during active patient efforts, is zero, while P_{aw} and $PEEP_{set}$ are determined by the clinician. Then, the

256   Lopez et al

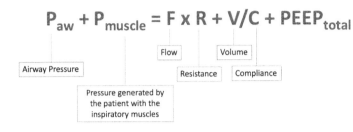

$$P_{aw} + P_{muscle} = F \times R + V/C + PEEP_{total}$$

Fig. 1. The equation of motion of mechanical ventilation.

resistance (R) and compliance (C) of the respiratory system will ultimately determine the flow (F), the delivered tidal volume (V), and the P_{plat}. On the other hand, for a sedated passive patient on volume control ventilation, F, TV, and $PEEP_{set}$ are determined by the clinician, and the patient's R and C will determine P_{aw} and P_{plat}. If a patient is actively inspiring on the ventilator, P_{mus} will be negative (<0). For an actively inspiring patient on pressure control ventilation, F and V increase further due to the additional effects of P_{mus}, with a consequent increase in P_{plat} due to higher volumes (V). Conversely, for an actively inspiring patient on volume control ventilation, P_{aw} will decrease, but P_{plat} will remain the same as V, and $PEEP_{set}$ is set by the clinician.

CARDIOPULMONARY INTERACTIONS DURING MECHANICAL VENTILATION
Effect of Positive Pressure and Mechanical Ventilation on Cardiovascular Function

Under positive pressure ventilation (PPV), when positive pressure is applied to the airways, it causes the pleural pressure to become positive. In general terms, PPV leads to a decrease in LV afterload, an increase in RV afterload, and a decrease in both LV and RV preload[15] (**Fig. 2**). PPV also improves myocardial mechanics of the LV by reducing wall tension and modulating afterload via elevation in aortic pressure that activates peripheral baroreceptors.[16] This phenomenon leads to a reduction in systemic vascular resistance (SVR) and LV afterload. Additionally, PPV increases transmural pressure in the LV, which, in combination with the decreased afterload, elevates cardiac output (CO).[17,18] PPV also promotes improved coronary blood flow by enhancing the pressure gradient between the aorta and coronary arteries.[19]

Changes in PPV can significantly impact RV preload, afterload, and myocardial perfusion. Systemic venous return to the right atrium is passive, with blood flow occurring as a result of a pressure gradient between the superior/IVC and right atrium. When PPV is applied, it increases the pressure within the right atrium, which in turn reduces the gradient between the extrathoracic and

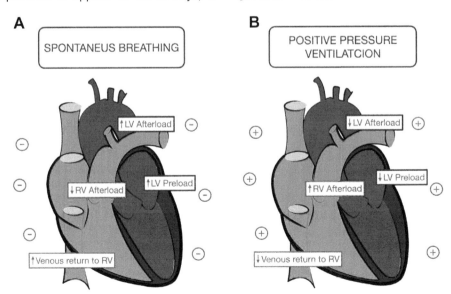

Fig. 2. Effect of pleural pressure on hemodynamics of the right ventricle (RV) and left ventricle (LV). (A) During spontaneous respiration, a negative pleural pressure occurs during inspiration. (B) Under positive pressure ventilation, the pleural pressure becomes positive.

intrathoracic circulation, leading to a decrease in venous return to the RV.[15] As explained previously, PVR is affected according to the lung volume in a U-shaped pattern.[16] In cases of atelectasis, where there is an increase in PVR due to hypoxia, an increase in PEEP can open alveoli and reverse this effect, thereby reducing the afterload on the RV. However, excessive PEEP can cause alveolar overdistension, compressing the extra-alveolar vessels and elevating PVR. This may redirect blood flow to poorly ventilated areas and creates a mismatch between ventilation and perfusion, resulting in hypoxemia and hypercapnia. High levels of PEEP tend to decrease the RV CO by reducing venous return and increasing afterload.[20] RV afterload can also be increased by increases on volume tidal and driving pressure.[21] Additionally, PPV leads to a decrease in preload on the LV due to reduced CO from the RV; consequently, ventricular interdependence can be potentiated, with RV overdistension and displacement of the interventricular septum toward the LV, subsequently diminishing CO.[22] Of note, the specific PEEP level to balance the concomitant prevention of atelectasis and optimization of pulmonary artery resistance (PVR) in patients with RV dysfunction should be individualized, as it is highly dependent on patients' pulmonary and chest wall compliance, body habitus, and loading conditions.

Hemodynamic Effects During Liberation from Mechanical Ventilation

In general, it is considered that a patient has approached "readiness for liberation from IMV" once minimal ventilator settings are achieved (eg, PEEP ≤ 8 cmH$_2$O and Fio$_2$ ≤ 50%), the patient has a mental status that would allow him to participate in the liberation process, and the etiology of their respiratory failure has improved or resolved. In a patient with cardiovascular disease, it is important to consider electrical and hemodynamic instability and integrate patient's individual physiology (eg, LV and RV function) into the approach to liberation. Similarly, patient–ventilator cardiopulmonary interactions should be optimized, ensuring that volume status, synchrony, and vasoactive support, if any, are improved. Removal of PPV has the potential to put incredible stress on the cardiovascular system, especially for those with ongoing ischemia and/or ventricular dysfunction, particularly as removal of PPV can lead to high LV afterload.[23–25] In order to test whether the patient can tolerate such stress, removal of IMV is evaluated with a spontaneous breathing trial (SBT). There are several ways to approach SBT, providing varying degrees of support,[26]

which depending on the level of support may reverse many of the potentially favorable effects of PPV detailed earlier.

Withdrawal of positive pressure will increase RV preload and reduce RV afterload, which may be helpful in those with right ventricular failure or pulmonary hypertension (PH). In comparison, LV afterload and preload can abruptly increase once positive pressure is discontinued.[27] Compared to full ventricular support, transition to unassisted spontaneous breathing (eg, T-piece) can increase the pulmonary capillary wedge pressure (PCWP) by upward of 41%.[28] Therefore, optimization of ventricular filling pressures with diuretics and extubation to noninvasive positive pressure will allow for a more successful liberation from IMV. Removal of positive pressure may also unmask worsening mitral regurgitation, a common etiology of weaning and extubation failure, by increasing LV afterload.[29] Alternatively, the increase in afterload may be potentially beneficial for certain pathologies, such as patients with left ventricular outflow tract obstructions, by reducing dynamic outflow tract obstruction, in such scenarios the opposite approach should take place, with avoidance of diuretics and inotropes, while preventing tachycardia and extubating to nasal cannula rather than to noninvasive mechanical ventilation.

MONITORING IN PATIENTS WITH RESPIRATORY FAILURE AND CARDIOVASCULAR DISEASE
Invasive Hemodynamic Monitoring

Invasive hemodynamic monitoring with pulmonary artery catheter (PAC) can be a very useful tool to guide therapeutic interventions in patients with cardiovascular disease undergoing IMV,[30] particularly when monitoring RV function.[31] Elevated RV filling pressures can lead to significantly compromised organ perfusion, attributed to a diminished gradient between mean arterial pressure (MAP) and central venous pressure (CVP), a key determinant of venous return.[32] In instances where RV failure coincides with or stems from LV failure, PCWP may exhibit an increase, which can be further exacerbated by displacement of the interventricular septum to the left.[33] The CVP waveform might display a prominent v-wave due to tricuspid regurgitation (TR) resulting from RV dilation, and in cases of restrictive RV physiology, such as constriction or significant right ventricular failure with ventricular interdependence, a "deep and plateau" waveform can be observed. Similarly, other important parameters of right ventricular dysfunction include a low right ventricular stroke work index, an elevated CVP to PCWP ratio, and a low pulmonary artery pulsatility index (PAPi). This last parameter, which is calculated as (systolic pulmonary artery pressure [PAP]−diastolic PAP)/CVP, has been validated to diagnose RV failure and RV shock in several conditions, including cardiogenic shock, inferior myocardial infarction, postventricular assist device implantation, and PH.[34] Notably, normal CO or PAP does not necessarily exclude the possibility of RV dysfunction.[22]

Another important application of the PAC relies on its ability to assist in PEEP titration in patients with RV dysfunction, especially when combined with echocardiographic assessment. For instance, in patients with severe hypoxia, slow increase in PEEP can be performed while closely monitoring CVP, pulmonary arterial diastolic pressures, and pulse pressure of the pulmonary artery and PAPi, along with septal positioning with real-time echocardiography. The objective would be to achieve an ideal balance between lung recruitment and hypoxia resolution and avoidance of worsening right heart hemodynamics. Furthermore, PAC can also assist in evaluating fluid responsiveness and filling pressures, not only by measuring CVP and PCWP values[35] but also by dynamic maneuvers. For instance, a rise in CVP following a fluid challenge, without a concurrent change in CO, suggests inadequate fluid responsiveness and should concern clinicians as a potential presence of RV dysfunction.[36]

Point-of-care Ultrasound in Respiratory Failure and Cardiovascular Disease

Echocardiographic assessment is a routine diagnostic modality part of the standard of care of patients admitted to the CICU, as it provides a detail and comprehensive assessment of biventricular and valvular function, as well as filling pressures and diastology. In the recent decades, the use of cardiac and noncardiac point-of-care ultrasound (POCUS) has become a key strategy to guide management in the critically ill patient, including patients with both cardiogenic and noncardiogenic pulmonary edema. Notably, in patients with acute lung injury, the concurrent inflammatory cascade can increase pulmonary vascular resistance, and may be further complicated by the application of PPV,[37] which has the potential of resulting in acute cor pulmonale.[38]

Bedside POCUS offers valuable insights into cardiopulmonary interactions. Evaluation of RV size to assess ventriculo-ventricular interaction and longitudinal function by the tricuspid annular plane systolic excursion (TAPSE) in case of dilation is important to estimate the potential impact of PPV. Systolic pulmonary arterial pressure

(sPAP) estimation using the tricuspid peak velocity is simple and practical; however, it may be limited by patient positioning and lung interpositions yielding suboptimal windows affecting Doppler acquisition. Additionally, sPAP may be largely underestimated in case of RV failure, related to the reduced force of contraction and therefore gradient creation. The ratio TAPSE/sPAP has been established as a marker of RV dysfunction in chronic PH[39]; however, its application in the acute settings has not been yet established. Similarly, the presence of a presystolic a-wave (pulmonary forward flow in correspondence of atrial contraction) is reflective of RV restrictive compliance and increased end-diastolic pressure, serving as a marker of diastolic dysfunction, and it has been described to be associated with higher $Paco_2$, PEEP, and inspiratory peak pressure.[40] However, its role in acute settings has not been systematically evaluated.

In terms of lung POCUS, the identification and quantification of B-lines with lung ultrasound (LUS) holds extremely high accuracy in defining the deaeration of the lung parenchyma and allows the clinician to estimate the extent of congestion in heart failure and myocardial infarction patients.[41–43] Additionally, the balance between lung recruitment and overdistension can also be assessed by LUS,[44] through the characterization of lung morphology,[45] which integrated with assessment of ventricular interdependence can provide useful information when pursuing PEEP titration. Lastly, diaphragmatic ultrasound allows the evaluation of diaphragmatic thickness and thickening fraction. Their alteration has been associated with total ventilation time and rate of weaning failure reflecting the ability of the diaphragmatic muscle mass to cope with the increased WOB due to the sudden cessation of PPV.[46] However, its role has been best characterized in medical intensive care units and less in the CICU. In summary, an ultrasound-integrated approach with POCUS, invasive hemodynamics, and ventilatory parameters (blood gas analysis and ventilation mechanics) is extremely useful for a comprehensive assessment or respiratory failure and hemodynamic response to PPV.[38,47]

Noninvasive Blood Pressure Monitoring

There is a growing field of hemodynamic monitoring technology designed to minimize invasiveness and maximize access to hemodynamic data at the bedside. The available studies evaluating the accuracy of measuring hemodynamic parameters in critically ill, intubated patients are limited.[48–51] Pulse contour analysis, both noninvasive or minimally invasive, uses proprietary algorithms to reconstruct arterial wave forms from peripheral arteries to calculate the MAP and CO utilizing the area under the systolic curve. This is ideally performed in patients who are completely passive on the ventilator in order to minimize wide variations in stroke volume measurements related to large changes in intrathoracic pressure with patient's respiratory efforts, especially if dyssynchrony is also present. Pulse contour analysis has not demonstrated interchangeability with gold standard thermodilution methods in critically ill patients by neither peripheral arterial nor finger cuff measurements.[48,52–54] Another major consideration when considering the use of minimally invasive devices is the pathophysiology of cardiogenic shock, which is highly variable and multifactorial, along with the limitations of these devices in such clinical scenarios. The physiologic responses in early circulatory failure include an increase in both SVR and venous congestion, which leads to the clinical findings of cool, mottled extremities, along with the evidence of increased extravascular lung water, and peripheral edema. Consequently, noninvasive methods to estimate CO have limited validity valid in situations requiring vasoactive medications, high SVR, and significant peripheral edema.

The value of these devices in the CICU patient population may be for the evaluation of fluid responsiveness and extravascular lung water by either thoracic bioimpedance or bioreactance or by transpulmonary thermodilution when using Pulse Index Continous Cardiac Output (PiCCO).[55–57] Of note, elevations in extravascular lung water will limit hemodynamic assessment by thoracic bioimpedance but can predict weaning failure from mechanical ventilation in patients with left ventricular ejection fraction (LVEF) less than 40%.[58] Similarly, thoracic bioreactance utilizes electrodes also placed on the chest wall to measure the phase shift of oscillating signals transmitted across the thorax. Although this technology has not been validated in patients with CS, it may not be limited by the elevations in extravascular lung water. While it is not directly interchangeable with invasive hemodynamics as the gold standard in CS, there is evidence to support its use in the evaluation of fluid responsiveness.[57] Another modality is transpulmonary thermodilution, which uses both thermodilution with a central venous line and a thermistor, along with a central arterial pulse waveform analysis. While this device provides a fairly accurate estimation of the CO, with a percent error of approximately 27%, it can be interchangeable with the PAC in patients with CS for assessment of the CO.[59] Similarly, this technology also offers the ability to measure extravascular lung water and correlated with B-lines on lung ultrasound,[60] but as with any other

noninvasive monitors, it does not provide an accurate and specific assessment of the filling pressures for the LV or the RV. In summary, some of the noninvasive monitoring technologies can assist in assessing CO and extravascular lung water; however, their role in patients with cardiovascular disease undergoing IMV is limited, given their inability to assess intracardiac filling pressures and right ventricular function.

CARDIOPULMONARY INTERACTIONS DURING VENTILATION IN SPECIFIC SITUATIONS
Cardiogenic Shock

The incidence of respiratory failure and the need for PPV in patients with CS rages between 50% and 88%,[61,62] and based on substudies of the TRIUMPH and CULPRIT-SHOCK trials, delays in initiation of invasive mechanical (IM) PPV in patients with CS are associated with increased mortality.[63,64] In terms of modes of IMV, no differences have been observed between volume-controlled continuous mechanical ventilation (VC-CMV) and pressure-controlled continuous mechanical ventilation (PC-CMV), however as mentioned in prior sections of this article, SIMV mode is not recommended as it can lead to swings in intrathoracic pressure, increased afterload, and ventilator dyssynchrony, thereby increasing myocardial oxygen consumption and worsening myocardial mechanics.[64]

PEEP titration should be individualized based on the hemodynamic profile and oxygen saturation of each patient. Observational studies suggest that PEEP can have a beneficial effect in patients with left ventricular dysfunction, improving CO,[65–68] decreasing PCWP, and mitigating mitral regurgitation.[69,70] Therefore, initiating PEEP at 5 cmH_2O and titrating it for optimal hemodynamics, gas exchange, and bedside ultrasound are recommended. However, in preload-sensitive states such as RV dysfunction, pericardial tamponade, pulmonary embolism with cor pulmonale, hypovolemia, or obstructive hypertrophic cardiomyopathy, higher levels of PEEP may have a negative hemodynamic impact.[71] In these cases, starting with a PEEP range of 3 to 5 cmH_2O and titrating to oxygen saturation greater than 92% with closely hemodynamic and POCUS monitoring are preferred to maintain adequate oxygenation and prevent atelectasis. In regard to tidal volume, as opposed to the acute respiratory distress syndrome (ARDS) literature, there are limited data assessing the impact of low tidal volume ventilation in patients with cardiovascular disease. A small nonrandomized study demonstrated higher mortality with TV above 9.3 mL/kg of ideal body weight[72];

however, the small sample size makes this study was underpowered for hard clinical outcomes and therefore it is difficult to draw conclusions from it. Therefore, tidal volume should be maintained between 6 and 10 mL/kg and titration along with respiratory rate to Pco_2 levels while preventing plateau pressures over 30 mmH_2O. Fio_2 should be titrated to ensure proper gas exchange, with a target oxygen saturation greater than 92% and prevention of hyperoxemia (Pao_2 <120 mm Hg; **Table 1**).

Mechanical Ventilation in the Patient Undergoing Venoarterial Extracorporeal Membrane Oxygenation

Venoarterial extracorporeal membrane oxygenation (VA-ECMO) provides oxygenation by removing deoxygenated blood from the patient's venous system, passing it through an oxygenator in the ECMO circuit, and returning oxygenated blood back into the arterial system. The oxygenator also facilitates gas exchange by removing carbon dioxide (CO_2) and adding oxygen to the blood. Thus, during VA-ECMO support, the impact of mechanical ventilation parameters on oxygenation and CO_2 removal is limited.[73] Additionally, there is a decrease in pulmonary arterial flow, leading to an alteration in the ventilation–perfusion ratio. As a result, maintaining normal alveolar ventilation in this context may result in overventilation of the lungs. The Extracorporeal Life Support Organization (ELSO) guidelines aim to rest the lung in patients supported with VA-ECMO.[74] In order to minimize ventilator-induced lung injury, the ventilation strategy often involves using lung-protective ventilation strategies. These strategies include limiting tidal volumes, maintaining PEEP to prevent alveolar collapse, and avoiding high inspiratory pressures.[75,76] However, mechanical ventilation data in VA-ECMO are limited, with randomized studies primarily focusing on venovenous ECMO with severe respiratory failure. Observational studies have shown that the use of lung-protective ventilation during the first 24 hours is associated with improved survival in CS patients requiring VA-ECMO.[77,78] Higher PEEP (recommended between 5 and 15 cmH_2O) may have a beneficial effect on hemodynamics by unloading the LV.[62,74] It is reasonable to maintain the lowest tolerable Fio_2 to target SaO_2 greater than 90% while avoiding hyperoxemia (Pao_2 > 300 mm Hg) as it has been associated with increased mortality.[79,80] Extubation during VA-ECMO circulatory

Table 1
Proposal for adjusting initial parameters of mechanical ventilation in patients with cardiogenic shock

Ventilator Parameters	Initial Ventilator Settings	Monitoring
Ventilatory mode	PC-CMV or VC-CMV (avoid modes that require patient effort)	Maintain synchrony
Tidal volume	6–10 mL/kg of IBW	• Plateau pressure <28–30 mm Hg • Driving pressure <15 mm Hg • Adjust to $Paco_2$
Respiratory rate	12–16 breaths/min	• Adjust to $Paco_2$ • Avoid autoPEEP
PEEP	LV dysfunction: • Start PEEP 5 cmH_2O (8–10 cmH_2O if PCWP > 18 mm Hg) "Preload dependent" states[a]: • Start PEEP 3–5 cmH_2O	• Title according to hemodynamic response (preferably invasive), gas exchange, and bedside ultrasound. • In LVAD or ECMO monitor LV unloading • Control plateau pressure <28–30 mm Hg • Avoid autoPEEP
Fio_2	Start at 100%, but adjusts rapidly according to SaO_2	• SaO_2 > 92% • Avoid hyperoxia (especially after cardiac arrest)

Abbreviations: ECMO, extracorporeal membrane oxygenation; IBW, ideal body weight; LV, left ventricle; LVAD, left ventricular assist device; PC-CMV, pressure-controlled mechanical ventilation; PEEP, positive end-expiratory pressure; VC-CMV, volume-controlled mechanical ventilation.
[a] Right ventricle dysfunction, cardiac tamponade, constrictive pericarditis, hypovolemia, obstructive hypertrophic cardiomyopathy.

support has been associated with reduced incidence of ventilator-associated pneumonia and mortality.[81] Patients eligible for liberation from mechanical ventilation while on VA-ECMO should be carefully selected due to the risk of sudden changes in blood pressure and blood flow resulting from the cessation of PPV.

Right Ventricular Failure and Pulmonary Hypertension

PH is common in the CICU and independently associated with a higher risk of death.[82] Thus, caring for these patients, it is important to understand cardiopulmonary interactions, particularly as it relates to sedation, intubation, and PPV. PPV is often discouraged in patients with PH and RV failure due to the potential for hemodynamic worsening when intrathoracic pressure is increased. The RV adapts to chronically elevated afterload with RV hypertrophy resulting in increased myocardial oxygen demand and simultaneous reduction in RV myocardial coronary blood flow. Patients with progressive PH often present to the CICU with worsening RV failure characterized by right atrial, RV and tricuspid annular dilation, reduced RV stroke volume, and advanced TR. The overloaded right heart and ventricular interdependence further compromises LV filling and stroke volume, causing systemic hypoperfusion and hypotension, RV ischemia and worsening RV failure. Severe RV failure often occurs in group 1 PH, though it may result from PH of any cause.[83]

In severe RV failure, rapid hemodynamic deterioration may be precipitated by small increases in RV afterload brought on by PPV-mediated compression of pulmonary vasculature. Additionally, PEEP can worsen hypoxemia and hypercapnia if compression of extra-alveolar vessels causes shunting of blood to poorly ventilated areas. The presence of atelectasis, hypoxemia, hypercapnia,

and acidosis (both respiratory and metabolic) can increase pulmonary vascular resistance and afterload but can be improved or resolved with the use of PPV, potentially improving hemodynamics.[15] Additionally, reduction in preload and LV afterload with PPV may improve hemodynamics especially when PH is caused by left heart disease. A comprehensive understanding of the severity of RV abnormalities and the cause of PH is helpful to predict the response to PPV (**Fig. 3**).

In patients with severe RV dysfunction, sedation, endotracheal intubation, and initiation of PPV is particularly hazardous. Preload and MAP should be optimized prior to sedation for intubation. A technique of awake, spontaneously breathing, semirecumbent positioned intubation over a bronchoscope to minimize risks of hemodynamic decompensation has been described.[84]

Cardiopulmonary Resuscitation

Cardiopulmonary resuscitation (CPR) often includes chest compression and ventilation; however, when comparing compressions with and without ventilation yields mixed data.[85–91] Compression-only CPR increases bystander willingness to begin CPR[92–94]; thus, it is an acceptable strategy to encourage early compressions.[95] Given the likely benefits of pairing CPR with ventilation, it is recommended for willing bystanders and health care providers[88,95] because longer duration of CPR without ventilation eventually depletes arterial oxygen stores.[96] When ventilation is attempted, there are equivalent outcomes for continuous asynchronous breaths compared to pausing compressions for breaths.[97] It is thus a 2b recommendation to deliver breaths in an asynchronous manner.[95] Notably, it has been observed that overventilation during CPR is common[98–100] and can lead to decreased coronary perfusion, gastric inflation with aspiration, increased intrathoracic pressure, decreased

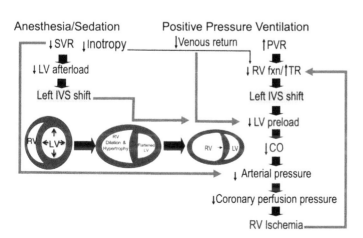

Anesthesia/Sedation   Positive Pressure Ventilation

Fig. 3. Mechanism of worsening right ventricle (RV) failure in positive pressure ventilation (PPV). CO, cardiac output; IVS, interventricular septum; LV, left ventricle; PVR, pulmonary vascular resistance; SVR, systemic vascular resistance; TR, tricuspid regurgitation. (*Courtesy of* and *adapted from* Teresa De Marco, MD, San Francisco, California.)

venous return, and ultimately decreased survival.[98,99] Therefore, providers in charge of ventilatory efforts during CPR should be mindful about maintaining slow and sustained breaths mimicking physiologic breathing.

Management of oxygenation and ventilation after return of spontaneous circulation varies depending on the etiology of the arrest and underlying comorbid conditions. For example, an arrhythmogenic cardiac arrest may be managed with basic ventilation immediately postarrest, whereas cardiac arrest secondary to respiratory failure may require advanced ventilation strategies, bronchoscopy, other procedural interventions, or additional imaging. There are some data that mild hypoventilation with increased $Paco_2$ may increase cerebral blood flow[101,102] in the postarrest period[103,104]; however, recent data from a randomized controlled trial in cardiac arrest patient showed no difference in neurologic outcomes between patients managed with normocapnia ($Paco_2$ 34–45 mm Hg) and mild therapeutic hypercapnia ($Paco_2$ 50–55 mmHg) goals.[105] Thus, ventilation targeting normal $Paco_2$ is recommended in most cases by the American Heart Association postarrest care guidelines.[106] The use of hyperventilation to correct metabolic acidosis should be avoided as it may induce cerebral vasoconstriction and therefore affect cerebral perfusion.[107–110] In regard of oxygenation targets, it is well established that hypoxia (Pao_2 usually <60 mm Hg) is deleterious[27–29] but optimal targets for Pao_2 are remain nebulous. In terms of hyperoxia, there are variable data, but nonrandomized studies have demonstrated that severe hyperoxia, particularly if Pao_2 greater than 300 mm Hg, is associated with worse outcomes cardiac arrest patients, particularly in terms of neurosurvival.[109–114] The 2015 postcardiac arrest guidelines suggest maintaining an arterial saturation over 94%.[106] The more recent BOX trial suggests that no difference between a restrictive versus liberal oxygenation target, however, the liberal oxygenation group targeted a Pao_2 98 to 105 mm Hg,[115] but this study did not assess the effect of hyperoxemia (usually defined as Pao_2 > 120 mm Hg) in cardiac arrest outcomes.

BEDSIDE TROUBLESHOOTING AND CLINICAL SCENARIOS
Airway Management in the Patient with Cardiovascular Disease

The decision to perform endotracheal intubation in a patient with cardiovascular disease should incorporate a careful assessment of the risk and benefits of intubation and the effects of PPV. The preintubation assessment should consider the underlying cardiac condition, hemodynamic status, right and left ventricular function, baseline pulmonary function, and other therapies such as mechanical circulatory support.[62] As such, the clinician should integrate such elements to decide on the timing of intubation, intubation approach, choice of induction agents, neuromuscular blockade, and selection of analgosedation postintubation. For instance, in patients with CS, early intubation and early initiation of mechanical ventilation are associated with better survival when compared to delayed initiation of IMV.[63,64] However, in patients with severe preload-sensitive conditions, such as PH, severe RV failure, or cardiac tamponade, the preference is to delay or avoid intubation and initiation of IMV.[15,83] If avoiding intubation is not possible, it is recommended to pursue awake intubation with minimal or no sedation by a clinician with expertise in such an approach.[15,84]

Regarding sedative selection, clinicians should consider agents with minimal impact on sympathetic tone and hemodynamics. Most induction agents will decrease the sympathetic tone and a decrease in preload, leading to hypotension. Etomidate at a lower dose may decrease the hemodynamic effects. Ketamine can be considered, recognizing that it may lead to severe hypertension (not a good choice in aortic dissection, acute pulmonary edema, or cardiac dysfunction). These agents are followed by the neuromuscular agent of choice to improve intubation conditions. The technique used will depend on the expertise of the center, although recent evidence may favor the use of video-assisted laryngoscope to minimize timing and intubation attempts.[116]

In patients who are already hypotensive at baseline, premedication with vasopressors can allow the clinician to improve hemodynamic parameters in preparation for intubation, targeting a MAP above 65 mm Hg before induction.[15,62] Correcting acidosis and hypoxia as much as possible before intubation and having readily invasive blood pressure monitoring and POCUS available to perform a comprehensive evaluation if hemodynamic instability ensues quickly should also be considered.

Autopositive End-Expiratory Pressure in the Cardiac Intensive Care Unit

An important parameter to monitor in patients undergoing IM-PPV is autoPEEP,[117] particularly in the presence of cardiovascular conditions given its potential for significant hemodynamic instability.[15,16] At the beginning of exhalation, P_{alv} starts at P_{plat} but gradually decreases exponentially toward set PEEP. Expiratory flow then results due to a pressure gradient between P_{alv} and P_{aw}, with P_{aw} being simply the set PEEP during exhalation. For passive exhalation, the amount of air remaining in the lungs depends on the expiratory time constant, a combination of resistance, and compliance (**Fig. 4**) of the respiratory system. In certain patients, incomplete exhalation of the inspired volume can progressively lead to air trapping with each subsequent breath, resulting in autoPEEP (also known as intrinsic PEEP).[12] Notably, patients with high resistance, high compliance, or both (eg, chronic obstructive pulmonary disease) need longer exhalation time and are therefore more prone to developing autoPEEP. Since autoPEEP can cause barotrauma or hemodynamic collapse, it should be carefully monitored in all patients but especially in those with obstructive lung disease, particularly if there is concomitant tachypnea or increased WOB.

If autoPEEP is not detected and addressed in a timely fashion, it has the potential to cause catastrophic hemodynamic consequences. The equation of motion dictates the potential impact of autoPEEP on pressure control versus volume control ventilation. If autoPEEP develops for a patient on pressure control ventilation, according to the equation, the F and TV must decrease since P_{aw} and $PEEP_{set}$ will remain constant, which are set by the clinician in pressure control. Thus, the consequence of autoPEEP for a patient on pressure control ventilation could be worsening respiratory acidosis caused by a decrease in tidal volume and flow. The worsening respiratory acidosis could, in turn, result in hemodynamic compromise. In contrast, if autoPEEP increases for a patient on volume control ventilation, according to the same equation, the P_{aw} and P_{plat} must increase since frequency (F), tidal volume (TV), and $PEEP_{set}$ will remain constant, which are set by the clinician in volume control. Thus, the consequence of autoPEEP for a patient on volume control ventilation, in contrast to pressure control,

could be hyperinflation and increased intrathoracic pressures. In turn, the increase in intrathoracic pressure may lead to a decrease in venous return and subsequently, hemodynamic compromise[118] (**Fig. 5**). Moreover, as more air is trapped and autoPEEP increases, patient will need to work more vigorously to trigger each breath, which can lead to triggering asynchrony, increased WOB, agitation, tachypnea, and tachycardia, which in turn, may further increase autoPEEP in a vicious cycle (**Fig. 6**). For these reasons, clinicians should be proactively vigilant about autoPEEP.[12]

Identifying and managing autopositive end-expiratory pressure

As opposed to other IM-PPV settings and parameters, such as peak pressures or minute ventilation, the mechanical ventilator does not have a specific alarm for autoPEEP. Moreover, patients with autoPEEP may not have evident hypoxemia or hypercarbia, and its only manifestation may be hemodynamic instability along with respiratory distress and patient–ventilator asynchrony due to air trapping. In cooperative patients, autoPEEP may be assessed by performing an end-expiratory hold. However, many patients who are not sufficiently sedated may not cooperate with the breath hold. If so, active patient efforts (P_{mus}) may interfere with this technique for assessing autoPEEP. An esophageal balloon can estimate autoPEEP in patients who are not cooperative with the end-expiratory pause maneuver. If patient does not cooperate with this maneuver and an esophageal balloon is not available, the clinician should look for indirect signs of autoPEEP such as ineffective triggering, as evidenced by failed inspiratory efforts to initiate a breath or a persistent end expiratory flow and a lack of return to the baseline of the expiratory limb of the flow curve (**Fig. 7**). Similarly, asymmetric areas under the flow time curves can be seen, particularly as a

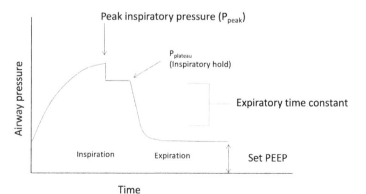

Peak inspiratory pressure (P_{peak})

$P_{plateau}$ (Inspiratory hold)

Expiratory time constant

Airway pressure

Inspiration   Expiration   Set PEEP

Time

Fig. 4. Pressure–time curve demonstrating the relationship between peak pressure (P_{peak}), plateau pressure ($P_{plateau}$), and positive end-expiratory pressure (PEEP) as well as the expiratory time constant as an exponential decay in pressure during passive exhalation due to recoil from thoracic wall and lung parenchyma.

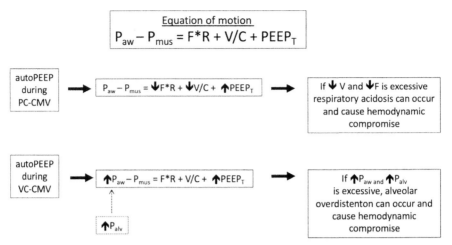

Fig. 5. Effect of autoPEEP on volume control ventilation (VC-CMV) and pressure control ventilation (PC-CMV). As autoPEEP increases, a compensatory effect will occur on F, V, P_{airway} and P_{alv}. If autoPEEP is not addressed hemodynamic compromise will ultimately occur by respiratory acidosis (if PC-CMV) or alveolar overdistension (if VC-CMV). C = compliance; F = flow; P_{airway} = airway pressure; P_{alv} = alveolar pressure; V = volume.

sign of obstructive airway disease, which should alert the clinician that the patient may be prone to developing autoPEEP. If autoPEEP is detected, it should be promptly addressed, and the strategies suggested in **Box 2** should be employed.

Decrease Lung Compliance in Cardiovascular Disease

Few data exist on the pathophysiological mechanisms of reduced lung compliance in cardiovascular

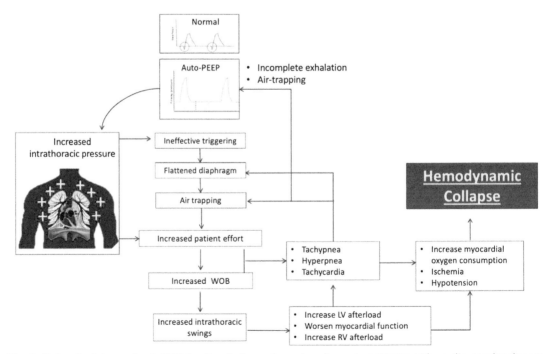

Fig. 6. Pathophysiology of autoPEEP leading to hemodynamic collapse in patients with cardiovascular disease. Note how the increase baseline dictated by autoPEEP (yellow area) represents a higher pressure to overcome by the patient to trigger breaths. As work of breathing increases and the patient becomes more dyssynchronous and tachypneic, autoPEEP will worsen with the potential of leading to hemodynamic collapse. LV, left ventricle; RV, right ventricle; WOB, work of breathing.

Identifying AutoPEEP on Ventilator Curves

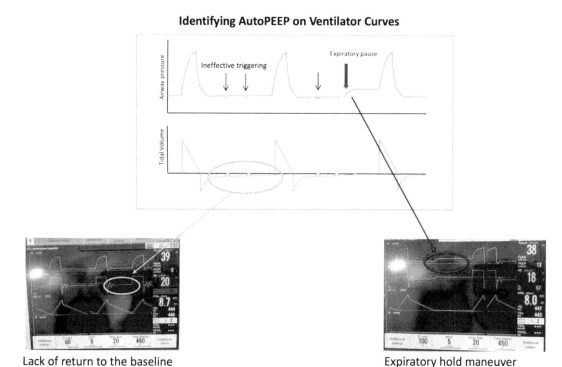

Lack of return to the baseline   Expiratory hold maneuver

Fig. 7. Detection of autoPEEP on volume control ventilation by assessing ventilator curves. Note the ineffective triggering efforts by the patient (*black arrows*) as well as the lack of return to the baseline in the volume/time curve (*yellow circle*). An expiratory hold maneuver is applied allowing to quantify total PEEP, from which subtracting set PEEP will provide you with the amount of autoPEEP.

disease, probably due to the difficulty in its noninvasive assessment. Impaired lung compliance is associated with several pulmonary alterations in cardiac disease, including impaired alveolar gas diffusion and worsening of ventilation–perfusion match,[119] contributing to exertional dyspnea. This has been reported, for example, in heart failure with preserved ejection fraction,[120,121] where patients may be more likely to cease exercising because pulmonary limitation and not because of impaired CO reserve, as happens in heart failure with reduced ejection fraction.[122]

Many factors causing reduced lung compliance have been hypothesized, with potentially different contributions according to distinct cardiovascular conditions: increased PCWP, increased PVR, and alteration in surface forces in alveoli. The pathophysiologic alteration most strictly linked to this phenomenon is pulmonary edema; in this context, liquid-filled alveoli induce mechanical stress on air-filled alveoli, hence reducing overall lung compliance.[123] Assessing lung compliance is more feasible in ventilated patients, where monitoring tidal volume and airway pressures aids its calculation, and it is not uncommon to observe elevated plateau pressures in pulmonary edema that significantly improved as volume status and CO is optimized.

Esophageal Pressure Monitoring in Cardiovascular Patient

Esophageal pressure (P_{es}) monitoring is valuable for assessing heart–lung interactions and gaining insights into the cardiopulmonary system. It involves inserting a catheter into the esophagus to obtain the esophageal pressure, which is a surrogate of the pleural pressure. Measuring P_{es} allows evaluation of intrathoracic pressure, transpulmonary, and transvascular pressures[124] The main use of P_{es} is calculating trans-structural pressure. That is the difference in pressure between the inside and outside of a structure. For the critical care patient, the 2 main uses are to calculate the transpulmonary pressure (P_{TP}) and the transvascular pressure.

The P_{TP} is calculated by subtracting P_{es} from the airway pressure (P_{AW}), $P_{TP} = P_{AW} - P_{es}$. This allows partitioning of the pressure required to distend the lung versus the one to distend the chest wall and abdomen. Thus, P_{TP} is the pressure required to distend the lung parenchyma. In patients with ARDS and low lung compliance,[125,126] clinicians calculating P_{TP} can make a more precise adjustment of mechanical ventilation parameters (eg, PEEP), which may lead to improving oxygenation,

Box 2
Strategies to manage autopositive end-expiratory pressure

1. Maximize expiratory time by lowering respiratory rate: This will have a direct effect in the inspiration to expiration time relationship (I:E time), which can also be directly adjusted in the ventilator but that would ultimately depend on respiratory rate. Other maneuvers such as increasing inspiratory flow or decreasing the set inspiratory time (eg, changing the flow pattern from a descending ramp to rectangular) may also increase the expiratory time, but to a lesser degree compared to decreasing the respiratory rate.

2. Optimize sedation: This may help mitigate potential patient discomfort due to auto-PEEP and also slow the patient's respiratory rate to avoid patient overbreathing the ventilator.

3. Optimize resistance: A decrease in the resistance will facilitate expiratory flow and thereby mitigate air trapping and autoPEEP. This can be potentially achieved with bronchodilators, corticosteroids, antibiotics, and secretion management.

4. Increase the set PEEP: This maneuver can facilitate patient triggering of assisted or spontaneous breaths by decreasing the pressure gradient that needs to be overcome by the inspiratory efforts to trigger a breath. However, the set PEEP should not be more than 75% to 85% of the total PEEP.[128,129]

5. Lastly, if none of the aforementioned maneuvers are effective or if the patient is rapidly decompensating with impending hemodynamic collapse, disconnecting the patient from the ventilator and compressing on their chest will relieve air trapping and resolve autoPEEP. However, the risk of alveolar derecruitment with this maneuver needs to be considered within the clinical context.

by recruiting alveoli and preventing barotrauma. This is often used in patients with obesity or restrictive chest disorders where chest wall compliance is reduced, and a significantly elevated plateau pressure is observed. In these patients, the plateau pressure may be elevated, but the P_{TP} is not; thus, an esophageal pressure measurement may allow increasing ventilator settings beyond usual thresholds.

P_{es} provides valuable insights into variations in transmural pressure across pulmonary vascular structures and cardiac chambers during the respiratory cycle. This aids in diagnosing and managing conditions like PH, cardiac tamponade, or right ventricular dysfunction.[127] Additionally, P_{es} enables assessment of ventricular interdependence, revealing complex interactions between heart chambers.[117] However, limitations exist in esophageal pressure measurement due to factors such as patient positioning, respiratory effort, and lung disease affecting accuracy. Interpreting esophageal pressure requires expertise in cardiovascular and respiratory system interactions.[124–127] Consequently, routine use is not recommended; it is reserved for specific cases where the accurate assessment of lung distending pressures is crucial, such as in obesity, abdominal compartment syndrome, chest wall deformities, or large pleural effusion.

CLINICS CARE POINTS

- Positive pressure ventilation produces hemodynamic changes: a decrease in LV afterload, an increase in RV afterload, and a decrease in both LV and RV preload.

- In patients with severe preload-sensitive conditions, such as pulmonary hypertension, severe RV failure, or cardiac tamponade, the preference is to delay or avoid intubation and the initiation of invasive mechanical ventilation. If intubation is necessary, high levels of PEEP should be avoided as they may have a negative hemodynamic impact.

- During induction for sedation, consider agents with minimal impact on sympathetic tone and hemodynamics. In patients who are already hypotensive at baseline, premedication with vasopressors can allow the clinician to improve hemodynamic parameters in preparation for intubation, targeting a mean arterial pressure above 65 mm Hg before induction and optimizing preload should be considered.

- An important parameter to monitor in patients undergoing invasive mechanical positive pressure ventilation is autoPEEP, particularly in the presence of cardiovascular conditions, given its potential for significant hemodynamic instability.

- During the removal of positive pressure, be cautious of the increase in afterload to the left ventricle, which can lead to elevated filling pressures, especially in patients with ventricular dysfunction, or may also unmask worsening mitral regurgitation, a common etiology of extubation failure.

DISCLOSURE

Dr Solomon receives research support from the National Institutes of Health Clinical Center intramural research funds.

REFERENCES

1. Morrow DA, Fang JC, Fintel DJ, et al. Evolution of critical care cardiology: transformation of the cardiovascular intensive care unit and the emerging need for new medical staffing and training models: a scientific statement from the American Heart Association. Circulation 2012;126(11):1408–28.
2. Katz JN, Shah BR, Volz EM, et al. Evolution of the coronary care unit: clinical characteristics and temporal trends in healthcare delivery and outcomes. Crit Care Med 2010;38(2):375–81.
3. Bohula EA, Katz JN, Van Diepen S, et al. Demographics, care patterns, and outcomes of patients admitted to cardiac intensive care units: the critical care cardiology trials network prospective North American Multicenter Registry of cardiac critical Illness. JAMA Cardiol 2019;4(9):928–35.
4. Metkus TS, Miller PE, Alviar CL, et al. Advanced respiratory support in the contemporary cardiac ICU. Crit Care Explor 2020;2(9):e0182.
5. Jentzer JC, van Diepen S, Barsness GW, et al. Changes in comorbidities, diagnoses, therapies and outcomes in a contemporary cardiac intensive care unit population. Am Heart J 2019;215:12–9.
6. Banner MJ. Respiratory muscle loading and the work of breathing. J Cardiothorac Vasc Anesth 1995;9(2):192–204.
7. Cabello B, Mancebo J. Work of breathing. Intensive Care Med 2006;32(9):1311–4.
8. West JB, Dollery CT, Naimark A. Distribution of blood flow in isolated lung; relation to vascular and alveolar pressures. J Appl Physiol 1964;19(4):713–24.
9. Disselkamp M, Adkins D, Pandey S, et al. Physiologic approach to mechanical ventilation in right ventricular failure. Ann Am Thorac Soc 2018; 15(3):383–9.
10. Magder S. Heart-Lung interaction in spontaneous breathing subjects: the basics. Ann Transl Med 2018;6(18):348.
11. Condos WR, Latham RD, Hoadley SD, et al. Hemodynamics of the Mueller maneuver in man: right and left heart micromanometry and Doppler echocardiography. Circulation 1987;76(5):1020–8.
12. Keller M, Applefeld W, Acho M, et al. How I Teach auto-PEEP Applying the physiology of expiration. ATS Sch 2021;2(4):610–24.
13. Downs JB, Klein EF, Desautels D, et al. Intermittent mandatory ventilation: a new approach to weaning patients from mechanical ventilators. Chest 1973; 64(3):331–5.
14. Marini JJ, Smith TC, Lamb VJ. External work output and force generation during synchronized intermittent mechanical ventilation. Effect of machine assistance on breathing effort. Am Rev Respir Dis 1988;138(5):1169–79.
15. Alviar CL, Miller PE, McAreavey D, et al. Positive pressure ventilation in the cardiac intensive care Unit. J Am Coll Cardiol 2018;72(13):1532–53.
16. Cheifetz IM. Cardiorespiratory interactions: the relationship between mechanical ventilation and hemodynamics. Respir Care 2014;59(12):1937–45.
17. Pang D, Keenan SP, Cook DJ, et al. The effect of positive pressure airway support on mortality and the need for intubation in cardiogenic pulmonary edema: a systematic review. Chest 1998;114(4): 1185–92.
18. Feihl F, Broccard AF. Interactions between respiration and systemic hemodynamics. Part II: practical implications in critical care. Intensive Care Med 2009;35(2):198–205.
19. Feihl F, Broccard AF. Interactions between respiration and systemic hemodynamics. Part I: basic concepts. Intensive Care Med 2009; 35(1):45–54.
20. Mahmood SS, Pinsky MR. Heart-lung interactions during mechanical ventilation: the basics. Ann Transl Med 2018;6(18):349.
21. Slobod D, Assanangkornchai N, Alhazza M, et al. Right ventricular loading by lung inflation during controlled mechanical ventilation. Am J Respir Crit Care Med 2022;205(11):1311–9.
22. Haddad F, Doyle R, Murphy DJ, et al. Right ventricular function in cardiovascular disease, part II: pathophysiology, clinical importance, and management of right ventricular failure. Circulation 2008; 117(13):1717–31.
23. Scharf SM, Bianco JA, Tow DE, et al. The effects of large negative intrathoracic pressure on left ventricular function in patients with coronary artery disease. Circulation 1981;63(4):871–5.
24. Rasanen J, Nikki P, Heikkila J. Acute myocardial infarction complicated by respiratory failure. The effects of mechanical ventilation. Chest 1984;85(1):21–8.
25. Lemaire F, Teboul JL, Cinotti L, et al. Acute left ventricular dysfunction during unsuccessful weaning from mechanical ventilation. Anesthesiology 1988; 69(2):171–9.
26. Ouellette DR, Patel S, Girard TD, et al. Liberation from mechanical ventilation in critically ill Adults: an Official American College of chest Physicians/ American thoracic Society clinical Practice guideline: inspiratory pressure augmentation during spontaneous breathing trials, Protocols minimizing sedation, and noninvasive ventilation immediately after extubation. Chest 2017;151(1):166–80.
27. Andi Shahu MM, Soumya Banna M, Willard Applefeld M, et al. Liberation from mechanical

ventilation in the cardiac intensive care Unit. JACC (J Am Coll Cardiol): Advances 2023;2(1):100173.

28. Cabello B, Thille AW, Roche-Campo F, et al. Physiological comparison of three spontaneous breathing trials in difficult-to-wean patients. Intensive Care Med 2010;36(7):1171–9.

29. Ruiz-Bailén M, Cobo-Molinos J, Castillo-Rivera A, et al. Stress echocardiography in patients who experienced mechanical ventilation weaning failure. J Crit Care 2017;39:66–71.

30. Tehrani BN, Truesdell AG, Psotka MA, et al. A Standardized and comprehensive approach to the management of cardiogenic shock. JACC Heart Fail 2020;8(11):879–91.

31. Hrymak C, Strumpher J, Jacobsohn E. Acute right ventricle failure in the intensive care Unit: assessment and management. Can J Cardiol 2017;33(1):61–71.

32. Bootsma IT, Boerma EC, Scheeren TWL, et al. The contemporary pulmonary artery catheter. Part 2: measurements, limitations, and clinical applications. J Clin Monit Comput 2022;36(1):17–31.

33. Naeije R, Badagliacca R. The overloaded right heart and ventricular interdependence. Cardiovasc Res 2017;113(12):1474–85.

34. Lim HS, Gustafsson F. Pulmonary artery pulsatility index: physiological basis and clinical application. Eur J Heart Fail 2020;22(1):32–8.

35. Eskesen TG, Wetterslev M, Perner A. Systematic review including re-analyses of 1148 individual data sets of central venous pressure as a predictor of fluid responsiveness. Intensive Care Med 2016; 42(3):324–32.

36. Pinsky M, Kellum J, Bellomo R. Central venous pressure is a stopping rule, not a target of fluid resuscitation. Available at: Critical Care and Resuscitation 2014;16(4):245–6 www.jficm.anzca.edu.au/aaccm/journal/publi-.

37. Price LC, McAuley DF, Marino PS, et al. Pathophysiology of pulmonary hypertension in acute lung injury. Am J Physiol Lung Cell Mol Physiol 2012;302(9):L803.

38. Repessé X, Charron C, Vieillard-Baron A. Acute cor pulmonale in ARDS: rationale for protecting the right ventricle. Chest 2015;147(1):259–65.

39. Schmeisser A, Rauwolf T, Groscheck T, et al. Pressure-volume loop validation of TAPSE/PASP for right ventricular arterial coupling in heart failure with pulmonary hypertension. Eur Heart J Cardiovasc Imaging 2021;22(2):168–76.

40. Tavazzi G, Bergsland N, Alcada J, et al. Early signs of right ventricular systolic and diastolic dysfunction in acute severe respiratory failure: the importance of diastolic restrictive pattern. Eur Heart J Acute Cardiovasc Care 2020;9(6):649–56.

41. Imanishi J, Maeda T, Ujiro S, et al. Association between B-lines on lung ultrasound, invasive haemodynamics, and prognosis in acute heart failure patients. Eur Heart J Acute Cardiovasc Care 2023;12(2):115–23.

42. Picano E, Scali MC, Ciampi Q, et al. Lung ultrasound for the Cardiologist. JACC Cardiovasc Imaging 2018;11(11):1692–705.

43. Araujo GN, Silveira AD, Scolari FL, et al. Admission bedside lung ultrasound reclassifies mortality prediction in patients with ST-Segment-elevation myocardial infarction. Circ Cardiovasc Imaging 2020;13(6):E010269.

44. Bouhemad B, Brisson H, Le-Guen M, et al. Bedside ultrasound assessment of positive end-expiratory pressure-induced lung recruitment. Am J Respir Crit Care Med 2011;183(3):341–7.

45. Constantin JM, Grasso S, Chanques G, et al. Lung morphology predicts response to recruitment maneuver in patients with acute respiratory distress syndrome. Crit Care Med 2010;38(4):1108–17.

46. Kim WY, Suh HJ, Hong SB, et al. Diaphragm dysfunction assessed by ultrasonography: influence on weaning from mechanical ventilation. Crit Care Med 2011;39(12):2627–30.

47. Corradi F, Brusasco C, Vezzani A, et al. Computer-aided Quantitative ultrasonography for detection of pulmonary edema in mechanically ventilated cardiac surgery patients. Chest 2016;150(3):640–51.

48. Compton FD, Zukunft B, Hoffmann C, et al. Performance of a minimally invasive uncalibrated cardiac output monitoring system (Flotrac/Vigileo) in haemodynamically unstable patients. Br J Anaesth 2008;100(4):451–6.

49. Li-ping Q, Hong-wei L, Chang-ming H, et al. Safety and efficacy of pulse-induced contour cardiac output monitoring in elderly patients with coronary artery disease and severe heart failure at coronary care units. Front Cardiovasc Med 2022;9. https://doi.org/10.3389/FCVM.2022.910898.

50. Peyton PJ, Chong SW. Minimally invasive measurement of cardiac output during surgery and critical care: a meta-analysis of accuracy and precision. Anesthesiology 2010;113(5):1220–35.

51. Saraceni E, Rossi S, Persona P, et al. Comparison of two methods for cardiac output measurement in critically ill patients. Br J Anaesth 2011;106(5):690–4.

52. Grensemann J, Defosse JM, Willms M, et al. Validation of radial artery-based uncalibrated pulse contour method (PulsioFlex) in critically ill patients: a observational study. Eur J Anaesthesiol 2017; 34(11):723–31.

53. Hadian M, Kim HK, Severyn DA, et al. Cross-comparison of cardiac output trending accuracy of LiDCO, PiCCO, FloTrac and pulmonary artery catheters. Crit Care 2010;14(6).

54. Saugel B, Hoppe P, Nicklas JY, et al. Continuous noninvasive pulse wave analysis using finger cuff technologies for arterial blood pressure and cardiac output monitoring in perioperative and intensive

care medicine: a systematic review and meta-analysis. Br J Anaesth 2020;125(1):25–37.

55. Segal E, Katzenelson R, Berkenstadt H, et al. Transpulmonary thermodilution cardiac output measurement using the axillary artery in critically ill patients. J Clin Anesth 2002;14(3):210–3.

56. Galarza L, Mercado P, Teboul JL, et al. Estimating the rapid haemodynamic effects of passive leg raising in critically ill patients using bioreactance. Br J Anaesth 2018;121(3):567–73.

57. Chopra S, Thompson J, Shahangian S, et al. Precision and consistency of the passive leg raising maneuver for determining fluid responsiveness with bioreactance non-invasive cardiac output monitoring in critically ill patients and healthy volunteers. PLoS One 2019;14(9).

58. Fathy S, Hasanin AM, Raafat M, et al. Thoracic fluid content: a novel parameter for predicting failed weaning from mechanical ventilation. J Intensive Care 2020;8(1).

59. Friesecke S, Heinrich A, Abel P, et al. Comparison of pulmonary artery and aortic transpulmonary thermodilution for monitoring of cardiac output in patients with severe heart failure: validation of a novel method. Crit Care Med 2009;37(1):119–23.

60. Volpicelli G, Skurzak S, Boero E, et al. Lung ultrasound predicts well extravascular lung water but is of limited usefulness in the prediction of wedge pressure. Anesthesiology 2014;121(2):320–7.

61. Vallabhajosyula S, Kashani K, Dunlay SM, et al. Acute respiratory failure and mechanical ventilation in cardiogenic shock complicating acute myocardial infarction in the USA, 2000-2014. Ann Intensive Care 2019;9(1).

62. Alviar CL, Rico-Mesa JS, Morrow DA, et al. Positive pressure ventilation in cardiogenic shock: review of the evidence and practical Advice for patients with mechanical circulatory support. Can J Cardiol 2020;36(2):300–12.

63. Van Diepen S, Hoohman JS, Stebbins A et al. Association between delays in mechanical ventilation initiation and mortality in patients with refractory cardiogenic shock. JAMA Cardiol 2020;5(8):965–7.

64. Rubini Giménez M, Elliott Miller P, Alviar CL, et al. Outcomes associated with respiratory failure for patients with cardiogenic shock and acute myocardial infarction: a Substudy of the CULPRIT-SHOCK trial. J Clin Med 2020;9(3).

65. Suter PM, Fairley HB, Isenberg MD. Optimum end-expiratory airway pressure in patients with acute pulmonary failure. N Engl J Med 1975;292(6):284–9.

66. Grace MP, Greenbaum DM. Cardiac performance in response to PEEP in patients with cardiac dysfunction. Crit Care Med 1982;10(6):358–60.

67. Kontoyannis DA, Nanas JN, Kontoyannis SA, et al. Mechanical ventilation in conjunction with the intra-aortic balloon pump improves the outcome of patients in profound cardiogenic shock. Intensive Care Med 1999;25(8):835–8.

68. Mathru M, Rao TL, El-Etr AA, et al. Hemodynamic response to changes in ventilatory patterns in patients with normal and poor left ventricular reserve. Crit Care Med 1982;10(7):423–6.

69. Patzelt J, Zhang Y, Seizer P, et al. Effects of mechanical ventilation on heart geometry and mitral valve leaflet coaptation during percutaneous edge-to-edge mitral valve repair. JACC Cardiovasc Interv 2016;9(2):151–9.

70. Bellone A, Barbieri A, Ricci C, et al. Acute effects of non-invasive ventilatory support on functional mitral regurgitation in patients with exacerbation of congestive heart failure. Intensive Care Med 2002; 28(9):1348–50.

71. Wiesen J, Ornstein M, Tonelli AR, et al. State of the evidence: mechanical ventilation with PEEP in patients with cardiogenic shock. Heart 2013;99(24): 1812–7.

72. Shorofsky M, Jayaraman D, Lellouche F, et al. Mechanical ventilation with high tidal volume and associated mortality in the cardiac intensive care unit. Acute Card Care 2014;16(1):9–14.

73. Andrei S, Nguyen M, Berthoud V, et al. Determinants of arterial pressure of oxygen and carbon dioxide in patients supported by Veno-arterial ECMO. J Clin Med 2022;11(17).

74. Lorusso R, Shekar K, MacLaren G, et al. ELSO Interim guidelines for venoarterial extracorporeal membrane oxygenation in adult cardiac patients. ASAIO J 2021;67(8):827–44.

75. Schmidt M, Pellegrino V, Combes A, et al. Mechanical ventilation during extracorporeal membrane oxygenation. Crit Care 2014;18(1).

76. Guglin M, Zucker MJ, Bazan VM, et al. Venoarterial ECMO for adults: JACC scientific Expert Panel. J Am Coll Cardiol 2019;73(6):698–716.

77. Rali AS, Tran LE, Auvil B, et al. Modifiable mechanical ventilation targets are associated with improved survival in ventilated VA-ECLS patients. JACC Heart Fail 2023. https://doi.org/10.1016/J.JCHF.2023.03.023.

78. Tonna JE, Selzman CH, Bartos JA, et al. The association of modifiable mechanical ventilation settings, blood gas changes and survival on extracorporeal membrane oxygenation for cardiac arrest. Resuscitation 2022;174:53–61.

79. Thomas A, van Diepen S, Beekman R, et al. Oxygen Supplementation and hyperoxia in critically ill cardiac patients: from pathophysiology to clinical Practice. JACC Advances 2022;1(3): 100065.

80. Jentzer JC, Miller PE, Alviar C, et al. Exposure to arterial hyperoxia during extracorporeal membrane oxygenator support and mortality in patients with cardiogenic shock. Circ Heart Fail 2023;16(4):E010328.

81. Montero S, Huang F, Rivas-Lasarte M, et al. Awake venoarterial extracorporeal membrane oxygenation for refractory cardiogenic shock. Eur Heart J Acute Cardiovasc Care 2021;10(6):585–94.

82. Jentzer JC, Wiley BM, Reddy YNV, et al. Epidemiology and outcomes of pulmonary hypertension in the cardiac intensive care unit. Eur Heart J Acute Cardiovasc Care 2022;11(3):230–41.

83. Barnett CF, O'Brien C, De Marco T. Critical care management of the patient with pulmonary hypertension. Eur Heart J Acute Cardiovasc Care 2022; 11(1):77–83.

84. Johannes J, Berlin DA, Patel P, et al. A technique of awake bronchoscopic endotracheal intubation for respiratory failure in patients with right heart failure and pulmonary hypertension. Crit Care Med 2017; 45(9):e980–4.

85. Kitamura T, Iwami T, Kawamura T, et al. Bystander-initiated rescue breathing for out-of-hospital cardiac arrests of noncardiac origin. Circulation 2010; 122(3):293–9.

86. Ogawa T, Akahane M, Koike S, et al. Outcomes of chest compression only CPR versus conventional CPR conducted by lay people in patients with out of hospital cardiopulmonary arrest witnessed by bystanders: nationwide population based observational study. BMJ 2011;342(7792):321.

87. Svensson L, Bohm K, Castrèn M, et al. Compression-only CPR or standard CPR in out-of-hospital cardiac arrest. N Engl J Med 2010;363(5):434–42.

88. Rea TD, Fahrenbruch C, Culley L, et al. CPR with chest compression alone or with rescue breathing. N Engl J Med 2010;363(5):423–33.

89. SOS-KANTO Study Group. Cardiopulmonary resuscitation by bystanders with chest compression only (SOS-KANTO): an observational study. Lancet 2007;369(9565):920–6.

90. Bobrow BJ, Spaite DW, Berg RA, et al. Chest compression-only CPR by lay rescuers and survival from out-of-hospital cardiac arrest. JAMA 2010;304(13):1447–54.

91. Panchal AR, Bobrow BJ, Spaite DW, et al. Chest compression-only cardiopulmonary resuscitation performed by lay rescuers for adult out-of-hospital cardiac arrest due to non-cardiac aetiologies. Resuscitation 2013;84(4):435–9.

92. Lubrano R, Cecchetti C, Bellelli E, et al. Comparison of times of intervention during pediatric CPR maneuvers using ABC and CAB sequences: a randomized trial. Resuscitation 2012;83(12): 1473–7.

93. Sekiguchi H, Kondo Y, Kukita I. Verification of changes in the time taken to initiate chest compressions according to modified basic life support guidelines. Am J Emerg Med 2013;31(8):1248–50.

94. Marsch S, Tschan F, Semmer NK, et al. ABC versus CAB for cardiopulmonary resuscitation: a prospective, randomized simulator-based trial. Swiss Med Wkly 2013;143.

95. Panchal AR, Bartos JA, Cabañas JG, et al. Part 3: adult basic and advanced life support: 2020 American heart association guidelines for cardiopulmonary resuscitation and Emergency cardiovascular care. Circulation 2020;142:S366–468.

96. Berg RA, Hilwig RW, Kern KB, et al. "Bystander" chest compressions and assisted ventilation independently improve outcome from piglet asphyxial pulseless "cardiac arrest." Circulation 2000; 101(14):1743–8.

97. Nichol G, Leroux B, Wang H, et al. Trial of continuous or Interrupted chest compressions during CPR. N Engl J Med 2015;373(23):2203–14.

98. Aufderheide TP, Lurie KG. Death by hyperventilation: a common and life-threatening problem during cardiopulmonary resuscitation. Crit Care Med 2004;32(9 Suppl).

99. Aufderheide TP, Sigurdsson G, Pirrallo RG, et al. Hyperventilation-induced hypotension during cardiopulmonary resuscitation. Circulation 2004; 109(16):1960–5.

100. O'Neill JF, Deakin CD. Do we hyperventilate cardiac arrest patients? Resuscitation 2007;73(1):82–5.

101. Buunk G, Van Der Hoeven JG, Meinders AE. Cerebrovascular reactivity in comatose patients resuscitated from a cardiac arrest. Stroke 1997;28(8): 1569–73.

102. Cold GE. Cerebral blood flow in acute head injury. The regulation of cerebral blood flow and metabolism during the acute phase of head injury, and its significance for therapy. Acta Neurochir Suppl 1990;49:1–64. https://pubmed.ncbi.nlm.nih.gov/ 2275429/. [Accessed 25 June 2023].

103. Kågström E, Smith MLL, Siesgö BK. Cerebral circulatory responses to hypercapnia and hypoxia in the recovery period following complete and incomplete cerebral ischemia in the rat. Acta Physiol Scand 1983;118(3):281–91.

104. Safar P, Xiao F, Radovsky A, et al. Improved cerebral resuscitation from cardiac arrest in dogs with mild hypothermia plus blood flow promotion. Stroke 1996;27(1):105–13.

105. Eastwood G, Nichol AD, Hodgson C, et al. Mild hypercapnia or normocapnia after out-of-hospital cardiac arrest. N Engl J Med 2023. https://doi.org/10. 1056/NEJMOA2214552.

106. Callaway CW, Donnino MW, Fink EL, et al. Part 8: post-cardiac arrest care: 2015 American heart association guidelines Update for cardiopulmonary resuscitation and Emergency cardiovascular care. Circulation 2015;132(18 Suppl 2):S465–82.

107. Roberts BW, Kilgannon JH, Chansky ME, et al. Association between postresuscitation partial pressure of arterial carbon dioxide and neurological

outcome in patients with post-cardiac arrest syndrome. Circulation 2013;127(21):2107–13.

108. Lee BK, Jeung KW, Lee HY, et al. Association between mean arterial blood gas tension and outcome in cardiac arrest patients treated with therapeutic hypothermia. Am J Emerg Med 2014; 32(1):55–60.

109. Ihle JF, Bernard S, Bailey MJ, et al. Hyperoxia in the intensive care unit and outcome after out-of-hospital ventricular fibrillation cardiac arrest. Crit Care Resusc 2013;15(3):186–90.

110. Kilgannon JH, Jones AE, Shapiro NI, et al. Association between arterial hyperoxia following resuscitation from cardiac arrest and in-hospital mortality. JAMA 2010;303(21):2165–71.

111. Vaahersalo J, Bendel S, Reinikainen M, et al. Arterial blood gas tensions after resuscitation from out-of-hospital cardiac arrest: associations with long-term neurologic outcome. Crit Care Med 2014;42(6): 1463–70.

112. Bellomo R, Bailey M, Eastwood GM, et al. Arterial hyperoxia and in-hospital mortality after resuscitation from cardiac arrest. Crit Care 2011;15(2).

113. Janz DR, Hollenbeck RD, Pollock JS, et al. Hyperoxia is associated with increased mortality in patients treated with mild therapeutic hypothermia after sudden cardiac arrest. Crit Care Med 2012; 40(12):3135–9.

114. Elmer J, Scutella M, Pullalarevu R, et al. The association between hyperoxia and patient outcomes after cardiac arrest: analysis of a high-resolution database. Intensive Care Med 2015;41(1):49–57.

115. Schmidt H, Kjaergaard J, Hassager C, et al. Oxygen targets in comatose Survivors of cardiac arrest. N Engl J Med 2022;387(16):1467–76.

116. Prekker ME, Driver BE, Trent SA, et al. Video versus direct laryngoscopy for Tracheal intubation of critically ill Adults. N Engl J Med 2023. https://doi.org/10.1056/NEJMOA2301601/SUPPL_FILE/NEJMOA2301601_DATA_SHARING

117. Luecke T, Pelosi P. Clinical review: positive end-expiratory pressure and cardiac output. Crit Care 2005;9(6):607–21.

118. Pinsky MR. Cardiopulmonary interactions: physiologic basis and clinical applications. In: Annals of the American Thoracic Society. American Thoracic Society 2018;15:S45–8.

119. Laghi F, Goyal A. Auto-PEEP in respiratory failure. Minerva Anestesiol 2012;78(2):201–21.

120. Ranieri VM, Giuliani R, Cinnella G, et al. Physiologic effects of positive end-expiratory pressure in patients with chronic obstructive pulmonary disease during acute ventilatory failure and controlled mechanical ventilation. Am Rev Respir Dis 1993; 147(1):5–13.

121. Sullivan MJ, Higginbotham MB, Cobb FR. Increased exercise ventilation in patients with chronic heart failure: Intact ventilatory control despite hemodynamic and pulmonary abnormalities. Circulation 1988; 77(3):552–9.

122. Obokata M, Olson TP, Reddy YNV, et al. Haemodynamics, dyspnoea, and pulmonary reserve in heart failure with preserved ejection fraction. Eur Heart J 2018;39(30):2810–21.

123. Andrea R, López-Giraldo A, Falces C, et al. Lung function abnormalities are highly frequent in patients with heart failure and preserved ejection fraction. Heart Lung Circ 2014;23(3):273–9.

124. Woods PR, Olson TP, Frantz RP, et al. Causes of breathing inefficiency during exercise in heart failure. J Card Fail 2010;16(10):835–42.

125. Perlman CE, Lederer DJ, Bhattacharya J. Micromechanics of alveolar edema. Am J Respir Cell Mol Biol 2010;44(1):34–9.

126. Mauri T, Yoshida T, Bellani G, et al. Esophageal and transpulmonary pressure in the clinical setting: meaning, usefulness and perspectives. Intensive Care Med 2016;42(9):1360–73.

127. Talmor D, Sarge T, Malhotra A, et al. Mechanical ventilation guided by esophageal pressure in acute lung injury. N Engl J Med 2008;359(20):2095–104.

128. Beitler JR, Sarge T, Banner-Goodspeed VM, et al. Effect of titrating positive end-expiratory pressure (PEEP) with an esophageal pressure-guided strategy vs an empirical high PEEP-Fio2 strategy on death and Days free from mechanical ventilation among patients with acute respiratory distress syndrome: a randomized clinical trial. JAMA 2019; 321(9):846–57.

129. Repessé X, Vieillard-Baron A, Geri G. Value of measuring esophageal pressure to evaluate heart-lung interactions-applications for invasive hemodynamic monitoring. Ann Transl Med 2018; 6(18):351.

Emergencies in Pulmonary Hypertension

Sanjeeb Bhattacharya, MD

KEYWORDS

• Pulmonary hypertension • Critical care • Emergencies • PAH

KEY POINTS

- Complex etiologies: Pulmonary hypertension is a complex disease with diverse underlying causes, making its management challenging.
- Critical care challenge: Patients with pulmonary arterial hypertension (WHO Group 1) pose significant challenges in critical care settings due to high morbidity and mortality risks.
- Multidisciplinary approach: Effective management necessitates a multidisciplinary team at specialized pulmonary hypertension care facilities for thorough evaluation and prompt initiation of treatment.
- Acute right heart failure focus: In cases of acute decompensated right heart failure, the management strategy should prioritize optimizing preload and afterload, incorporating pulmonary vasodilator therapy.
- Tailored treatment of specialized situations: a careful assessment of specialized situations is crucial to tailor the treatment response appropriately for individuals with pulmonary arterial hypertension, ensuring comprehensive care.

INTRODUCTION

Pulmonary hypertension (PH) is a challenging disease with various underlying etiologies, making it difficult to diagnose and manage. It is defined by invasive hemodynamics with a mean pulmonary artery pressure greater than 20 mmHG. This is further delineated as precapillary, isolated postcapillary, or combined precapillary and postcapillary PH (**Table 1**). Diagnosis is made via insertion of a pulmonary artery catheter for hemodynamic profiling. Hemodynamics is essential to diagnosing the general diagnosis of PH; however, it is critical to further understand the underlying cause (base on the WHO Group) given the differences in treatments. Etiology range from left-sided heart disease-related PH, PH associated with lung disease (chronic obstructive pulmonary disease [COPD], intersitial lung disease [ILD], obstructive sleep apnea [OSA]), chronic thromboembolic disease, and so forth. Significant attention is given to the WHO Group 1 PH given high acuity of illness and lack of familiarity with

treatment (**Table 2**). Moreover, these patients provide unique challenges in the critical care setting that can be overwhelming to care givers. This review focuses on Group 1 PH patients and unique management in the critical care setting.

Pathophysiology of Right Ventricular Failure in Pulmonary Arterial Hypertension

Pulmonary arterial hypertension's pathophysiology is characterized by endothelial dysfunction, vascular inflammation, and vascular remodeling leading to increase in pulmonary pressures and pulmonary vascular resistance (PVR) with significant reduction in compliance.[1] This occurs from microscopic endothelial injury and proliferation, vascular fibrosis, and obstruction of small vessels by plexiform lesions creating disease from small-to-large pulmonary vessels.[2] This progressive vascular disease leads to worsening afterload upon the right ventricle (RV). The RV inherently is not designed to pump against high afterload

Section of Heart Failure and Cardiac Transplantation, Cleveland Clinic, 9500 Euclid Avenue, Suite J3-4, Cleveland, OH 44195, USA
E-mail address: BHATTAS3@ccf.org

Cardiol Clin 42 (2024) 273–278
https://doi.org/10.1016/j.ccl.2024.02.011

Table 1
Defining hemodynamics in pulmonary hypertension

	Precapillary PH	Isolated Postcapillary PH	Combined Precapillary and Postcapillary PH
Pulmonary Pressure	20 mm Hg	20 mm Hg	20 mm Hg
PCWP	<15 mm Hg	15 mm Hg	15 mm Hg
PVR	2 Wu	<2 Wu	2 Wu

Abbreviations: PCWP. pulmonary capillary wedge pressure; PH, pulmonary hypertension; Wu, wood unit.

states, but rather designed to pump against a highly compliant pulmonary system with low vascular resistance.[3] This is in contradiction to the interaction of the left ventricle and systemic circulation.

In PH, the RV faces pathophysiologic changes associated with the increased afterload. The RV hypertrophies initially to the response in afterload; however, persistent exposure to high afterload leads to progressive RV dilatation and dysfunction. This maladaptation leads to increase in right ventricular volume, pressure, wall stress, and myocardial oxygen demand. Owing to ventricular interdependence, the septum bulges toward the left ventricle leading to decreased left ventricular filling and cardiac output. Diastolic pressure decreases causing a decrease in right ventricular perfusion pressures (diastolic blood pressure: RV-end diastolic pressure) leading RV ischemia. There is a progressive increase in right atrial pressure leading to peripheral congestion.[4] This ultimately will lead to worsening RV failure and hemodynamic collapse (**Fig. 1**).

Epidemiology and Outcomes of Pulmonary Hypertension in Critical Care Setting

PH outcomes are poorly characterized in the critical care setting. Most studies have looked at characterizing patients based on estimated pulmonary pressures on echocardiogram. Early retrospective

Table 2
Etiology of Group 1 pulmonary hypertension

Group 1 Pulmonary Hypertension	Idiopathic
	Heritable
	Drugs/toxins
	Connective tissue associated
	HIV
	Portal hypertension
	Congenital heart disease
	Schistosomiasis
	Persistent PH of newborn
	Pulmonary veno-occlusive disease

studies by Stamm and colleagues assessed intensive care unit (ICU) admissions assessing outcomes comparing patients with PH to controls. PH was estimated by echocardiogram. Patients with PH portended a lower survival than patients without.[5] In a separate retrospective study reviewing admissions to the cardiac care unit, over 60% of admissions were characterized to have some degree of PH by echocardiogram. In-hospital mortality was closely tied to severity of RV dysfunction and elevation in right ventricular systolic pressure (RVSP).[6]

A retrospective analysis of pulmonary arterial hypertension (PAH) patients at Stanford evaluated hospital admissions. Patients' characteristics with PAH were predominantly young and female. There was a high likelihood of the primary outcome (defined as death or lung transplantation). Tachypnea, reduced estimated glomerular filtration rate, hyponatremia, and tricuspid regurgitation (TR) severity were predictors of the primary outcome within 90 days of admission. Although this did not specifically evaluate in the critical care setting, it revealed the gravity of admissions with PAH.[7]

The ASPIRE registry took a close look at PH referrals to a tertiary care center. Within the registry, ICU admissions were analyzed within their PH cohort. Of the cohort, 67% of patients were diagnosed with PAH (World Health Organization [WHO] Group 1). Most common reason for medical ICU admission for patients with PAH was related to right heart failure with respiratory failure following. ICU admission for PAH led to significantly reduced hospital (71%), 1 year (55%), and 5 year (32%) survival. Mortality was affected by acute physiology and chronic health evaluation (APACHE) score, lactate, oxygen saturation, and age. This analysis provides targeted insight to the high morbidity and mortality associated with ICU admissions in PAH.[8]

Medical Management of Pulmonary Hypertension in Intensive Care Unit

Given the complexity of these patients and the medications involved in the care of patients with

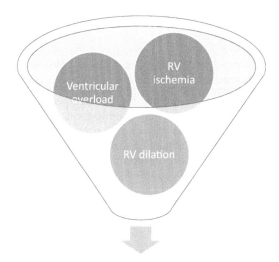

RV Failure

Fig. 1. Pathophysiology in PH leading to RV failure.

PH, speciality care should be provided in centers equipped for these patients. Early referral and longitudinal care at specialty PH centers led to improved outcomes.[9] In addition, a multidisciplinary team approach including critical care pharmacy, led to improve access to PH medications inpatient and when transitioning to outpatient care.[10]

Management of RV failure is tailored to improving RV function. Optimizing preload is extremely important. Avoiding excessive increases in preload is critical to avoid worsening RV wall stress, ventricular interdependence, and RV failure. Emphasis on decreasing RV afterload is imperative. Pulmonary vasodilators are initiated to target 3 critical pathways: prostanoids, endothelin-1 receptor blockers, and enhancing nitric oxide. Prostanoids involve intravenous epoprostenol and treprostinil, providing the most power impact on hemodynamics in patients with PAH. Prostacylins act on prostacyclin receptors increasing circulating cyclic adenosine monophosphate. These leads to vasodilation in the pulmonary vasculature as well as reversing endothelial proliferation while exerting an antithrombotic effect. Intravenous use in ICU setting for severe RV failure in PAH can lead to profound pulmonary vasodilation and reduction in PVR. Intravenous titration should be done cautiously in closely monitored ICU setting. Avoiding rapid titration is required to avoid systemic hypotension and minimize side effects.[11,12]

Endothelin-1 is produced by endothelial cells and if left unregulated, this acts a potent vasoconstrictor and leads to smooth muscle cell proliferation in PAH.[13] Endothelin-1 receptor antagonists prevent endothelin-1 from binding to endothelin receptor A and B, therefore mitigating the adverse remodeling and vasoconstrictive effects.[11] Upfront therapy with endothelin 1 receptor antagonists and PD5 inhibitors, has shown to improve in time to clinical failure events (combination of death, hospitalizations, disease progression, or inadequate long-term response).[14] It is unclear the acute hemodynamic effects of using ET-1 antagonists in oral form. Earlier studies have shown intravenous bosentan causing nonselective vasodilation with equal decrease in both PVR and systemic vascular resistance (SVR).[15]

Nitric oxide is a potent vasodilator especially in the pulmonary vasculature. Early studies have shown that there is a diminished expression of endothelial nitric oxide synthase which produces nitric oxide.[16,17] Inhaled nitric oxide is an effective pulmonary vasodilator and blunts effects of hypoxic-driven pulmonary vasoconstriction in PH patients.[18] Phosphodiesterase inhibitors such as sildenafil or tadalafil inhibit degradation of cyclic guanosine monophosphate-adenonsine monophophate (cGMP) which activates protein kinase G leading to vasodilation. Soluble guanylate cyclase stimulators, such as riociguat, directly activate soluble guanylate cyclase which enhance the effect of nitric oxide and cGMP production. It has been shown to have hemodynamic effect with reducing mean pulmonary artery (PA) pressure.[11] RESPITE trial showed improved efficacy of riociguat with endothelin (ET) antagonist for patients with poor clinical response to PD5 inhibitor and ET antagonist.[19]

Guidance is limited when utilizing vasopressor or inotropes for hemodynamics support in PH patients. In treatment of hypotension, vasopressin and norepinephrine may be preferentially used due to neutral or decreasing effect on PVR/SVR ratio. Phenylephrine does have a potent vasoconstrictive effect but on both systemic and pulmonary vascular, leading to its limited use in acute PH management. Inotropes such as dobutamine have been used to increase cardiac output without increasing PVR. Milrinone does have an effect on inotropy but can affect both SVR and PVR and should be used cautiously given risk for systemic hypotension.[20]

Airway Management in Pulmonary Hypertension

Pulmonary vascular is very sensitive to hypoxemia and hypercapnia. The correction of hypoxia and hypercapnia may require the use of more advanced ventilation strategies other than nasal cannula or high flow oxygen supplementation. Positive pressure ventilation (PPV) may be required to help with atelectasis and hypoxia. However, there can be deleterious effects on hemodynamics. PPV may decrease venous return as well as increase RV afterload by increasing transpulmonary pressures. Intubation and mechanical ventilation pose more immediate hemodynamic compromise, leading to RV preload, afterload, hypotension, and decrease in cardiac output related to hemodynamic effects of sedative medication and mechanical ventilation.[21] There are limited data on the use of awake bronchoscopic endotracheal intubation in patients with decompensated PH. Eight of 9 patients survived the first 24 hours but there were still complications of systemic hypotension.[22]

Management of Pericardial Effusion

Pericardial effusions can be commonly seen in patients with severe PAH. The possible underlying pathophysiology includes impaired cardiac venous drainage from the coronary sinus to right atrium, leading to leak into the pericardial space.[23] Pericardial effusions have been linked to disease severity and are part of the REVEAL risk calculator.[24] In a majority of cases, the presence of pericardial effusion is related to the severity of the PH. Thus, the direct treatment of PH with pulmonary vasodilators usually leads to resolution of the pericardial effusion. Less attention should be given to the direct treatment of the pericardial effusion as these typically are not causing the hemodynamic compromise. Vasquez and colleagues found a higher risk of mortality in patients with PH undergoing pericardiocentesis.[25] A possible explanation may be related to

worsening RV dilation, leading to increase ventricular interdependence.

Advanced Pulmonary Hypertension Support in Pulmonary Hypertension

In patients with refractory decompensated PH, advanced therapies may need to be considered. When considering more invasive supports, lung transplantation candidacy must be considered. In cases of palliation, balloon septostomy may be considered to unload the right heart and improve left ventricle (LV) filling and cardiac output. This should be done at an experienced center.[26] Potts shunt has been also described as a bridging technique to transplantations where an anastomosis is created from the left pulmonary artery to the descending thoracic aorta.[27]

There is less evidence in utilization of temporary mechanical support in PAH. Veno-arterial extracorporeal membrane oxygenation (VA-ECMO) has been a bridging tool for cardiogenic shock in PAH awaiting bilateral lung transplantation. There has been some cases of utilizing VA-ECMO as bridge to recovery in hopes to aggressively titrate medical therapy. However, data are limited, and pharmacokinetics of IV prostacyclins in VA-ECMO have been variable.[28] It is unknown how direct right atrial/vena caval to pulmonary artery devices behave in PAH. Concern is providing increase flow to a highly resistant vascular bed.

Management Algorithm

Given the complexities of patients with PAH, it is important to create a structure for effective management and treatment of these patients (**Fig. 2**).

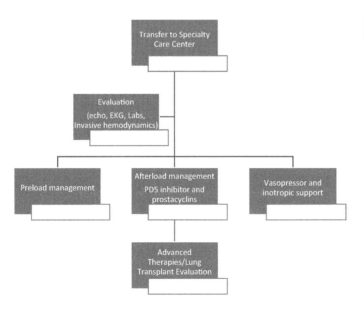

Fig. 2. Algorithm for management of PAH in ICU.

In patients with concern for decompensated PH, patients should be referred and transferred immediately to specialty care center where a comprehensive team is ready for management. This team should include critical care and cardiology trained in PH, PH pharmacist, and nurses experienced managing PH therapies. Upon arrival, prompt evaluation should be done including transthoracic echocardiography, laboratories including lactate assessment. Echocardiography can quickly and safely assess degree of RV dysfunction. If diagnosis is new, a workup for PAH includes (if undifferentiated diagnosis) rheumatologic serologies, V/Q scan, and CT of chest (if stable). If the diagnosis is known, it is important to continue all preexisiting PH therapies.

Invasive hemodynamic monitoring can be considered in patients who are stable. Supine positioning may reduce lung volumes and exacerbate atelectasis and further increase PVR.[29] If stable, the insertion of PA catheter can fully delineate hemodynamics in newly diagnose PAH patients. Ongoing monitoring may be achieved with central venous access to assess right atrial pressure and central venous oxygen saturations to guide hemodynamic management of these critically ill patients. Optimization of RV function should follow. Prompt initiation and titration of pulmonary vasodilator therapies should commence with close monitoring hemodynamics and end-organ function. Tailored use of inotropes and vasopressors should be utilized based on hemodynamic profiling. A careful attention to preload is required to avoid over- or under-diuresis.

Aggressively treating hypoxia is paramount to avoid hypoxic-induced pulmonary vasoconstriction. Care should be taken to avoid intubation and mechanical ventilation. If patients are continuing to fail medical therapy, patient should be evaluated for lung transplant candidacy. If more advanced PH therapies are required, a multidisciplinary team including proceduralist should be conducted to ensure proper patient selection. This includes atrial septostomy to utilization of VA-ECMO.

SUMMARY

Despite advances in therapies, mortality remains high for patients with PAH in the critical care setting. In addition, most recommendations on management are based on low-quality data or expert recommendations. More data are required on the unique challenges these patients face in the intensive care unit and how to tailor therapy to manage these patients safe and effectively. In addition, despite the increase in the number of temporary ventricular support platforms, VA-ECMO remains the main option for temporary mechanical support without much data on the other RV support devices. In light of these limitations, the evidence supports management at specialty care centers with a multidisciplinary team approach which can improve care and outcomes of these sick patients. Aggressive management in preload, afterload, and inotropy/vasoreactivity is required to acutely manage PH patients. If patients are refractory, then careful evaluation is required for advanced PH therapies.

CLINICS CARE POINTS

- Pulmonary Hypertension is a challenging disease and can have a high mortality rate in the critical care setting.

- Appropriate phenotypic diagnosis of pulmonary hypertension is critical leading to disease specific optimization of right ventricular preload and afterload.

- Advanced noninvasive and invasive mechanical ventrilation can be used cautiously to improve hypoexmia and/or hypercapnea.

- Pericardial effusions are related to disease severity in pulmonary arterial hypertension and rarely need pericardiocentesis.

- Temporary mechanical circulatory support can be used in pulmonary arterial hypertension in specific cases for bridge to recovery or to lung transplantation.

REFERENCES

1. Hassoun PM. Pulmonary arterial hypertension. N Engl J Med 2021;385(25):2361–76.
2. Schermuly RT, Ghofrani HA, Wilkins MR, et al. Mechanisms of disease: pulmonary arterial hypertension. Nat Rev Cardiol 2011;8(8):443–55.
3. Haddad F, Hunt SA, Rosenthal DN, et al. Right ventricular function in cardiovascular disease, Part I. Circulation 2008;117(11):1436–48.
4. Haddad F, Doyle R, Murphy DJ, et al. Right ventricular function in cardiovascular disease, Part II. Circulation 2008;117(13):1717–31.
5. Stamm JA, McVerry BJ, Mathier MA, et al. Doppler-defined pulmonary hypertension in medical intensive care unit patients: retrospective investigation of risk factors and impact on mortality. Pulm Circ 2011;1(1):95–102.
6. Jentzer JC, Wiley BM, Reddy YNV, et al. Epidemiology and outcomes of pulmonary hypertension in

the cardiac intensive care unit. Eur Heart J Acute Cardiovasc Care 2022;11(3):230–41.

7. Haddad F, Peterson T, Fuh E, et al. Characteristics and outcome after hospitalization for acute right heart failure in patients with pulmonary arterial hypertension. Circulation: Heart Fail 2011;4(6):692–9.

8. Bauchmuller K, Condliffe R, Southern J, et al. Critical care outcomes in patients with pre-existing pulmonary hypertension: insights from the ASPIRE registry. ERJ Open Research 2021;7(2):00046–2021.

9. Pi H, Kosanovich CM, Handen A, et al. Outcomes of pulmonary arterial hypertension are improved in a specialty care center. Chest 2020;158(1):330–40.

10. Martirosov AL, Smith ZR, Hencken L, et al. Improving transitions of care for critically ill adult patients on pulmonary arterial hypertension medications. Am J Health Syst Pharm 2020;77(12):958–65.

11. Tettey A, Jiang Y, Li X, et al. Therapy for pulmonary arterial hypertension: glance on nitric oxide pathway. Front Pharmacol 2021;12.

12. Gomberg-Maitland M, Olschewski H. Prostacyclin therapies for the treatment of pulmonary arterial hypertension. Eur Respir J 2008;31(4):891–901.

13. Rubin LJ, Badesch DB, Fleming TR, et al. Long-term treatment with sildenafil citrate in pulmonary arterial hypertension: the SUPER-2 study. Chest 2011; 140(5):1274–83.

14. Galiè N, Barberà JA, Frost AE, et al. Initial use of ambrisentan plus tadalafil in pulmonary arterial hypertension. N Engl J Med 2015;373(9):834–44.

15. Williamson DJ, Wallman LL, Jones R, et al. Hemodynamic effects of bosentan, an endothelin receptor antagonist, in patients with pulmonary hypertension. Circulation 2000;102(4):411–8.

16. Giaid A, Saleh D. Reduced expression of endothelial nitric oxide synthase in the lungs of patients with pulmonary hypertension. N Engl J Med 1995;333(4):214–21.

17. Förstermann U, Sessa WC. Nitric oxide synthases: regulation and function. Eur Heart J 2012;33(7): 829–37.

18. Klinger JR, Abman SH, Gladwin MT. Nitric oxide deficiency and endothelial dysfunction in pulmonary arterial hypertension. Am J Respir Crit Care Med 2013;188(6):639–46.

19. Hoeper MM, Simonneau G, Corris PA, et al. RESPITE: switching to riociguat in pulmonary arterial hypertension patients with inadequate response to phosphodiesterase-5 inhibitors. Eur Respir J 2017; 50(3):1602425.

20. Barnett CF, O'Brien C, De Marco T. Critical care management of the patient with pulmonary hypertension. European Heart Journal. Acute Cardiovascular Care 2022;11(1):77–83.

21. Alviar CL, Miller PE, McAreavey D, et al. Positive pressure ventilation in the cardiac intensive care unit. J Am Coll Cardiol 2018;72(13):1532–53.

22. Johannes J, Berlin DA, Patel P, et al. A technique of awake bronchoscopic endotracheal intubation for respiratory failure in patients with right heart failure and pulmonary hypertension. Crit Care Med 2017; 45(9):e980–4.

23. Vaidy A, O'Corragain O, Vaidya A. Diagnosis and management of pulmonary hypertension and right ventricular failure in the cardiovascular intensive care unit. Crit Care Clin 2024;40(1):121–35.

24. Benza RL, Gomberg-Maitland M, Miller DP, et al. The REVEAL registry risk score calculator in patients newly diagnosed with pulmonary arterial hypertension. Chest 2012;141(2):354–62.

25. Vasquez MA, Iskander M, Mustafa M, et al. Pericardiocentesis outcomes in patients with pulmonary hypertension: a nationwide analysis from the United States. Am J Cardiol 2024;210:232–40.

26. Khan MS, Memon MM, Amin E, et al. Use of balloon atrial septostomy in patients with advanced pulmonary arterial hypertension: a systematic review and meta-analysis. Chest 2019;156(1):53–63.

27. Esch JJ, Shah PB, Cockrill BA, et al. Transcatheter Potts shunt creation in patients with severe pulmonary arterial hypertension: initial clinical experience. J Heart Lung Transplant 2013;32(4):381–7.

28. Tsai M-T, Hsu CH, Luo CY, et al. Bridge-to-recovery strategy using extracorporeal membrane oxygenation for critical pulmonary hypertension complicated with cardiogenic shock. Interact Cardiovasc Thorac Surg 2015;21(1):55–61.

29. Katz S, Arish N, Rokach A, et al. The effect of body position on pulmonary function: a systematic review. BMC Pulm Med 2018;18(1):159.

The Pharmacologic Management of Cardiac Arrest

Amandeep Singh, MD*, Megan Heeney, MD,
Martha E. Montgomery, MD, MS

KEYWORDS

- Cardiac arrest medications • Epinephrine • Amiodarone • Lidocaine

KEY POINTS

- The foundation of cardiac arrest management is high-grade chest compressions.
- The preferred route for medications during cardiac arrest is the peripheral IV. Intraosseous access is acceptable in patients for whom peripheral IV access was unsuccessful.
- The use of epinephrine and the combination of vasopressin-steroids-epinephrine for cardiac arrest have been shown to improve short-term survival. Their effect on survival with favorable neurologic outcomes is less certain.
- Both amiodarone and lidocaine have been shown to increase survival to hospital admission in patients with pulseless ventricular tachycardia or ventricular fibrillation.
- The routine use of calcium, sodium bicarbonate, magnesium, or atropine in cardiac arrest is not supported and may cause harm.

INTRODUCTION

The cornerstone of cardiac arrest management is high-quality cardiopulmonary resuscitation (CPR) and early defibrillation in patients with pulseless ventricular tachycardia/ventricular fibrillation (pVT/VF) and high-quality CPR alone in patients with pulseless electrical activity (PEA) or asystole. Medications, particularly epinephrine, are nearly universally used in cardiac arrest codes; however, the data supporting their use are limited. These medications typically produce a short-term survival benefit (ie, return of spontaneous circulation [ROSC], survival to hospital admission or hospital discharge) but rarely produce meaningful long-term improvements (ie, survival at 90 days or longer or, more importantly, survival with favorable neurologic outcome).[1] This review will cover vascular access, vasopressors, antiarrhythmics, and other medications such as calcium, sodium bicarbonate, magnesium, and atropine that are commonly used during cardiac arrest care. Finally, we review the role of β-blockers for refractory pVT/VF and thrombolytics in cardiac arrest and fatal pulmonary embolism.

VASCULAR ACCESS

The preferred route for medications during cardiac arrest is the peripheral intravenous (IV); however, obtaining IV access can be challenging based on patient characteristics, operator experience, and the emergency nature of the situation. These factors may all contribute to a delay in administering pharmacologic treatments during cardiac arrest. Alternatives to IV access include intraosseous (IO) access, central venous access, and endotracheal routes. Of these choices, IO access has become the preferred second-line, and in some systems, first-line, route based on its relative

This article originally appeared in *Emergency Medicine Clinics*, Volume 41 Issue 3, August 2023.
Alameda Health System, Highland Hospital Emergency Department, 1411 East 31st Street, Oakland, CA 94602, USA
* Corresponding author.
E-mail address: amasingh@alamedahealthsystem.org

ease and higher first-attempt success than IV cannulation.

Given the observation that advanced cardiac life suport (ACLS) medications have not been shown to improve long-term survival or survival with favorable neurologic outcomes, it is unlikely that the choice of vascular route to give these drugs would have any influence on this outcome. Although it has been demonstrated that IO access provides faster vascular access and requires less time to epinephrine administration, trials fail to show improvement in long-term clinically important outcome.[2,3] A recent meta-analysis that included 9 retrospective observational studies and 111,746 patients with out-of-hospital cardiaac arrest (OHCA) did not find any association between type of vascular access (IO vs IV) and survival with favorable neurologic outcome.[4] IV access compared with IO access was associated with an improvement in survival to hospital admission but not to hospital discharge. It is important to note that retrospective studies show association, not causation, and that patient selection bias, namely that IO placement may indicate patient or arrest characteristics that are also risk factors for poor outcomes, is a significant confounder in the analyzed trials. Currently, IV access is the preferred route for initial vascular access, providing the most predictable medication response. In scenarios where IV access is not successful or feasible, the IO route can be attempted.[5,6]

VASOPRESSOR MEDICATIONS DURING CARDIAC ARREST
Epinephrine

Epinephrine is the only medication indicated for cardiac arrest management regardless of initial rhythm. While the α-adrenergic effects of epinephrine improve aortic diastolic pressure, thereby improving coronary and cerebral perfusion pressure and the likelihood of ROSC, its β-adrenergic effects may increase cardiac rate and contractility, which increase myocardial oxygen demand and may lead to arrhythmias. Furthermore, some animal models have shown that epinephrine may actually decrease cerebral microcirculatory blood flow during CPR leading to worse neurologic outcomes.[7,8]

The use of epinephrine in cardiac arrest has never been supported by high-quality, randomized data until the publication of two trials, The Prehospital Adrenaline for Cardiac Arrest (PACA) trial and The Prehospital Assessment of the Role of Adrenaline: Measuring the Effectiveness of Drug Administration in Cardiac Arrest (PARAMEDIC 2)

trial.[9,10] Prior observational studies on the use of epinephrine in cardiac arrest were subject to patient selection bias, confounding by unmatched or unmeasured variables, and resuscitation time bias.[11]

In the PACA trial, 601 OHCA patients, serviced by a single emergency ambulance company in Western Australia, were randomized in a double-blind manner to receive epinephrine 1 mg every 3 minutes (median total dose 5 mg, interquartile range [IQR] 3.0 mg to 7.0 mg) or normal saline placebo (median total dose 5 mL, IQR 3.0 mL to 8.0 mL). The prehospital administration of epinephrine resulted in improved rates of ROSC, but did not improve survival to hospital discharge.[9]

The PARAMEDIC 2 trial was a randomized, double-blind trial involving 8014 OHCA patients and 5 National Health Service ambulance services in the United Kingdom. The prehospital administration of epinephrine resulted in improved 30-day survival and survival at 3 months.[10] A subsequent analysis of these trial participants reported that this survival benefit persisted at a 1-year time point.[12] Given the poor overall rates of survival in this trial (expected 30-day survival rate 6.0% in placebo group and 7.5% in the epinephrine group; actual trial 30-day survival rate 2.4% in the placebo group and 3.2% in the epinephrine group), PARAMEDIC 2 was underpowered to detect meaningful differences in survival with favorable neurologic outcome. Analysis of the supplemental appendix of this trial reveals that survival with no disability or slight disability (ie, modified Rankin score of 0–2) was similar between the two groups at 3-month and 6-month follow-up.[12] A criticism of PARAMEDIC 2 is that epinephrine resulted in an increase in the proportion of survivors with moderate or severe disability (ie, modified Rankin score 3–5) at the time of hospital discharge. Although a substantial number of cardiac arrest survivors have significant care needs upon hospital discharge, over time, these needs decrease. At 6-month follow-up, the proportion of survivors with moderate or severe disability was similar between the two groups.[12] PARAMEDIC 2 established that epinephrine seems to increase the number of survivors with both a good and poor neurologic outcome. A cost-effectiveness analysis of PARAMEDIC 2 found that epinephrine administration during cardiac arrest is a cost-effective intervention with a societal benefit when organ donation and transplant recipients are taken into account.[13]

When combined, PACA and PARAMEDIC 2 demonstrate improvement in survival to hospital discharge but not in survival with favorable neurologic outcome in patients receiving prehospital epinephrine. This effect seems most pronounced in patients with nonshockable rhythms but is also seen, albeit with less statistical certainty, in patients with shockable rhythms.[14,15] In both shockable and nonshockable rhythms, survival to hospital discharge is most pronounced when epinephrine is given within the first 5 minutes of emergency medical service (EMS) arrival.[16]

Current guidelines support the use of epinephrine in cardiac arrest at a dose of 1 mg every 3 to 5 minutes.[17–20] For shockable rhythms, epinephrine is recommended to be administered if initial attempts with CPR and defibrillation are unsuccessful. With nonshockable rhythms, it is reasonable to administer epinephrine as soon as feasible.

Vasopressin-Steroids-Epinephrine Therapy

In 2009, Mentzelopoulos and colleagues hypothesized that the combination of vasopressin-steroids-epinephrine (VSE) given during and after cardiac resuscitation would improve ROSC in patients with cardiac arrest. They enrolled 100 in-hospital cardiac arrest (IHCA) cases into a single-center, prospective, double-blind randomized controlled trial (RCT) where patients received either vasopressin 20 IU plus epinephrine 1 mg per CPR cycle or saline placebo plus epinephrine 1 mg per CPR cycle. On the first CPR cycle, the study group patient received methylprednisolone 40 mg and controls received saline placebo. Following ROSC, postresuscitation shock was treated with stress-dose hydrocortisone 300 mg daily for up to 7 days, with gradual taper or saline placebo. Patients randomized to VSE had higher rates of ROSC and improved survival to hospital discharge compared with patients in the standard care group.[21] This study was followed up in 2013 by the same author group when they randomized 268 IHCA cases across 3 medical centers to either VSE or standard care. Again, rates of ROSC and survival to hospital discharge were higher in the VSE group.[22] Importantly, survival with favorable neurologic outcome was seen in the VSE group compared with standard care. In 2021, a third trial, the Vasopressin and Methylprednisolone for In-Hospital Cardiac Arrest trial, used a multicenter, prospective, double-blind RCT methodology to randomize 501 IHCA patients to VSE or standard care. In this trial, rates of ROSC were higher in the VSE group; however, 30-day survival and survival with favorable neurologic outcome showed no difference between the two groups.[23] Survival at 1 year was not different between the two groups.[24] When combined, these three RCTs with a total of 869 patients show that VSE improves ROSC for IHCA cases.[25] Further high-quality RCTs are needed to define the role of VSE in OHCA patients and its effect on long-term survival and neurologic outcome.

ANTIARRHYTHMIC MEDICATIONS DURING CARDIAC ARREST

Antiarrhythmic medications are indicated in patients with refractory pVT/VF. Refractory pVT/VF is defined as an initial rhythm of pVT or VF that is still present after three consecutive rhythm analyses and standard defibrillation separated by 2-minute intervals of CPR.

A systematic review in 2018 evaluated the efficacy of amiodarone, procainamide, lidocaine, magnesium, and bretylium for cardiac arrest due to pVT/VF.[26] Overall this review found no supporting evidence for association of these agents to the outcomes or survival to hospital discharge, survival with favorable neurologic outcome, or long-term survival.

Amiodarone

An initial bolus of 300 mg of amiodarone is recommended for adult patients in cardiac arrest who showed pVT/VF after three shocks have been administered; an additional 150 mg of amiodarone is recommended after the fifth shock.[5,6] The strength of this recommendation is based on two medium-sized RCTs that demonstrated amiodarone's superiority to placebo[27] and to lidocaine[28] with respect to survival to hospital admission. A follow-up RCT, Amiodarone, Lidocaine, or Placebo in Out-of-Hospital Cardiac Arrest (ALPS) trial, involving 3026 patients comparing amiodarone, lidocaine, and placebo for shock-refractory pVT/VF confirmed antiarrhythmic therapy (either amiodarone or lidocaine) was superior to placebo for survival to hospital admission. In this trial, antiarrhythmic therapy did not show improvement in survival to hospital discharge or survival with favorable neurologic outcome compared with placebo.[29]

Several interesting exploratory analyses of the ALPS trial have been published. One analysis evaluated the efficacy of antiarrhythmic therapy in the subgroup of cardiac arrest patients that initially had a nonshockable rhythm and subsequently developed a shockable rhythm. Although not statistically significant, more patients in the antiarrhythmic-treated group survived to hospital discharge.[30] A second subgroup analysis evaluated the efficacy of antiarrhythmic therapy in the subgroup of patients based on vascular access (ie, IV vs IO administration). When adjusted for common confounders (ie, age, sex, cardiac cause, public location, EMS witnessed, bystander witnessed, bystander CPR, EMS arrival time, advanced life support (ALS) arrival time, time to study drug, and study site), IV administration of amiodarone was associated with survival to hospital admission, survival to hospital discharge, and survival with favorable neurologic outcome. These associations were less pronounced in patients receiving lidocaine and were not seen in the patients who received IO amiodarone or IO lidocaine.[31] Time to treatment was assessed in a third exploratory analysis. The probability of achieving ROSC was highest in patients that received antiarrhythmic within the first 10 minutes from the time of the 911 call and decreased over time.[32] Finally, a Bayesian reanalysis of the ALPS trial was performed. Bayesian analysis provides a probabilistic estimate of treatment effect by incorporating prior knowledge of the potential effects with the trial data to generate probability distributions that represent the entire range of effect consistent with the prior knowledge and the study data. The Bayesian reanalysis of ALPS concluded that amiodarone is "highly likely" to improve survival and neurologic outcome compared with placebo.[33]

Procainamide

Procainamide was previously recommended for shock-refractory cardiac arrest; however, its use has fallen out of favor because of its slow infusion rate, side effects profile, and the development of newer agents that initially seemed promising for the treatment of pVT/VF. With the results of the Procainamide versus Amiodarone for the Acute Treatment of Tolerated Wide QRS Tachycardia (PROCAMIO) trial, an RCT that studied stable patients with VT and showed fewer adverse events at 40 minutes after procainamide infusion compared with amiodarone[34] and the failure of amiodarone or lidocaine to show meaningful long-term survival benefit in cardiac arrest patients, there has been some renewed interest in using procainamide for pVT/VF. While no RCTs have evaluated procainamide for shock-refractory cardiac arrest, two retrospective studies have failed to show improved survival outcomes in patients who received procainamide for this indication.[35,36]

Lidocaine

Lidocaine 100 mg may be used as an alternative to amiodarone for refractory pVT/VF cardiac arrest patients; an additional 50 mg is recommended after the fifth shock.[5,6] Observational data suggest an association between patients that receive lidocaine for refractory pVT/VF and improved 1-year survival,[37] as well as improved survival with favorable neurologic outcome.[38] When more rigorously tested in RCTs, lidocaine has not been shown to be superior to amiodarone or to placebo with respect to survival to hospital discharge or survival with favorable neurologic outcome.[26,28,29] A Bayesian reanalysis of the ALPS trial concluded that lidocaine is 'moderately likely' to improve survival and neurologic outcome compared with placebo.[33]

OTHER MEDICATIONS
Corticosteroids (Without Vasopressin)

Global ischemia during cardiac arrest triggers the activation of multiple inflammatory systems leading to a sepsis-like syndrome.[39,40] Furthermore, low circulating cortisol and poor adrenocortical reserve complicate the postarrest period.[41,42] Corticosteroid use during and/or after cardiac arrest may help treat these issues[43] and has been studied in a handful of cohort trials and small RCTs. Neither the American Heart Association (AHA) in 2020 nor the European Resuscitation Council in 2021 recommend the routine use of corticosteroids for cardiac arrest[5,6]; however, in the past 2 years, at least four additional RCTs have been published.[23,24,44,45] When combined with the results of prior analyses,[46] corticosteroids given during and after cardiac arrest seem to increase the rate of ROSC but have unclear effects on longer-term survival or survival with favorable neurologic outcomes.

Calcium

Calcium is an inotropic agent that has vasopressor effects and may counter the proarrhythmic effects of hyperkalemia. Two small trials involving a total of 163 OHCA patients in PEA or asystole identified a trend favoring calcium over placebo with respect to ROSC.[47,48] Calcium is commonly thought to be a benign medication that may help in undifferentiated cardiac arrest. A recent contemporary review of hospitals that participate in the AHA's Get with the Guidelines Resuscitation database noted that the rate of calcium administration for IHCA has steadily increased over the period of 2001 to 2016.[49] On the basis of these observations, the Calcium for Out-of-Hospital Cardiac Arrest trial randomized 397 OHCA patients to receive either 5 to 10 mmol calcium chloride administered immediately after the first and second dose of epinephrine or saline placebo. The trial was stopped early on the recommendation of the independent safety committee because of safety concerns in the calcium group. Statistically, there was no difference between the groups with respect to the primary outcome of sustained ROSC or the secondary outcomes of 30-day survival, 90-day survival, or 90-day survival with favorable neurologic outcome—although in all these groups, it appeared that the patients that received calcium did consistently worse.[50] A subsequent analysis of these trial participants reported similar results when analyzing 1-year outcomes.[51] Interestingly, both the subgroup of patients with last known rhythm of PEA and the subgroup of patients with ECG characteristics potentially associated with hyperkalemia and/or ischemia also seemed to show lack of benefit or harm from calcium administration.[52] On the basis of these data, calcium should not be routinely administered for cardiac arrest unless there is high suspicion for arrest due to, or complicated by, hyperkalemia, hypocalcemia, hypermagnesemia, or overdose of calcium-channel-blocking drugs.

Sodium Bicarbonate

Although sodium bicarbonate has been considered an important part of treatment for severe metabolic acidosis in cardiac arrest, recent cardiac arrest guidelines have strongly discouraged its routine use.[53] Despite the lack of compelling data, the use of sodium bicarbonate during IHCA has steadily increased from 2001 to 2016, with nearly 50% of inpatient codes receiving sodium bicarbonate in 2016.[49] Overall, the published data on sodium bicarbonate in cardiac arrest do not support the increased usage over this time. A systematic review and meta-analysis of 4 RCTs and 10 observational trials enrolling 28,412 OHCA patients found that routine administration of sodium bicarbonate was not associated with improved ROSC or survival to hospital discharge.[54] Observational data from one of the included trials suggest an association between administration of sodium bicarbonate and poor neurologic outcome, although interpretation of the data is limited as this medication may be more frequently used in a population of sicker patients as a "last resort" (ie, resuscitation time bias).[55] A similar observation between patients that received sodium bicarbonate and poor neurologic outcome was seen in a data set involving North American patients with OHCA.[56] Currently sodium bicarbonate is specifically recommended only in the following situations: hyperkalemia, sodium channel blocker toxicity. There are limited data to guide therapy with sodium bicarbonate in the population of patients with pre-exiting acidosis[57] and in patients with acidosis due to prolonged resuscitation.[58–60]

Magnesium

Magnesium is an essential electrolyte in regulating sodium, potassium, and calcium flow across cell membranes and cofactor for a variety of metabolically important reactions, particularly those involving adenosine triphosphate. A handful of small RCTs[61–64] and one observational study[65] have evaluated the role of magnesium infusion versus placebo in a total of 499 OHCA patients with both shockable and nonshockable initial rhythms. No difference was observed between the two groups in terms of ROSC or survival to hospital discharge.[66,67] Empiric treatment with magnesium is, therefore, not recommended for routine use in cardiac arrest.[54,68]

Magnesium is commonly used to treat torsade de pointes (ie, polymorphic VT associated with long QT interval); however, it generally acts to prevent the reinitiation of torsades rather than to pharmacologically convert polymorphic VT. Its use in this setting is based on limited data.[69,70] Episodes of torsades de pointes may be short-lived and self-terminate only to recur or may be sustained. Although defibrillation is the treatment of choice for sustained episodes or episodes associated with hemodynamic instability, magnesium sulfate is recommended to prevent recurrences.[54,68] A reasonable approach to prevent torsade de pointes recurrence is to give 2 to 4 g of MgSO4 followed by an infusion at 1 g/h titrated to achieve a serum magnesium level of 3.5 to 5.0 mg/dL.

Atropine

Atropine is a potent anticholinergic that reverses cholinergic-mediated decreases in heart rate and blood pressure. No prospective controlled clinical trials have evaluated the role of atropine in asystole or bradycardia PEA cardiac arrest leading to its removal from cardiac arrest guidelines in 2010.[53] In a cohort study involving 7448 patients with either PEA or asystole, the use of atropine in addition to standard therapy when compared to standard therapy alone was not associated with improved 30-day survival with favorable neurologic outcome.[71] An analysis of the AHA's Get with the Guidelines Resuscitation database for IHCAs noted that the removal of atropine from cardiac arrest guidelines in 2010 did not impact ROSC, survival to hospital discharge, or survival with favorable neurologic outcome.[72] Atropine remains a viable option for acute symptomatic bradycardia in the nonarrest situation.

Beta-Blockers for Shock-Resistant Pulseless Ventricular Tachycardia/Ventricular Fibrillation

Although β-blockers have been proposed for the treatment of refractory pVT/VF, there are no high-quality trials that have supported their use in this setting. A systematic review and meta-analysis on the use of β-blockers for refractory pVT/VF identified 3 observational studies involving a total of 115 patients.[73] When the data from these trials were combined, the addition of β-blockers demonstrated improvements in sustained ROSC, survival to hospital admission, survival to hospital discharge, and survival with favorable neurologic outcome. These trials were judged to be at moderate or serious risk of bias, and the certainty of the overall conclusion is low. A subsequent sequential analysis of these trials concluded that additional studies are required before making a recommendation for the use of β-blockers for refractory pVT/VF.[74]

Thrombolytic Therapy for Cardiac Arrest

Acute myocardial infarction and pulmonary embolism are potentially reversible causes of cardiac arrest that may benefit from systemic thrombolytic therapy. The use of thrombolytics during cardiac arrest has been examined both in the treatment of undifferentiated cardiac arrest and specifically for patients with fulminant pulmonary embolism.

Three RCTs have evaluated the role of thrombolytics in undifferentiated cardiac arrest.[75–77] When analyzed together, no difference in the rates of ROSC or survival to hospital discharge was seen with the administration of thrombolytics.[78] Thirty-day survival and neurologic outcome was evaluated in one of these trials and similarly showed no difference between patients receiving thrombolytics or placebo.[77]

Approximately 2% to 5% of cardiac arrest cases are due to fulminant pulmonary embolism.[79] Although no RCTs have evaluated the role of thrombolytics in patients with pulmonary embolism, a handful of observational trials have yielded mixed, but generally favorable, results with respect to ROSC.[79–84] A relatively large retrospective study from the French National Cardiac Arrest Registry compared the outcomes in 58 patients with confirmed PE who received thrombolytics during CPR to 188 patients with confirmed PE who did not receive thrombolytics during CPR. Thrombolytic use was associated with an increase in 30-day survival and showed a favorable trend in neurologic outcome.[85] Based on the total of the data, it is reasonable to consider thrombolytic therapy when acute PE is a known or highly suspected cause of cardiac arrest.[5,6] If the patient has arrested or is peri-arrest, thrombolytics should be given promptly during CPR. Although not standardized, it is recommended that CPR be continued for at least 60 to 90 minutes after the thrombolytics are given and before terminating resuscitation efforts.[6,86]

SUMMARY

The pharmacologic management of cardiac arrest is continuing to evolve. Recent trials have increased our understanding of the role of epinephrine, VSE, amiodarone, and lidocaine in cardiac arrest. These agents increase short-term survival, a necessary step on the way to giving patients a chance at long-term survival, and several of them have point estimates slightly favoring survival with favorable neurologic outcome. Adjunct medications commonly used in cardiac arrest management include calcium, sodium bicarbonate, and magnesium. These agents should only be used in specific settings and not routinely in cardiac arrest cases. Atropine has not been established as an effective medication in cases of PEA or asystole. The use of β-blockers for refractory pVT/VF may be used on a case-by-case basis but currently lacks high-quality data supporting its use. Finally, thrombolytics should not be used in undifferentiated cardiac arrest but may have a role in cases where acute PE is known or highly suspected as the cause of cardiac arrest.

CLINICS CARE POINTS

- Medications given during cardiac arrest may be delivered via intravenous (IV) access, intraosseous (IO) access, central venous catheter (CVC), or endotracheal tube (ETT).

- The preferred route for giving medications during cardiac arrest is the peripheral IV. Intraosseous access is acceptable in patients where peripheral IV access has been unsuccessful.

- Epinephrine is commonly used in both shockable and nonshockable arrest situations and has recently been shown to produce a long-term benefit in the number of cardiac arrest survivors with both a good and poor neurologic outcome.

- The combination of vasopressin-steroids-epinephrine has been shown to improve ROSC; however, future high-quality RCTs are needed to define its effect on long-term survival and neurologic outcome.

- Antiarrhythmic therapy with amiodarone and lidocaine for refractory pVT/VF has been shown to improve survival to hospital admission and may result in higher rates of favorable neurologic outcome than placebo.

- The routine use of calcium, sodium bicarbonate, and magnesium cannot be recommended at this time.

- Atropine has not been established as an effective medication in PEA arrest or asystole.
- There is insufficient evidence to make a recommendation on the use of β-blockers in refractory pVT/VF.
- Thrombolytics have not been shown to improve any meaningful outcome in undifferentiated cardiac arrest. Their use can be considered when acute PE is known or highly suspected as the cause of cardiac arrest.

DISCLOSURE

The authors have nothing to disclose.

REFERENCES

1. Olasveengen TM, Sunde K, Brunborg C, et al. Intravenous drug administration during out-of-hospital cardiac arrest: a randomized trial. JAMA 2009; 302(20):2222–9.
2. Tan BKK, Chin YX, Koh ZX, et al. Clinical evaluation of intravenous alone versus intravenous or intraosseous access for treatment of out-of-hospital cardiac arrest. Resuscitation 2021;159:129–36.
3. Reades R, Studnek JR, Garrett JS, et al. Comparison of first-attempt success between tibial and humeral intraosseous insertions during out-of-hospital cardiac arrest. Prehosp Emerg Care 2011;15(2): 278–81.
4. Hsieh YL, Wu MC, Wolfshohl J, et al. Intraosseous versus intravenous vascular access during cardiopulmonary resuscitation for out-of-hospital cardiac arrest: a systematic review and meta-analysis of observational studies. Scand J Trauma Resusc Emerg Med 2021;29(1):44. PMID: 33685486; PMCID: PMC7938460.
5. Panchal AR, Bartos JA, Cabañas JG, et al. Adult Basic and Advanced Life Support Writing Group. Part 3: Adult Basic and Advanced Life Support: 2020 American Heart Association Guidelines for Cardiopulmonary Resuscitation and Emergency Cardiovascular Care. Circulation 2020;142(16_suppl_2):S366–468. Epub 2020 Oct 21. PMID: 33081529.
6. Soar J, Böttiger BW, Carli P, et al. European Resuscitation Council Guidelines 2021: Adult advanced life support. Resuscitation 2021;161:115–51 [Erratum in: Resuscitation. 2021 Oct;167:105-106. PMID: 33773825].
7. Ristagno G, Tang W, Huang L, et al. Epinephrine reduces cerebral perfusion during cardiopulmonary resuscitation. Crit Care Med 2009;37(4):1408–15. PMID: 19242339.
8. Ristagno G, Sun S, Tang W, et al. Effects of epinephrine and vasopressin on cerebral microcirculatory flows during and after cardiopulmonary resuscitation. Crit Care Med 2007;35(9):2145–9.
9. Jacobs IG, Finn JC, Jelinek GA, et al. Effect of adrenaline on survival in out-of-hospital cardiac arrest: A randomised double-blind placebo-controlled trial. Resuscitation 2011;82(9):1138–43. Epub 2011 Jul 2. PMID: 21745533.
10. Perkins GD, Ji C, Deakin CD, et al, PARAMEDIC2 Collaborators. A Randomized Trial of Epinephrine in Out-of-Hospital Cardiac Arrest. N Engl J Med 2018;379(8):711–21. PMID: 30021076.
11. Andersen LW, Grossestreuer AV, Donnino MW. Resuscitation time bias"-A unique challenge for observational cardiac arrest research. Resuscitation 2018;125:79–82. Epub 2018 Feb 6. PMID: 29425975; PMCID: PMC6080954.
12. Haywood KL, Ji C, Quinn T, et al. Long term outcomes of participants in the PARAMEDIC2 randomised trial of adrenaline in out-of-hospital cardiac arrest. Resuscitation 2021;160:84–93. Epub 2021 Jan 30. PMID: 33524488.
13. Achana F, Petrou S, Madan J, et al, PARAMEDIC2 Collaborators. Cost-effectiveness of adrenaline for out-of-hospital cardiac arrest. Crit Care 2020;24(1): 579.
14. Gavin D, Kenna C, Ji C, et al. The effects of adrenaline in out of hospital cardiac arrest with shockable and non-shockable rhythms: Findings from the PACA and PARAMEDIC-2 randomised controlled trials. Resuscitation 2019;140:55–63. Epub 2019 May 19. PMID: 31116964.
15. Kempton H, Vlok R, Thang C, et al. Standard dose epinephrine versus placebo in out of hospital cardiac arrest: A systematic review and meta-analysis. Am J Emerg Med 2019;37(3):511–7. Epub 2019 Jan 11. PMID: 30658877.
16. Okubo M, Komukai S, Callaway CW, et al. Association of Timing of Epinephrine Administration With Outcomes in Adults With Out-of-Hospital Cardiac Arrest. JAMA Netw Open 2021;4(8):e2120176.
17. Berg KM, Soar J, Andersen LW, et al. Adult Advanced Life Support Collaborators. Adult Advanced Life Support: 2020 International Consensus on Cardiopulmonary Resuscitation and Emergency Cardiovascular Care Science With Treatment Recommendations. Circulation 2020; 142(16_suppl_1):S92–139. Epub 2020 Oct 21. PMID: 33084390.
18. Nolan JP, Sandroni C, Böttiger BW, et al. European Resuscitation Council and European Society of Intensive Care Medicine guidelines 2021: post-resuscitation care. Intensive Care Med 2021;47(4): 369–421. Epub 2021 Mar 25. PMID: 33765189; PMCID: PMC7993077.
19. Holmberg MJ, Issa MS, Moskowitz A, et al. International Liaison Committee on Resuscitation Advanced Life Support Task Force Collaborators.

Vasopressors during adult cardiac arrest: A systematic review and meta-analysis. Resuscitation 2019; 139:106–21. Epub 2019 Apr 10. PMID: 30980877.

20. Panchal AR, Berg KM, Hirsch KG, et al. American Heart Association Focused Update on Advanced Cardiovascular Life Support: Use of Advanced Airways, Vasopressors, and Extracorporeal Cardiopulmonary Resuscitation During Cardiac Arrest: An Update to the American Heart Association Guidelines for Cardiopulmonary Resuscitation and Emergency Cardiovascular Care. Circulation 2019; 140(24):e881–94.

21. Mentzelopoulos SD, Zakynthinos SG, Tzoufi M, et al. Vasopressin, epinephrine, and corticosteroids for in-hospital cardiac arrest. Arch Intern Med 2009; 169(1):15–24.

22. Mentzelopoulos SD, Malachias S, Chamos C, et al. Vasopressin, steroids, and epinephrine and neurologically favorable survival after in-hospital cardiac arrest: a randomized clinical trial. JAMA 2013; 310(3):270–9.

23. Andersen LW, Isbye D, Kjærgaard J, et al. Effect of Vasopressin and Methylprednisolone vs Placebo on Return of Spontaneous Circulation in Patients With In-Hospital Cardiac Arrest: A Randomized Clinical Trial. JAMA 2021;326(16):1586–94.

24. Granfeldt A, Sindberg B, Isbye D, et al. Effect of vasopressin and methylprednisolone vs. placebo on long-term outcomes in patients with in-hospital cardiac arrest a randomized clinical trial. Resuscitation 2022;175:67–71. Epub 2022 Apr 28. PMID: 35490936.

25. Abdelazeem B, Awad AK, Manasrah N, et al. The Effect of Vasopressin and Methylprednisolone on Return of Spontaneous Circulation in Patients with In-Hospital Cardiac Arrest: A Systematic Review and Meta-analysis of Randomized Controlled Trials. Am J Cardiovasc Drugs 2022;22(5):523–33. Epub 2022 Mar 22. PMID: 35314927.

26. Ali MU, Fitzpatrick-Lewis D, Kenny M, et al. Effectiveness of antiarrhythmic drugs for shockable cardiac arrest: A systematic review. Resuscitation 2018;132: 63–72. Epub 2018 Sep 1. PMID: 30179691.

27. Kudenchuk PJ, Cobb LA, Copass MK, et al. Amiodarone for resuscitation after out-of-hospital cardiac arrest due to ventricular fibrillation. N Engl J Med 1999;341(12):871–8.

28. Dorian P, Cass D, Schwartz B, et al. Amiodarone as compared with lidocaine for shock-resistant ventricular fibrillation. N Engl J Med 2002;346(12):884–90. in: N Engl J Med 2002;347(12):955. PMID: 11907287.

29. Kudenchuk PJ, Brown SP, Daya M, et al. Resuscitation Outcomes Consortium Investigators. Amiodarone, Lidocaine, or Placebo in Out-of-Hospital Cardiac Arrest. N Engl J Med 2016;374(18): 1711–22.

30. Kudenchuk PJ, Leroux BG, Daya M, et al. Resuscitation Outcomes Consortium Investigators. Antiarrhythmic Drugs for Nonshockable-Turned-Shockable Out-of-Hospital Cardiac Arrest: The ALPS Study (Amiodarone, Lidocaine, or Placebo). Circulation 2017;136(22):2119–31. Epub 2017 Sep 13. PMID: 28904070; PMCID: PMC5705566.

31. Daya MR, Leroux BG, Dorian P, et al. Resuscitation Outcomes Consortium Investigators. Survival After Intravenous Versus Intraosseous Amiodarone, Lidocaine, or Placebo in Out-of-Hospital Shock-Refractory Cardiac Arrest. Circulation 2020;141(3):188–98.

32. Rahimi M, Dorian P, Cheskes S, et al. Effect of Time to Treatment With Antiarrhythmic Drugs on Return of Spontaneous Circulation in Shock-Refractory Out-of-Hospital Cardiac Arrest. J Am Heart Assoc 2022; 11(6):e023958.

33. Lane DJ, Grunau B, Kudenchuk P, et al. Bayesian analysis of amiodarone or lidocaine versus placebo for out-of-hospital cardiac arrest. Heart 2022; 108(22):1777–83.

34. Ortiz M, Martín A, Arribas F, et al, PROCAMIO Study Investigators. Randomized comparison of intravenous procainamide vs. intravenous amiodarone for the acute treatment of tolerated wide QRS tachycardia: the PROCAMIO study. Eur Heart J 2017; 38(17):1329–35.

35. Markel DT, Gold LS, Allen J, et al. Procainamide and survival in ventricular fibrillation out-of-hospital cardiac arrest. Acad Emerg Med 2010;17(6):617–23.

36. Huebinger R, Harvin JA, Chan HK, et al. Procainamide for shockable rhythm cardiac arrest in the Resuscitation Outcome Consortium. Am J Emerg Med 2022;55:143–6. Epub 2022 Feb 24. PMID: 35325787.

37. Huang CH, Yu PH, Tsai MS, et al. Acute hospital administration of amiodarone and/or lidocaine in shockable patients presenting with out-of-hospital cardiac arrest: A nationwide cohort study. Int J Cardiol 2017;227:292–8. Epub 2016 Nov 9. PMID: 27843049.

38. Wagner D, Kronick SL, Nawer H, et al. Comparative Effectiveness of Amiodarone and Lidocaine for the Treatment of: In-Hospital Cardiac Arrest. Chest 2022. S0012-3692(22)04039-9.

39. Bro-Jeppesen J, Kjaergaard J, Wanscher M, et al. Systemic Inflammatory Response and Potential Prognostic Implications After Out-of-Hospital Cardiac Arrest: A Substudy of the Target Temperature Management Trial. Crit Care Med 2015;43(6): 1223–32. PMID: 25756419.

40. Bro-Jeppesen J, Johansson PI, Kjaergaard J, et al. Level of systemic inflammation and endothelial injury is associated with cardiovascular dysfunction and vasopressor support in post-cardiac arrest patients. Resuscitation 2017;121:179–86. Epub 2017 Sep 23. PMID: 28947390.

41. Hékimian G, Baugnon T, Thuong M, et al. Cortisol levels and adrenal reserve after successful cardiac arrest resuscitation. Shock 2004;22(2):116–9.

42. Kim JJ, Lim YS, Shin JH, et al. Relative adrenal insufficiency after cardiac arrest: impact on postresuscitation disease outcome. Am J Emerg Med 2006; 24(6):684–8.

43. Roberts BW, Trzeciak S. Systemic inflammatory response after cardiac arrest: potential target for therapy? Crit Care Med 2015;43(6):1336–7. PMID: 25978161.

44. Rafiei H, Bahrami N, Meisami AH, et al. The effect of epinephrine and methylprednisolone on cardiac arrest patients. Ann Med Surg (Lond) 2022;78:103832.

45. Mentzelopoulos SD, Pappa E, Malachias S, et al. Physiologic effects of stress dose corticosteroids in in-hospital cardiac arrest (CORTICA): A randomized clinical trial. Resusc Plus 2022;10:100252.

46. Penn J, Douglas W, Curran J, et al. Efficacy and safety of corticosteroids in cardiac arrest: a systematic review, meta-analysis and trial sequential analysis of randomized control trials. Crit Care 2023; 27(1):12.

47. Stueven HA, Thompson B, Aprahamian C, et al. The effectiveness of calcium chloride in refractory electromechanical dissociation. Ann Emerg Med 1985; 14(7):626–9.

48. Stueven HA, Thompson B, Aprahamian C, et al. Lack of effectiveness of calcium chloride in refractory asystole. Ann Emerg Med 1985;14(7):630–2.

49. Moskowitz A, Ross CE, Andersen LW, et al. American Heart Association's Get With The Guidelines – Resuscitation Investigators. Trends Over Time in Drug Administration During Adult In-Hospital Cardiac Arrest. Crit Care Med 2019;47(2):194–200. PMID: 30407950; PMCID: PMC6336500.

50. Vallentin MF, Granfeldt A, Meilandt C, et al. Effect of Intravenous or Intraosseous Calcium vs Saline on Return of Spontaneous Circulation in Adults With Out-of-Hospital Cardiac Arrest: A Randomized Clinical Trial. JAMA 2021;326(22):2268–76.

51. Vallentin MF, Granfeldt A, Meilandt C, et al. Effect of calcium vs. placebo on long-term outcomes in patients with out-of-hospital cardiac arrest. Resuscitation 2022;179:21–4. Epub 2022 Jul 30. PMID: 35917866.

52. Vallentin MF, Povlsen AL, Granfeldt A, et al. Effect of calcium in patients with pulseless electrical activity and electrocardiographic characteristics potentially associated with hyperkalemia and ischemia-substudy of the Calcium for Out-of-hospital Cardiac Arrest (COCA) trial. Resuscitation 2022;181:150–7. Epub 2022 Nov 18. PMID: 36403820.

53. Neumar RW, Otto CW, Link MS, et al. Part 8: adult advanced cardiovascular life support: 2010 American Heart Association Guidelines for Cardiopulmonary Resuscitation and Emergency Cardiovascular Care. Circulation 2010;122(18 Suppl 3):S729–67 [Erratum in: Circulation. 2011 Feb 15;123(6):e236. Erratum in: Circulation. 2013;128(25):e480. PMID: 20956224].

54. Alshahrani MS, Aldandan HW. Use of sodium bicarbonate in out-of-hospital cardiac arrest: a systematic review and meta-analysis. Int J Emerg Med 2021; 14(1):21.

55. Kawano T, Grunau B, Scheuermeyer FX, et al. Prehospital sodium bicarbonate use could worsen long term survival with favorable neurological recovery among patients with out-of-hospital cardiac arrest. Resuscitation 2017;119:63–9. Epub 2017 Aug 10. PMID: 28802878.

56. Touron M, Javaudin F, Lebastard Q, et al, RéAC Network. Effect of sodium bicarbonate on functional outcome in patients with out-of-hospital cardiac arrest: a post-hoc analysis of a French and North-American dataset. Eur J Emerg Med 2022;29(3): 210–20. Epub 2022 Mar 16. PMID: 35297385.

57. Mclean H, Wells L, Marler J. The Effect of Prearrest Acid-Base Status on Response to Sodium Bicarbonate and Achievement of Return of Spontaneous Circulation. Ann Pharmacother 2022;56(4):436–40. PMID: 34353142.

58. Vukmir RB, Katz L, Sodium Bicarbonate Study Group. Sodium bicarbonate improves outcome in prolonged prehospital cardiac arrest. Am J Emerg Med 2006;24(2):156–61.

59. Weng YM, Wu SH, Li WC, et al. The effects of sodium bicarbonate during prolonged cardiopulmonary resuscitation. Am J Emerg Med 2013;31(3): 562–5. Epub 2012 Dec 12. PMID: 23246112.

60. Ahn S, Kim YJ, Sohn CH, et al. Sodium bicarbonate on severe metabolic acidosis during prolonged cardiopulmonary resuscitation: a double-blind, randomized, placebo-controlled pilot study. J Thorac Dis 2018;10(4):2295–302.

61. Fatovich DM, Prentice DA, Dobb GJ. Magnesium in cardiac arrest (the MAGIC trial). Resuscitation 1997; 35:237–41.

62. Thel MC, Armstrong AL, McNulty SE, et al. on behalf of the Duke Internal Medicine Housestaff. Randomised trial of magnesium in in-hospital cardiac arrest. Lancet 1997;350:1272–6.

63. Hassan TB, Jagger C, Barnett DB. A randomised trial to investigate the efficacy of magnesium sulphate for refractory ventricular fibrillation. Emerg Med J 2002; 19:57–62.

64. Allegra J, Lavery R, Cody R, et al. Magnesium sulfate in the treatment of refractory ventricular fibrillation in the prehospital setting. Resuscitation 2001;49:245–9.

65. Miller B, Craddock L, Hoffenberg S, et al. Pilot study of intravenous magnesium sulfate in refractory cardiac arrest: safety data and recommendations for future studies. Resuscitation 1995;30(1):3–14. PMID: 7481101.

66. Reis AG, Ferreira de Paiva E, Schvartsman C, et al. Magnesium in cardiopulmonary resuscitation: critical review. Resuscitation 2008;77(1):21–5. Epub 2007 Nov 26. PMID: 18037222.

67. Chen F, Lin Q, Chen G, et al. Does intravenous magnesium benefit patients of cardiac arrest? A meta-analysis. Hong Kong J Emerg Med 2012;19(2): 103–9.

68. Panchal AR, Berg KM, Kudenchuk PJ, et al. American Heart Association Focused Update on Advanced Cardiovascular Life Support Use of Antiarrhythmic Drugs During and Immediately After Cardiac Arrest: An Update to the American Heart Association Guidelines for Cardiopulmonary Resuscitation and Emergency Cardiovascular Care. Circulation 2018;138:e740–9.

69. Tzivoni D, Banai S, Schuger C, et al. Treatment of torsade de pointes with magnesium sulfate. Circulation 1988;77:392–7.

70. Manz M, Pfeiffer D, Jung W, et al. Intravenous treatment with magnesium in recurrent persistent ventricular tachycardia. N Trends Arrhythmias 1991;7: 437–42.

71. Survey of Survivors After Out-of-hospital Cardiac Arrest in KANTO Area, Japan (SOS-KANTO) Study Group. Atropine sulfate for patients with out-of-hospital cardiac arrest due to asystole and pulseless electrical activity. Circ J 2011;75(3):580–8. Epub 2011 Jan 8. PMID: 21233578.

72. Holmberg MJ, Moskowitz A, Wiberg S, et al. American Heart Association's Get With The Guidelines®-Resuscitation Investigators. Guideline removal of atropine and survival after adult in-hospital cardiac arrest with a non-shockable rhythm. Resuscitation 2019;137:69–77.

73. Gottlieb M, Dyer S, Peksa GD. Beta-blockade for the treatment of cardiac arrest due to ventricular fibrillation or pulseless ventricular tachycardia: A systematic review and meta-analysis. Resuscitation 2020; 146:118–25. Epub 2019 Nov 29. PMID: 31790759.

74. Manogaran M, Yang SS. Data for beta-blockade in ACLS - A trial sequential analysis. Resuscitation 2020;150:191–2. Epub 2020 Feb 27. PMID: 32114073.

75. Abu-Laban RB, Christenson JM, Innes GD, et al. Tissue plasminogen activator in cardiac arrest with pulseless electrical activity. N Engl J Med 2002; 346(20):1522–8. N Engl J Med. 2003;349(15):1487. PMID: 12015391.

76. Fatovich DM, Dobb GJ, Clugston RA. A pilot randomised trial of thrombolysis in cardiac arrest (The TICA trial). Resuscitation 2004;61(3):309–13. PMID: 15172710.

77. Böttiger BW, Arntz HR, Chamberlain DA, et al. TROICA Trial Investigators; European Resuscitation Council Study Group. Thrombolysis during resuscitation for out-of-hospital cardiac arrest. N Engl J Med 2008;359(25):2651–62.

78. Alshaya OA, Alshaya AI, Badreldin HA, et al. Thrombolytic therapy in cardiac arrest caused by cardiac etiologies or presumed pulmonary embolism: An updated systematic review and meta-analysis. Res Pract Thromb Haemost 2022;6(4):e12745.

79. Kürkciyan I, Meron G, Sterz F, et al. Pulmonary embolism as a cause of cardiac arrest: presentation and outcome. Arch Intern Med 2000;160(10): 1529–35.

80. Sharifi M, Berger J, Beeston P, Bay C, Vajo Z, Javadpoor S. "PEAPETT" investigators. Pulseless electrical activity in pulmonary embolism treated with thrombolysis (from the "PEAPETT" study). Am J Emerg Med 2016;34(10):1963–7.

81. Yousuf T, Brinton T, Ahmed K, et al. Tissue Plasminogen Activator Use in Cardiac Arrest Secondary to Fulminant Pulmonary Embolism. J Clin Med Res 2016;8(3):190–5.

82. Peppard SR, Parks AM, Zimmerman J. Characterization of alteplase therapy for presumed or confirmed pulmonary embolism during cardiac arrest. Am J Health Syst Pharm 2018;75(12):870–5.

83. Summers K, Schultheis J, Raiff D, et al. Evaluation of Rescue Thrombolysis in Cardiac Arrest Secondary to Suspected or Confirmed Pulmonary Embolism. Ann Pharmacother 2019;53(7):711–5.

84. de Paz D, Diez J, Ariza F, et al. Emergency Thrombolysis During Cardiac Arrest Due to Pulmonary Thromboembolism: Our Experience Over 6 Years. Open Access Emerg Med 2021;13:67–73.

85. Javaudin F, Lascarrou JB, Le Bastard Q, et al. Research Group of the French National Out-of-Hospital Cardiac Arrest Registry (GR-RéAC). Thrombolysis During Resuscitation for Out-of-Hospital Cardiac Arrest Caused by Pulmonary Embolism Increases 30-Day Survival: Findings From the French National Cardiac Arrest Registry. Chest 2019;156(6):1167–75. Epub 2019 Aug 2. PMID: 31381884.

86. Böttiger BW, Wetsch WA. Pulmonary Embolism Cardiac Arrest: Thrombolysis During Cardiopulmonary Resuscitation and Improved Survival. Chest 2019; 156(6):1035–6.

Cardiac Arrest in Special Populations

Ravi W. Sumer, MD, MS[a],*, William A. Woods, MD, MS[b]

KEYWORDS

- Cardiac arrest • Anaphylaxis • Drowning • Hypothermia • Pregnancy • Left ventricular assist device
- Special populations

KEY POINTS

- Tailored resuscitation: Cardiac arrest in special populations may require customized approaches, considering the unique circumstances to optimize patient outcomes.
- Identifying reversible causes: Quick detection and treatment of reversible causes, such as electrolyte imbalances, hypothermia, or poisoning, are crucial to enhance patient recovery.
- Specialized techniques: Certain scenarios may demand distinct procedural skills, which should be used judiciously and only for select patients.

This article reviews cardiac arrest in special populations where modifications to standard resuscitation can improve outcomes. Best practices in cardiac arrest depend on continuous high-quality chest compressions, appropriate ventilatory management, early defibrillation of shockable rhythms, and identification and treatment of reversible causes. Some of the situations presented here include recommended interventions before cardiac arrest to prevent deterioration in a critically ill patient. Certain situations include utilization of specialized skill sets and knowledge to apply the appropriate intervention. The decision to apply modifications should ultimately be made by the clinician considering the patient's history, presentation, and evidence for such modifications described in the following text.

ELECTRICAL INJURIES

Electrical injuries represent a special situation in the study of cardiac arrest where the sudden exposure to electrical energy induces cardiac arrest with, hopefully, a higher survival rate with rapid access to effective resuscitation. The literature on electrical injuries is often subdivided into lightning versus manmade sources of electrical exposure—with further subdivision of manmade sources into "high voltage" (>1000 V) and "low voltage" (<1000 V) exposures.

The pathophysiology of lightning injuries is typically broken down into several exposure types: direct strike, contact potential, side flash, step voltage, and upward streamer.[1] The investigators differ on the significance of various explanations about how the physics of electricity exposure contribute to the risks of injury. For instance, recommendation exists regarding the direction a victim is facing at the time of lightning strike, yet not data exist to confirm high- or low-risk body positions.

For the clinician, the most time sensitive conditions associated with electrical injuries include cardiac arrest or arrhythmias, respiratory arrest, and traumatic injuries. Other factors that may interfere with emergency care include scene safety for rescuers and water exposure to the victim that can hamper resuscitation conditions or result in patient hypothermia.

After assuring scene safety for rescuers, rapid access to basic life support (BLS) care pending arrival of advanced cardiovascular life support

This article originally appeared in *Emergency Medicine Clinics*, Volume 41 Issue 3, August 2023.
[a] Department of Emergency Medicine, 4601 Dale Road, Modesto, CA 95356-8713, USA; [b] Department of Emergency Medicine, University of Virginia Health System, PO Box 800699, Charlottesville, VA 22908-0699, USA
* Corresponding author. 4601 Dale Road, Modesto, CA 95356-8713.
E-mail addresses: ravi.n.wettasinghe@kp.org; raviwet@gmail.com

(ACLS) level care is mandatory for the patient in cardiac arrest. Lightning strikes may induce respiratory depression independent of and lasting longer than cardiac arrhythmias or cardiac arrest.[1] Thus, respiratory support should be emphasized as well as chest compressions during BLS efforts awaiting ACLS resources. ACLS protocols should be followed when resources are available.

Regardless of the type of electrical exposure, prudence suggests that rescuers should take precautions that the victim may have significant traumatic injuries—whether spinal injuries or intracranial injuries. However, data suggest that these injuries are rare in survivors of lightning stikes.[2]

In aggregate data, electrical injuries due to man-made sources are much more common than lightning exposures. Interestingly, in one series, the incidence of prehospital cardiac arrhythmia was comparable between high- and low-voltage exposures.[3] In that series, those with high-voltage injuries required prehospital intubation more commonly in these, primarily, industrial exposures.[3] For those reaching the hospital alive, 1% to 3% may experience significant arrhythmias. Hospitalized cardiac monitoring is currently prudent in those with high-risk injuries (ECG abnormalities, loss of consciousness, prehospital dysrhythmias, or those who required chest compressions).[3–5] Emergency department measurements of serum troponin are currently not adequate to predict all of those patients who will have a clinically significant arrhythmia.[5]

ANAPHYLAXIS

Anaphylaxis is considered a special resuscitation situation as the acute reason for the treatment of sudden cardiovascular collapse differs from traditional treatments for cardiac arrest. The sudden onset of life-threatening symptoms is most commonly due to drugs, food, and venoms.[6] Traditionally, symptoms present in one or more of four organ systems—dermatologic, gastrointestinal, respiratory, and cardiovascular. The authors differ on the definition of anaphylaxis,[7] which demonstrates the difficulty studying a condition, that is, on the one hand, common (with a lifetime prevalence presumed to be 0.05% to 2.0%)[8] but on the other hand varied in the numerous combinations of presenting signs and symptoms.[9] In addition, once anaphylaxis has occurred, a biphasic reaction may occur between 1 and 72 hours after initial resolution in between less than 1% and 20% of patients.[6] The clinical challenge is that many patients with anaphylaxis may survive with less than maximal treatment, whereas a delay in

treatment is presumed to place a patient at higher risk of fatal anaphylaxis.[6]

In describing the epidemiology, anaphylaxis accounts for a very small percentage of out of hospital cardiac arrests (0.03% in Japan)[10] with approximately 200 patients per year in the United States suffering fatal anaphylaxis[11] yet hospitalization rates are increasing.[7,12] It is impossible to predict which patients will have a biphasic reaction, but those at higher risk include those with a more severe initial presentation, cutaneous signs and symptoms, and wide pulse pressure and those with longer times until the first dose of epinephrine administration.[6]

Published treatment recommendations emphasize the early administration of epinephrine as rapidly as possible in the event of an anaphylactic reaction.[6,13–15] The overriding goal of these recommendations is to prevent any delays in epinephrine administration—such as trials of antihistamines and/or corticosteroids or patient apprehension surrounding using an auto-injector. Reasonable careful emergency physicians may vary in their indications for epinephrine dosing within the controlled environment of the emergency department, but liberal criteria should be emphasized in educating patients and out of hospital clinicians on indications for epinephrine administered intramuscularly in the lateral thigh (preferred route of administration). Subcutaneous administration of epinephrine is not recommended as the effectiveness is unknown.[6] In addition, if symptoms fail to resolve briskly in the first aid setting, it is not unreasonable to recommend a second dose of epinephrine.[16]

In cases of critically ill patients with anaphylaxis, early aggressive BLS and ALS are recommended.[13] Airway intervention may be indicated with the expectation that the patient in anaphylaxis may have a difficult airway due to obstructive airway edema. The emergency physician should be prepared to use adjunctive methods to secure the airway. Epinephrine is the therapy of choice for the cardiovascular collapse from vasogenic shock. Intermittent bolus doses followed by continuous infusion should be anticipated with dosing as frequently as every 5 to 15 minutes having been reported.[17] Intraosseous doses are presumed to be as effective as similar intravenous dosing.[13] Volume expansion with intravenous crystalloid is also believed to have a role in the treatment of anaphylactic shock.[18] There are insufficient data to describe the role of antihistamines and corticosteroids in cases of cardiac arrest due to anaphylaxis.[13]

Controversy exists in the observation period for those who have brisk resolution of symptoms.

Observation period of 1 hour is not considered unreasonable for those with brisk resolution of symptoms with all of the following: no risk factors for potential biphasic reaction, no high-risk comorbid conditions, and no social determinants of health limiting the ability to access care (lack of access to epinephrine, poor self-management skills, and so forth).[6] Prolonged observation, potentially including hospital admission, may be warranted in those who do not meet the above criteria.

ASTHMA

Asthma as a cause of cardiac arrest presents an often preventable scenario if appropriate resuscitation measures are taken early during an asthma exacerbation.[19] The centers for disease control and prevention (CDC) noted 3518 asthma deaths in the United States in 2016.[20] Adults were nearly five times more likely than children to die from asthma.[20] Non-Hispanic blacks were two to three times more likely to die from asthma compared with other ethnicity groups.[20] Overall in hospital mortality in the United States from asthma is 0.5% in patients older than 5 year old.[21] Approximately 5% of asthma hospitalizations in the United States among patients older than 5 year old result in mechanical ventilation.[21]

The pathophysiology of severe asthma exacerbations includes bronchoconstriction, airway inflammation, and mucus plugging. Patients with fatal asthma exacerbations have dramatic hypercarbia and respiratory acidosis.[19] Initially, patients with an asthma exacerbation may demonstrate hypoxia with hypocarbia. Pneumothorax is not common in those with asthma exacerbations, but can occur, and can occur as a tension pneumothorax.[22]

Treatment includes aggressive use of oxygen, identification of pneumothoraxes, and medical management with albuterol, ipratropium, magnesium, corticosteroids, and mechanical ventilation as necessary.[23–25] Continuous nebulized bronchodilators may be more clinically effective than intermittent nebulized treatments in those with severe bronchospasm.[23] The addition of anticholinergics, especially in severe asthma exacerbations, to beta agonists in the emergency department is considered beneficial.[24] The early administration of systemic corticosteroids is indicated for all severe, all moderate, and most mild exacerbations of asthma.[14,25] Intravenous magnesium can reduce the need for hospital admission in severe asthma, but current data do not support a mortality benefit.[13]

The role of intravenous terbutaline is unclear but is actively being investigated.[26–28] At this time, the role of ketamine (a dissociative anesthetic with bronchodilatory properties) is unknown.[29] The role of heliox and inhaled anesthetics (isoflurane) remains unclear.[14]

For cardiac arrest due to asthma, there are no BLS modifications. ACLS modifications include the recognition and management of possible auto-positive end-expiratory pressure (PEEP) and pneumothoraxes. Auto-PEEP can cause excess pressure on the airways and vessels within the chest. This can prevent adequate ventilation, decrease cardiac output, and ultimately lead to circulatory collapse.[30] If an asthma patient is intubated, auto-PEEP can be countered by using a low tidal volume and low respiratory rate ventilation strategy to prolong exhalation time.[13,31]

If significant auto-PEEP is suspected, the bag valve mask or ventilator can be temporarily disconnected for compression of the chest wall in effort to remove air trapping. There is limited published experience in the manual external compression of children to reverse air trapping, but limited evidence suggests that its use can lead to improvement in hypercapnia with decreased respiratory failure.[32]

Before respiratory arrest in the severe asthmatic, noninvasive ventilation strategies with either high-flow nasal cannula or bilevel positive airway pressure (BiPAP) can potentially prevent intubation and mechanical ventilation.[33] High auto-PEEP in asthma can increase the likelihood of developing a pneumothorax or pneumomediastinum, which is associated with greater morbidity and mortality.[22] Care should be taken to screen for a pneumothorax via lung examination or chest radiographs and manage it with needle decompression followed by chest tube.

One study reviewing the use of extracorporeal life support (ECLS) as a salvage treatment in severe status asthmaticus found that survival to hospital discharge for asthma patients undergoing ECLS (83.3%) was significantly greater than matched non-asthmatics (50.8%).[34] The investigators note that this may be related to the younger age of asthmatics, reversibility of status asthmaticus, single organ involvement, and potential earlier initiation of ECLS in asthma patients. It can be considered as a salvage therapy; however, survival advantage is not clear.[34]

DROWNING

Drowning is defined as "the process of experiencing respiratory impairment from submersion or immersion in liquid."[35] Terms no longer used to subcategorize drowning include "wet," "dry," "freshwater," "saltwater," "near," "active," and "passive."[36] Drowning is worthy of a discussion of special situations because many who experience submersion/immersion do not require specialized care and the rescue of the drowning victim may place rescuers at personal risk. In addition, the CDC estimates that there are nearly 4000 drowning deaths per year in the United States.[35] Death rates from accidental drowning are highest in young children. In children aged 1 to 4 year old in the United States, drowning was the leading cause of death in 2020.[37] Drowning continues to have racial differences with death rates higher in non-Hispanic Black persons and American Indian or Alaska Native persons.[38]

Drowning may occur in water too deep for rescuers to stand to protect themselves. In water rescue should only be attempted by those with adequate training, ability, and equipment.[39] Once rescued, Szpilman created a flowchart giving recommendations for the level of care required by victims.[36] In this flowchart, advanced medical attention and oxygen is not usually required for those victims that are awake with a cough with normal lung auscultation and with no coexisting conditions. Rescuers should initiate and maintain respiratory support in those with who have a palpable pulse but no visible respiratory effort. Closed chest compressions should be initiated for those found without respiratory effort, without a palpable pulse, with a submersion time of less than 60 minutes and without other obvious physical signs of death.[36] For those requiring resuscitation efforts, survival rates are improved for those that are younger victims, had a witnessed event, had a shockable rhythm on automated external defibrillator (AED) arrival, and had early cardiopulmonary resuscitation (CPR) (including bystander CPR).[40–42]

Skilled rescuers should consider the following information. Data are not clear, but it is suspected that compression only CPR is likely of less value in drowning victims than in witnessed adult cardiac arrest.[43] Thus, the use of compressions-only resuscitation should be limited to untrained bystanders.[39,43] Skilled rescuers should prioritize early, aggressive respiratory support.[13,36,39] In contrast to typical recommendations for adult cardiac arrest victims, resuscitation efforts should not be delayed to allow time for the application of an AED.[39] Although specialty recommendations state that an AED can be used on a wet victim, drowning victims less commonly present with rhythms responsive to defibrillation.[39] Most common rhythms encountered include sinus tachycardia, bradycardia, and pulseless electrical activity.[39] The risk of cervical spine injury is so low, especially in those without a preceding high-risk event that resuscitation efforts should not be delayed in low-risk patients due to concerns for cervical spine injury.[13,36,39]

Once a victim reaches the emergency department care is continued and a disposition decision must be reached. The patient who is asymptomatic after 4 to 6 hours of observation, even if the person had rales and some respiratory symptoms initially, can be safely discharged.[39] For the victim that arrives in continued cardiac arrest, there are no definitive data to guide the emergency physician on when resuscitation efforts have become futile. Researchers have not been able to identify factors such as laboratory values, body temperature, duration of submersion, or duration of resuscitation efforts that offer reliable predictors of futility.

As drowning is such a significant cause of mortality with increasing racial disparity, it is worth considering the barriers to drowning prevention. Challenges include enforcing physical access to pools as well as increasing water safety.[44] Additional challenges include prioritizing and retention of resuscitation skills among rescuers. In one study from Brazil, resuscitation efforts were performed in only one of every 112,000 lifeguarding actions, reflecting the challenge of emphasizing a skill that is rarely used, even in those in a high-risk occupation.[45]

HYPOTHERMIA

Hypothermic cardiac arrest patients present a difficult scenario where patients can present with clinical signs of irreversible cardiac arrest, yet still be salvageable. When body temperature falls below 30°C, life is difficult to detect. There may be fixed dilated pupils, asystole on the electrocardiogram (ECG)/monitor, and impalpable pulses, yet multiple case reports demonstrated survival with good neurologic outcome in resuscitation of hypothermic cardiac arrest patients' hours after arrest.[46]

Hypothermia diminishes oxygen demands of the body by approximately 67% per 1°C of cooling, which protects oxygen-dependent organs including the brain and heart. There are mild, moderate, and severe forms of hypothermia with varying treatment for each. Cardiac arrest from hypothermia is associated with severe hypothermia (<30°C). The treatment of mild hypothermia (temperature > 34° C) involves removing wet clothes, limiting environmental heat loss, and passive rewarming. For moderate hypothermia (30–34° C), active external rewarming is often needed, such as forced warm air through a device like a Bair hugger.[47]

Managing cardiac arrest from severe hypothermia (<30° C) deviates from standard resuscitation with a focus on aggressive rewarming. Standard chest compressions and ventilation should continue after the identification of cardiac arrest. There is an association with severe hypothermia and arrhythmias triggered by movement, but the benefits of CPR outweigh these risks in a pulseless patient.[46] Defibrillation may be ineffective at low temperatures. Current AHA recommendations are for standard defibrillation for shockable rhythms during pulse checks. European Resuscitation Council guidelines recommend three defibrillation attempts in the profoundly hypothermic patient, and then no more until the patient reaches a core temperature over 30°C.[15]

The patient should be brought to at least 32°C before ceasing resuscitative efforts. Some patients respond to rewarming alone, as extreme temperatures alter physiologic processes necessary for successful resuscitation. Core temperature should be obtained by either esophageal measurement, rectal, or bladder temperature to monitor response to rewarming. Cardiac arrest from hypothermia should be treated with aggressive rewarming. Extracorporeal warming through warmed fluid, peritoneal, bladder, and thoracic lavage can be used as part of the resuscitation. If available, cardiac bypass with extracorporeal membrane oxygenation should be used for rapid rewarming. Warmed fluids and warmed humidified oxygen should be delivered if available.[46]

Prognostication should not be made for these patients until they have been rewarmed unless there are obvious signs of nonreversible processes such as rigor mortis or non-survivable trauma. Hypothermia associated cardiac arrest may be due to secondary causes such as opioid intoxication, trauma, or other primary cause of cardiac arrest. It is important to look for and treat underlying conditions while simultaneously treating hypothermia.

Consideration of the avalanche victim is warranted as the number of deaths continues to increase annually in the United States, with up to 40 deaths per year up to 2013.[48] Most avalanche victims die from either asphyxia, trauma, hypothermia, or some combination of the three. In cases where avalanche victims become hypothermic before developing cardiac arrest, they may benefit from aggressive rewarming alongside standard resuscitation techniques.[46] If they present with a snow-packed airway and burial time over 60 minutes, resuscitation will likely be futile.[49] This may be due to the arrest happening before the patient reaches a state of hypothermia while oxygen demands remain high. Avalanche victims who happen to be buried with an air pocket may survive up to 90 to 130 minutes before succumbing to slow asphyxia and hypothermia.[49] Similar to the hypothermic drowning patient, priority should be taken for rescue breaths and aggressive rewarming for the avalanche victim.

ELECTROLYTE ABNORMALITIES
Hyperkalemia

The presence of hyperkalemia should always be considered in cases of sudden cardiac arrest and/or arrhythmia.[15] Risk factors for hyperkalemia include renal failure, heart failure, diabetes mellitus, and rhabdomyolysis.[50] Severe hyperkalemia is defined as greater than 6.5 mmol/L.[14] The most recent Cochrane review on the topic is from 2005, where it supports inhaled beta agonists and intravenous (IV) insulin-and-glucose as first-line therapy.[51] In addition, the use of calcium is supported when arrhythmias are present.[51]

In one review of inpatients with hyperkalemia, of 406 cases of significant hyperkalemia 58 deaths occurred. Of those 58, 7 were due to hyperkalemia. In those seven, all had significant renal impairment (three patients also had acute pancreatitis and two had acute hepatic failure).[52]

A recent emergency department (ED)-based multicenter observational study noted a 2.7 hour median time to treatment of hyperkalemia.[53] ECG changes typical for hyperkalemia were only noted in 23% of all patients and 45% of those with a K+ greater than 7.0 mmol/L. Insulin/glucose was used in 64% of patients with hypoglycemia noted in 6% of all patients and 17% of those with a K+ greater than 7.0 mmol/L. Four hour response to medication therapy was a median level of 6.3 to 5.3 mmol/L while those underoing dialysis decreased from 6.2 to 3.8 mmol/L.[53]

The treatment of hyperkalemia can be separated into three categories (in order of urgency):[11]

1. Stabilize myocardial cell membrane (calcium chloride or calcium gluconate)
2. Shift potassium into the cells (sodium bicarbonate, glucose plus insulin, inhaled B2 agonists)
3. Promote potassium excretion (furosemide, kayexalate—standard use is discouraged,[13] dialysis)

The European guidelines recommend the early use of calcium in patients with significant hyperkalemia (regardless of presenting rhythm) to "protect the heart."[15] Dialysis should be arranged early for post-return of spontaneous circulation (ROSC) patients who arrested due to hyperkalemia to remove potassium from the body. Potassium-eliminating treatments such as Lasix and potassium-binding oral agents should be reserved for relatively stable patients, as their onset of action is slow.

Hypokalemia

Hypokalemia has been associated with ventricular fibrillation and torsades de pointes. The most common causes of hypokalemia are diarrhea and/or vomiting, diuretic therapy, and nutritional causes.[54]

Mortality after acute myocardial infarction is higher in those with hypokalemia. Risk of ventricular fibrillation or cardiac arrest was as high in those with potassium less than 3 mEq/L as greater than 5 mEq/L.[55]

Repletion of potassium by infusion in patients with polymorphic ventricular tachycardia or ventricular fibrillation in the setting of hypokalemia can be useful. The European guidelines recommend to restore potassium level "rate and route of replacement guided by clinical urgency."[15] One published recommendation is "2 mmol/min over 10 minutes followed by 10 mmol over 5 to 10 minutes."[50] IV bolus administration of potassium in cardiac arrest is not recommended (and may cause harm).[13]

Hypermagnesemia

Magnesium is excreted via the kidneys and the skin. Those at risk for hypermagnesemia are those with renal insufficiency especially if taking magnesium-containing medications or therapeutic complications such as pregnant women receiving intravenous magnesium. Another risk group is those with excessive laxative or enema use. There is a theoretic benefit to IV or intraosseous (IO) calcium boluses in cases of cardiac arrest with hypermagnesemia; however, there are no direct data supporting this use.[13]

Hypomagnesemia

Hypomagnesemia is common in hospitalized patients—it is mainly caused by gastrointestinal (GI) and renal disorders and may lead to secondary hypokalemia and hypocalcemia. Hypomagnesemia has been correlated with worse outcomes in critically ill patients.[56] IV magnesium is thought to prevent the reinitiation of torsades de pointes, it does not actually pharmacologically convert polymorphic ventricular tachycardia.[57] The first-line intervention for polymorphic ventricular tachycardia with cardiac arrest is high-quality CPR and defibrillation.[57] IV magnesium is not recommended during the routine use of ventricular fibrillation/ventricular tachycardia (VF/VT) in the absence of prolonged QT.[13] However, it is recommended in cases of prolonged QT interval.[13]

TOXIC EXPOSURES

The clinical course of a poisoned patient can rely on the quality of focused care delivered within the time immediately after an exposure. Fortunately, the poison or toxin can, in most cases, usually be quickly suspected if not certainly identified via a careful history, a focused physical examination, and rapidly available diagnostic studies. Once a toxin is suspected, the emergency physician must consider methods to limit the bioavailability and clinical effects of the toxin yet to be absorbed, consider any potential specific antidotes and methods to enhance elimination as able. In cases of critical illness following toxin exposure, the emergency physician must respond quickly, remembering principles specific to particular agents.

Rescuer safety must be considered in cases of toxic exposure—one would expect that the risk to rescuers is highest with the care of a critically ill patient where the toxin is not within the common experience of the providers. In the Tokyo subway sarin gas of March 1995, 23% of employees who responded to a post-event survey complained of acute poisoning symptoms.[58] Fortunately, none of these hospital team members required hospitalization. Some of the more significant exposures were those in a poorly ventilated area[58] and those caring for critically ill patients.[59] Some basic principles are available to consider in assessing the risk of secondary contamination.[59] Toxic gases should be lower risk because of rapid dispersal once the patient has been removed from the site of exposure. Liquids are a higher risk as patients or clothing may remain contaminated. The risk of liquids to rescuers is related to the volatility of the particular agent. "Volatility" may be considered the rate at which a liquid evaporates. Those of higher volatility are a more immediate risk at the time of exposure, but ideally disperse quickly. Those of lower volatility may persist, placing emergency department staff at risk. Even if patients are decontaminated they should still be considered at risk of exposing rescuers via exhaled breath in some highly volatile exposures and via emesis of ingested chemicals. Although rescuers must remain vigilant to team member risks, fortunately the published experience of rescuer secondary illness is very limited based on a review of published work.[60]

Determining the toxic agent is an important skill of the emergency physician. History obtained from as many sources as practical is imperative. The physical examination traditionally focuses on vital signs, mental status, pupil size, skin, and characteristic odors.[61] Laboratory studies that should be considered routine include rapid glucose measurement and serum electrolytes to assess bicarbonate levels and the anion gap. The electrocardiogram can be of value, especially in those that are hemodynamically unstable. Recent published work has demonstrated the findings identified in those with adverse cardiac events after toxin exposure to include QT prolongation, prominent R wave in lead aortic valve replacement (AVR), and prolonged QRS duration.[62] Evidence of acute myocardial ischemia was also frequently identified among those having acute cardiovascular events after ingestion. Risk factors for adverse cardiovascular events have been found to be a corrected QT interval greater than 500 msec, a serum bicarbonate level less than 20 mEq/L, and prior cardiac disease.[63]

Any review of critical toxic exposures in 2023 must include accidental opioid overdoses which is the leading cause of death in those between 25 and 64 years of age.[64] According to the CDC, in 2019, 70,630 overdose deaths occurred in the United States. Of those, 49,860 (70.6%) involved opioids, with the bulk (36,359 deaths) involving synthetic opioids, and 16,167 (22.9%) involved psychostimulants.[65] When considering adverse cardiac events after toxic ingestion, the most common agents are opioids and cocaine. Although the these classes account for the greatest number of events, if considering the proportion of ingestions that lead to adverse cardiac events, those with the highest frequency of deterioration include digoxin, angiotensin-converting enzyme inhibitors (ACE-I), beta blockers, diuretics, and calcium channel blockers.[63] Highest in-hospital mortality rates are associated with digoxin and ACE-I exposures. Toxicologic effects of pharmacologic agents (legal and illegal) result in the highest number of deaths. The highest number of deaths from non pharmacologic agents includes carbon monoxide, Freon and other propellants, and herbicides (glyphosphate).[66] Frequent pathways to cardiac arrest after toxic exposure include pathologic bradycardia and pathologic tachycardia which also includes conduction abnormalities, ventricular arrhythmias, and acute coronary syndromes. Respiratory arrest, as often seen in opioid overdose, also leads to cardiac arrest.

More common causes of toxic bradycardia include exposure to alpha-adrenergic agonists (eg, clonidine), beta-blocking agents, calcium channel blockers, cholinergic agents (eg, organophosphates), digoxin, and other cardioactive steroids and opioids. Activated charcoal may be considered in very narrow circumstances of a beta blocker or calcium channel blocker overdose in the awake and hemodynamically stable patient.

Potential interventions for pathologic bradycardia include atropine, naloxone, digoxin-specific antibody fragments, calcium and glucagon, high-dose insulin, and intravenous lipid emulsion. Atropine is a competitive antagonist of the muscarinic acetylcholine receptor. Typically, a first-line agent in symptomatic bradycardia, atropine, is often ineffective in restoring heart rate and cardiac output. Large doses of atropine may be useful in the control of bronchial secretions in cases of cholinesterase inhibitor poisoning. Atropine has a mild side effect profile with potential for delayed gastrointestinal motility, dry mouth, and urinary retention among common reactions. Naloxone has been used in the treatment of alpha-adrenergic agonist overdoses with some success in improving mental status, probably more effectively than hemodynamic status.[67]

Treatment with digoxin-specific antibody fragments can result in rapid improvement in the patient with symptomatic digoxin or other cardioactive steroid poisoning. Clinicians should consider liberal use of digoxin-specific antibody fragments in the symptomatic patient. Indications for treatment include acute large dose ingestions, chronic poisoning with end-organ involvement, elevated serum levels (any level of 15 ng/mL or greater or a level of at least 10 ng/mL measured 6 or more hours after ingestion), hemodynamic instability (including cardiogenic shock), hyperkalemia (serum potassium >5 mEq/L) in acute toxicity, and refractory bradydysrhythmia.[68] Empiric dosing for acute toxicity would start at 10 to 20 vials, but dosing can be adjusted for chronic toxicity, known ingested dose and/or known serum digoxin concentration.[68] In addition to digoxin-specific antibody fragments, lidocaine should be considered the first-line therapy for ventricular arrhythmias.[15]

Treatment of beta blocker overdoses continues to be controversial. Infrequently, patients may see benefit from atropine, calcium, and glucagon.[69] Euglycemic high-dose insulin, catecholamine infusions, and extracorporeal membrane oxygenation seem to have more of a survival benefit.[15,69] The first-line treatment of calcium channel blocker overdose should include calcium infusions, high-dose insulin euglycemic therapy, catecholamine infusions, and atropine.[15] Although intravenous lipid emulsion is considered a possible intervention for beta blocker and calcium channel blocker overdoses,[15] there are data questioning the efficacy and safety profile of this medication.[70] Thus, expert consultation could be considered in complex clinical cases.

Toxic tachycardia and vasoconstriction can occur after stimulant exposures such cocaine and amphetamine. Regardless of the ingestion, aggressive use of benzodiazepines should be considered. In addition to controlling resultant seizures and agitation, hypertension may also resolve. Hyperthermia can be managed with cooling methods, including cooling blankets. If hypertension persists, titratable vasodilators can be used—often with nitroglycerin, nitroprusside infusions, or alpha-adrenergic antagonists.[15,68] It is prudent to monitor for evidence of end-organ damage from vasoconstriction and manage as able with specific agents. Local care strategies for those with evidence of acute coronary syndromes may be best managed collaboratively with multidisciplinary teams.

Opioid overdoses require special consideration due to the severity of the crisis in the United States. In addition to taking steps to treat those acutely intoxicated, emergency physicians are in a unique position to assure best possible infrastructure to treat and prevent these fatalities. There are several risk factors for opioid-associated out-of-hospital cardiac arrest (OA-OHCA). These include concurrent using other recreational or medicinal sedatives, suffering from co-morbid medical conditions (eg, sleep apnea), being relatively opioid naïve or developing a loss of tolerance (eg, recent incarceration, inpatient hospitalization, or recent release from an abstinence-based treatment program), or having social factors resulting in isolation (ie, being alone when using opioids).[64] Keys to survival of the opioid poisoned patient include early administration of naloxone and respiratory support. Encouraging lay responders to perform a jaw thrust maneuver may reduce airway obstruction and hopefully provide a harmless painful stimuli promoting spontaneous respiration.[64] OA-OHCA is a unique clinical scenario where respiratory support should ideally be provided in addition to chest compressions, rather than relying on "compressions only" resuscitation due to the respiratory insufficiency and dramatic hypoxia evident in these cases. In cases of respiratory depression or respiratory arrest with intact pulses, trained providers may opt to start with lower doses of naloxone. Trying to find the lowest effective dose that restores respiratory effort and airway protective reflexes may be optimal to prevent the uncomfortable precipitated withdrawal, maintaining the therapeutic relationship between patient and rescuers.

For those patients in opioid-associated cardiac arrest, the role of naloxone is unclear. Thus, standard resuscitation without the use of naloxone is recommended.[64] In clinical situations (eg, unmonitored OA-OHCA) where rescuers are unable to reliably determine the presence of cardiac activity, naloxone can be administered.

The postresuscitation care of these patients requires careful attention from providers. Emergency physicians must remain vigilant when considering co-etiologies for out-of-hospital cardiac arrest in cases of suspected opioid overdose. The course of patients after immediate resuscitation can vary between patients. Complications can include post-obstructive pulmonary edema, rebound opioid depression after naloxone metabolism, additional side effects from coingestants, hypothermia due to environmental exposure, hypovolemia due to poor pre-arrest physical condition and sepsis due to aspiration or unsanitary parenteral drug administration practices.[64] Those patients that require intubation may present a challenge in identifying effective sedation medications and doses. These patients may have a tolerance to sedation medications and thus finding lower doses of short-acting agents that will facilitate earliest possible extubation may be challenging. With opioid, as well as all life threatening but reversible toxic insults, extracorporeal membrane oxygenation can provide a bridge therapy for further drug metabolism and treatment in appropriate cases.

The American Heart Association Scientific Statement on OA-OHCA includes five pages of recommendations for secondary prevention and rehabilitation to prevent the death of overdose survivors. These recommendations include recommendations ranging from brief counseling on safe practices (eg, not being alone while using opioids, using clean equipment and water) to increasing availability of naloxone and face shields and masks.[64]

For critically ill burn victims, smoke inhalation with carbon monoxide and cyanide poisoning should be assumed.[71,72] Carbon monoxide causes decreased oxygen carrying capacity by binding to hemoglobin. Cardiac arrest due to carbon monoxide poisoning is almost always fatal. Critically ill unresponsive burn patients should be mechanically ventilated with 100% oxygen. Studies on hyperbaric oxygen for carbon monoxide poisoning are conflicting, but its use can be considered due to the relative safety of hyperbaric oxygen. A Cochrane review published in 2011 found no strong evidence of clinical benefit using hyperbaric oxygen for carbon monoxide poisoning.[72]

Cyanide disrupts aerobic cellular metabolism. Several studies indicate that patients with life-threatening cyanide toxicity can have reversal of toxicity and improved outcomes with hydroxocobalamin. The addition of sodium thiosulfate, a cofactor for cyanide metabolism, has controversial effectiveness but can be given as adjunctive medication with hydroxycobalamin.[71]

TRAUMA

Traumatic circulatory arrest often happens in otherwise healthy patients who could respond to the early identification and treatment of reversible causes.[73] Hemorrhage control is a priority, especially for penetrating trauma. A circulation first "coronary artery bypass (CAB)" approach is of particular importance in the traumatic arrest patient, as a large proportion of early mortality results from blood loss.

The following interventions should be started simultaneously with chest compressions. Active bleeding should be quickly identified and managed through the use of direct pressure, tourniquets for extremities, packing of wounds, clamping of vessels, and/or suturing. The patient should be completely undressed and examined head to toe for any wounds with attention toward easily overlooked areas such as the perineum and axilla. Tension pneumothorax as a cause of arrest should be assumed and managed emergently with bilateral chest decompressions using either finger thoracostomies or chest tubes. The patient should undergo rapid sequence intubation to secure the airway and maximize oxygenation. If an unstable pelvic fracture is suspected, a pelvic binder should be placed. Two large bore IVs of at least 18 gauge should be placed with prompt resuscitation of blood products for hemorrhagic shock/arrest trauma patients. Blood should be given at a ratio of 1:1:1 packed red blood cells (RBCs), platelets, and plasma.[73]

A resuscitative thoracotomy can be considered in select patients with short arrest times when resources and skilled providers are available. The best outcomes for resuscitative thoracotomies are for patients who arrest in the hospital. For out-of-hospital cardiac arrest, better outcomes are seen in penetrating trauma over blunt trauma. Consider a resuscitative thoracotomy in penetrating injury patients who have had CPR for less than 15 minutes or blunt trauma patients that have arrested within 10 minutes.[74] In traumatic cardiac arrest, the procedure should be started as soon as possible in the emergency department without delay for transport to an operating room. A left-sided thoracotomy allows repair of cardiac defects (cardiac lacerations, tamponade), direct control of thoracic hemorrhage, internal cardiac massage, and cross-clamping of the aorta. If the penetrating injury is in the right chest, a clamshell thoracotomy should be done to control potential right-sided thoracic hemorrhage. This procedure is technically challenging and should only be done by prepared practitioners with the availability of a surgeon to assist with the procedure and assume care of the patient if return of spontaneous circulation is achieved.

The prognosis for out of hospital traumatic cardiac arrest patients is generally poor. If an out of hospital traumatic arrest patient shows no signs of life (no respirations, cardiac activity on the monitor, blood pressure or pulses) has been in cardiac arrest for an extended time, or fails to respond to initial CPR, it is reasonable to withhold or terminate resuscitation.[75] Ultimately, physician discretion on resuscitative efforts should be made for each individual case depending on the potential reversible, or irreversible, causes of cardiac arrest.

OBESITY

Obese patients in cardiac arrest present a special situation where there are mechanical barriers to high-quality resuscitation and common comorbidities, which often lead to worse outcomes.[76] Obesity is defined as excess fat tissue with a body mass index greater than 30 kg/m^2. Obesity-related conditions that contribute to sudden cardiac arrest include diabetes, heart disease, stroke, and cancers.[77] In one prospective study of 1326 Japanese out-of-hospital cardiac arrest patients, neurologic outcomes were worse in obese patients. The investigators noted that longer periods of chest compressions, often more difficult in obese patients, may have contributed.[78]

The prevalence of obesity in the United States is approximately 40%.[77] In a population-based review of sudden cardiac arrest in Oregon, those aged 35 to 59 were more likely to be obese (48.1%) than those at least 60 year old (33%).[79] Another Oregon-based study identified obesity in 50% of those aged 25 to 34 year old with sudden cardiac arrest.[80] In resuscitating an obese cardiac arrest patient, standard resuscitation algorithms apply but often require adjustments to increase effectiveness.

Obese patients have reduced chest wall compliance due to increased overlying soft tissue.[81] For the obese patient, increase the depth of chest compressions to 6 cm. Giving quality compressions in an obese patient requires more force and fatigue more quickly develops. Rescuers performing chest compressions should rotate more frequently to counteract fatigue.[81]

Regarding defibrillation, there is concern that the attenuation of energy with increasing adipose tissue may lessen effect.[15] Thus, early energy dose-escalation or manual pressure (paddles or manual pressure augmentation technique) may improve the success rates of electrical energy.[15] IV access can be challenging in the obese patient. Veins in the antecubital fossa or neck may be the easiest to access. If unsuccessful after two or more IV attempts, one should use an appropriately sized interosseous needle or an ultrasound-guided line. Standard resuscitation medication doses should be used (epinephrine, calcium, and atropine).[82] Evidence for drug dose changes is lacking, with sources varying on recommendations for sedatives and paralytics.[83]

One should anticipate that endotracheal intubation and ventilation will be challenging. Obese patients desaturate more quickly due to lower functional residual capacity and increased oxygen consumption.[84] Ventilation with a bag-mask device should be minimized and done by experienced personnel using a two-person technique with a two-handed bilateral jaw thrust.[82] Early endotracheal intubation is recommended to minimize the duration of oxygenation and ventilation via a bag valve mask.[15]

Intubation should be done with the goal of first past success, using advanced airway modalities such as hyper-angulated video laryngoscopes as needed to increase chances of first pass success. For the obese patient, the use of a "ramped" (more upright) position can improve airway positioning. One should consider a supraglottic device as a backup. If faced with a "can't intubate, can't ventilate" scenario, one should proceed without delay to a cricothyrotomy. When doing this procedure on a rapidly deteriorating obese patient, one needs apply attention toward clearly identifying the cricothyroid membrane because it can be more challenging with increased surrounding soft tissue. Once an airway is secured, obese patients may benefit from lower tidal volumes (5–6 mL/kg ideal body weight) used in acute respiratory distress syndrome, as their lung volumes are decreased and under higher pressure.[83]

PREGNANCY

Cardiac arrest in pregnancy presents a challenging scenario with the potential resuscitation of the mother and the baby as two patients. This population is usually younger and healthier than most cardiac arrest patients, and they may respond to special resuscitative efforts with a good outcome. Owing to the low frequency of pregnant cardiac arrest cases, teams are often inexperienced and reliant on guidelines and simulations to perform the indicated interventions. If the patient is known to be less than 20 weeks pregnant, or the uterus lies distinctly below the umbilicus (at which level 20 weeks is estimated), standard resuscitation protocols are indicated. There is no evidence that defibrillation in pregnancy negatively affects the fetus. No defibrillator pad position change is indicated in the gravid patient and standard placement can be used.[85] Standard ACLS medications are indicated, and epinephrine can be given every 3 to 5 minutes.

If the patient is known or estimated to be over 20 weeks, further action beyond standard resuscitation algorithms is indicated due to physiologic changes.[86] On notification of the arrival of a gravid patient in cardiac arrest with a potentially viable pregnancy, obstetric and neonatal response teams should be activated to assist in management of the mother and potentially the neonate. Neonatal resuscitation equipment should be prepared as well as a warmer alongside adult resuscitation equipment. Time-sensitive interventions should continue at the initial location of the patient in the hospital, without delay for transport to an operating room or obstetric floor.

Throughout pregnancy, cardiac output increases 30% to 50% because of increased stroke volume and heart rate. Heart rate increases by 15 to 20 bpm. By weeks 12 to 14 of gestation, the uterus puts pressure on the abdominal aorta and vena cava, causing an increase in afterload and decrease in venous return. The fetus shunts from 50 mL/min to approximately 1000 mL/min of blood and receives up to 20% of cardiac output.[86]

Fundal height can estimate gestational age in singleton pregnancies between weeks 16 and 36. The distance from the symphysis to the fundus roughly correlates to the week of gestation. Alternatively, common landmarks can be used as rough estimates. At 12 weeks gestational age, the uterus is palpable above the pubic symphysis. At 20 weeks gestation, the uterus is palpable at the level of the umbilicus. These are rough estimates and may be poor predictors of gestational age. The fundus may reach the umbilicus between 15 and 19 weeks of gestation, and after 36 weeks gestation, the fundal height can lower as the fetal head engages the pelvis. Other factors that affect fundal height include twin pregnancy, fetal lie, and increased body mass index (BMI). If it is difficult to estimate fundal height, a bedside ultrasound can assist in determining approximate gestational age. Fetal viability begins at approximately 23 weeks gestation.[87]

A 30° tilt helps an unstable pregnant patient by allowing gravity to take pressure off the great vessels by displacing the uterus, but this should not be used in cardiac arrest as it can decrease the quality of chest compressions. Left lateral displacement of the uterus helps prevent aortocaval blockage. This can be done with one or two hands. With one hand, the dominant hand can be used from the patient's right side to displace the uterus to the left. Care should be taken to apply force laterally and not downward to avoid inadvertent aortocaval compression. From the patient's left side, one can cup the uterus with both hands and lift it up and leftward. For first responders to such a case, there should be at least four people to have enough hands for uterine displacement, chest compressions, airway management, and defibrillation until further assistance arrives. IV placement is preferred above the diaphragm to bypass potential compression of the vena cava by the uterus.

Pregnant patients are more prone to hypoxia, and so oxygenation should be prioritized as a potential cause of cardiac arrest. Functional residual capacity decreases by 10% to 25% during pregnancy as the uterus elevates the diaphragm. Oxygen demands also increase to a level 20% to 33% above baseline to maintain maternal and fetal metabolic demands. To compensate, respiratory rates increases causing a mild respiratory alkalosis. The airway of gravid patients may be smaller, more edematous, and friable, making it more difficult. The most experienced practitioner should attempt intubation, and a smaller endotracheal (ET) tube size, 6.0 to 7.0 should be considered. If intubation is not successful after two tries, a supraglottic device should be used to prevent further trauma/edema. As with all difficult airways, if the patient is unable to be intubated and ventilated, a surgical airway is indicated.[88]

A perimortem cesarean delivery (PMCD) should be considered and decided on early in the pregnant cardiac arrest patient past 20 weeks gestation. If decided upon, current guidelines recommend that it be done within 4 minutes of the arrest with a goal of fetus delivery in 1 minute from the start of the procedure. The procedure requires at a minimum a scalpel. It can be done through a Pfannenstiel or vertical incision. Time should not be spent waiting for specialized surgical equipment or prepping the abdomen. Antiseptic solution may be poured on the abdomen if desired. The vertical incision provides better visualization and is preferable for those inexperienced with the procedure. The incision, through multiple cuts, should quickly reach the level of the uterus and proceed with delivery of the fetus. The fetus should be handed off to the neonatal resuscitation team, and then, the placenta should be delivered. The uterus can then be packed or closed with a running locking stitch using absorbable suture. It is reasonable to defer wound closure to surgical or obstetric colleagues if the one performing the procedure is not surgically trained. If the resuscitation is successful, prophylactic antibiotics should be given.[89]

A review of all published cases of PMCD from 1980 to 2010 showed that PMCD led to a clear maternal survival benefit in 19 of 60 cases (31.7%), and there were no cases in which PMCD may have been deleterious to maternal survival. In practice, the time to delivery is often delayed upward to 30 minutes, with better outcomes being reported for cases delivered less than 10 minutes of arrest.[87] The procedure must be decided on and done rapidly, and transport to an operating room during maternal cardiac arrest would likely worsen outcomes. Chest compressions during stretcher transportation are often ineffective, and such transportation would delay time to procedure completion, increasing anoxic injury to both the mother and fetus.

Following delivery of the fetus and placenta, incision wounds should be packed and closing of incisions should be deferred to obstetric/surgical services with care of the neonate handed off to neonatal intensive care unit team. The stress of maternal cardiac arrest results in most neonates delivered by PMCD requiring active resuscitation. Neonatal resuscitation should follow the most recent American Heart Association (AHA) recommendations.

There are certain risks involved for the newborn during maternal resuscitation in cardiac arrest. The greatest risk for the fetus is the lack of perfusion, and resuscitative measures for the mother are aimed at restoring maternal and fetal perfusion. Maternal health is prioritized because fetal circulation depends on it. Embryogenesis is mostly complete by 12 weeks, so most medications are unlikely to have teratogenic effects if given after the first trimester. Medications may have toxic effects, such as opioids, and each medication given in the post-arrest period should be considered based on their risks and benefits. If the mother has return of spontaneous circulation without delivery of the fetus, fetal monitoring should be initiated promptly to assess for signs of distress and need for emergent delivery.[89]

LEFT VENTRICULAR ASSIST DEVICE

Care of the patient with a left ventricular assist device (LVAD) must be considered within the skill set of every emergency physician as the use and role of LVADs continues to expand. The LVAD was initially considered a bridge to transplantation but is becoming more often a destination therapy for patients with advanced heart failure. Although ventricular assist devices can be used to support right, left, or both ventricles, the LVAD is most common and will be the focus of this review.

The LVAD is a mechanical device that supports systemic circulation where blood enters the device via an inflow cannula positioned at the apex of the left ventricle. Blood flows into the pumping chamber, typically a continuous flow pump, which drives blood into the outflow cannula into the ascending aorta. A battery-powered system controller is worn by the patient and maintains connection to the pumping chamber via a percutaneously tunneled driveline. The external controller has data visible including battery alarms and device warning alarms.

The clinical assessment of the patient with an LVAD is complicated by the continuous flow of the device. Blood pressure and heart rate are assessed differently in the LVAD patient. If a patient is awake and alert, some degree of cerebral blood flow can be assumed. Perfusion status can be assumed based on mental status, patient's pallor, extremity perfusion (warm vs cold), and capillary refill.[90] Determine mean arterial pressure via a Doppler device noting the cuff pressure where Doppler flow is first identified. Mean arterial pressure (MAP) in left ventricular assist device (LVAD) patients is generally between 70 and 90 mm HG. MAP greater than 90 mm HG may be reasonable to avoid in those with a new hemorrhagic stroke.[91] In the unconscious and/or unstable patient, invasive blood pressure monitoring with an arterial line may be preferred. The physician should also auscultate to identify a device "hum" assuring device function.

In addition to routine diagnostic studies (complete blood count, electrolytes, and hepatic function studies), the initial diagnostic studies should include lactate dehydrogenase (LDH), plasma free hemoglobin, haptoglobin, electrocardiogram, and chest radiograph. A chest x-ray can assess pump position and integrity of the driveline if previous images are available. A targeted x-ray of the driveline can be obtained to assess integrity of the wires.[90] Patients with an LVAD should be expected to have a perfusing rhythm on their ECG. The emergency physician should attempt to read any device warnings on the system controller, as this may lead to clues for the etiology of the patient's current condition.

Common acute conditions in the patient with an LVAD include bleeding, sepsis, acute neurologic events, and device-specific complications. A brief discussion about the emergency department considerations for each of the following in patients that present away from an LVAD center follow.

Bleeding is a common presentation in those with an LVAD, with gastrointestinal bleeding being the most common source. Gastrointestinal bleeding is a relatively common complication felt to be due to a combination of coagulopathy, acquired von Willebrand disease and continuous non-pulsatile blood flow.[92] Although bleeding can occur anywhere throughout the GI tract, upper sources are most common.[92] In case of substantial hemorrhage, a reading on the control unit may signal a low output state. Resuscitation should proceed as normal for patients with hemodynamically significant hemorrhage. However, if time allows, discussion with VAD consultants is desirable early in the resuscitation.[90] Limiting exposure to antigens during transfusion may be desirable in those with an LVAD as a bridge to transplantation. In addition, aggressive volume resuscitation can increase pulmonary artery pressure and impede right ventricle function.

Sepsis is a risk for all patients with indwelling devices. Patients with an LVAD possess a unique risk of infection at the site of the percutaneous driveline as well as with pocket infections and infections of the device components. Although it is important to restore adequate intravascular volume, the rate of infusion must be tempered with the need to prevent acute right ventricular overload. Vasoactive infusions can be used to support systemic vascular resistance or right ventricular contractility as needed. Milrinone should be avoided unless recommended by the LVAD center.

Acute neurologic events continue to be a source of morbidity and mortality for patients with an LVAD. The greatest challenge for the emergency physician is to determine if the unresponsive patient with an LVAD has inadequate flow which has led to prolonged poor cerebral perfusion and thus brain death or if the patient has adequate cerebral perfusion but another active condition as the primary etiology for the altered mental status. As for all unresponsive patients, it is important to consider those noncardiac causes of altered mental status (hypoglycemia, hypoxia, or overdose).[93] When trying to ascertain if a patient with an LVAD has adequate cerebral perfusion pressure, current recommendations are that if the mean arterial pressure is above 50 mm Hg and/or the end-tidal CO_2 is greater than 20 mm Hg, at least minimally acceptable cerebral perfusion can be assumed and external chest compressions should not be initiated.[93] If a cause for altered mental status cannot be identified, proceeding through an aggressive stroke evaluation is warranted. In cases of ischemic stroke, early consultation with an LVAD specialist is required as thrombolysis may be ineffective due to the differing composition of thrombi in these patients.[91] With an elevated risk of hemorrhagic transformation in these patients, endovascular therapy is unproven but may be preferred over thrombolysis.[91] Expert consultation is warranted in cases of hemorrhagic stroke as reversal of anticoagulation is a complicated decision in patients with an LVAD. Blood pressure control to decrease mean arterial pressure below 90 mm Hg is not unreasonable.[91] A declaration of death is difficult in the unresponsive patient with a functioning LVAD. Liberal consultation and aggressive neuroimaging should be considered.[91]

Device-specific complications can be as simple as exchanging a battery to pump failure, or as complicated as driveline thrombosis. In cases of pump failure or driveline thrombosis, early expert consultation is recommended. Thrombosis may be suggested by elevations in serum LDH, elevated free hemoglobin, increased bilirubin, and/or reduced haptoglobin levels.[90] Systemic thrombolysis should not be routinely performed without contacting the implanting center and without evidence of subacute stoke on head CT.[90] There are no recommended acute interventions currently for emergency physicians to perform in the event of device thrombosis, especially in the absence of expert consultation.

Emergency physicians should perform indicated resuscitation procedures as needed.[94] Closed chest compressions, external defibrillation, and cardioversion can be performed with an indwelling LVAD while maintaining contact between the controller and the pump.[90,91,93] Chest tube placement might be safer if positioned more laterally than normal. Pericardiocentesis should only be performed after careful consideration. Emergency physicians should anticipate that bedside ultrasound windows of the pericardial space will be difficult to visualize. Remember that some devices are designed to be placed within the pericardial space. Arrhythmias should be aggressively treated with medical management and defibrillation/cardioversion to preserve right ventricular function.

PULMONARY EMBOLISM

Pulmonary embolism (PE) as a cause of cardiac arrest is associated with a rapid onset and poor prognosis. In massive PE, 90% of cardiac arrests occur within 1 to 2 hours of symptoms onset. Circulatory arrest occurs due to obstruction of the pulmonary arteries leading to right heart failure and distention. This right heart failure leads to decreased left heart preload and cardiac output. The rapid onset of cardiovascular collapse due to PE often necessitates cardio PE before a diagnosis being made.[95]

If the patient does not have a known history of PE, the presence of risk factors and relevant clinical along with point of care echo findings of right heart strain in pulseless electrical activity (PEA) arrest can indicate a likely massive PE.[96] An EKG can help with the diagnosis by excluding acute coronary syndrome and showing signs of right heart strain as a marker for PE. If the patient is stable for transport, a CT pulmonary angiography can confirm the diagnosis.[15]

Common risk factors for PE to consider include prior PE/deep vein thrombosis (DVT), recent surgery or immobilization, active cancer, signs of DVT, hormone replacement therapy or oral contraceptive pill (OCP) use, and long-distance flights.[15] Of patients with the following three characteristics, PE is very likely (true positive rate of 53%): age less than 65 years, witnessed arrest, presence of PEA as the first rhythm.[97] Of patients with sudden cardiac arrest of uncertain etiology, PE accounts for about 10%.[98] Approximately half of all patients with cardiac arrest due to PE present in PEA.[13] Low end-tidal carbon dioxide ($ETCO_2$) during high-quality chest compressions may support the diagnosis of PE but this is a nonspecific sign.[15]

If the patient has a known or highly suspected PE as a cause of cardiac arrest, the administration of thrombolytics may have a benefit.[13] Heparin should be initiated if the diagnosis of PE is confirmed or highly suspected. If the decision is made to use thrombolytics, the duration of CPR should continue for additional time after administration of thrombolytics to allow for adequate circulation. The investigators' recommendations vary on the duration of CPR following thrombolytics given in cardiac arrest cases. The 2021 European Resuscitation Council guidelines recommend 60 to 90 minutes of CPR following thrombolytics,[15] This is based on the limited evidence of good neurologic recovery after thrombolytics were used as a rescue therapy for PE after 90 minutes of CPR.[99] The routine use of tenecteplase in undifferentiated out-of-hospital cardiac arrest did not improve outcomes in randomized studies.[100]

There have been case reports of good outcomes with the use of percutaneous mechanical thrombectomy in patients requiring CPR with a known massive PE.[101] In patients with confirmed PE as the precipitant of cardiac arrest, thrombolysis, surgical embolectomy, and mechanical embolectomy are reasonable options.[13] Consider extracorporeal cardiopulmonary resuscitation, if available, as a last resort in select moribund PE cases that fail to respond to conventional CPR and thrombolytics.[102]

SUMMARY

All emergency providers should have some understanding of the resuscitation interventions for these special populations. The mainstay of resuscitation in cardiac arrest remains to be high-quality cardiopulmonary resuscitation, early defibrillation of shockable rhythms, and identification and treatment of reversible causes. Understanding the unique aspects of reversibility in these situations may provide invaluable information during high-pressured cardiac arrest resuscitation. This is not an exhaustive review of special populations in cardiac arrest. Each section was deliberately chosen as a situation where application of specific resuscitation modifications can lead to improved outcomes.

CLINICS CARE POINTS

Pearls

- The role of extracorporeal care in those victims of acute asthma events, drowning, pulmonary embolism, and hypothermia is an area of active research.

- Suggestions exist for which victims of drowning, electrical injury, anaphylaxis, and opioid overdose do not require hospitalization.

- For drowning patients, prioritize airway management and ventilation, as drowning often results in hypoxia and aspiration.

- Spinal injuries are uncommon in those victims of drowning and electrical injury.

- Recommendations for performing a perimortem cesarean delivery within 4 minutes of maternal cardiac arrest for pregnant patients past 20 weeks gestation are primarily based on expert consensus, observational studies, and case reports. In practice, this 4-minute time frame is often not met in practice, but outcomes favor earlier cesarean delivery.

Pitfalls

- In hypothermic patients, resuscitation may be ineffective until rewarming occurs. Avoid withholding resuscitation without attempting rewarming unless there are evident indications of a non-survivable injury.

- Focusing solely on chest compressions during traumatic arrest, without concurrently addressing active bleeding and other reversible causes.

- Delaying a resuscitative thoracotomy or perimortem cesarean when warranted can negatively impact patient outcomes. Evidence supports performing these procedures promptly in the emergency department, rather than waiting for the operating room.

- Difficulty obtaining a blood pressure in an LVAD patient. The assessment of blood pressure in LVAD patients can be challenging due to the continuous flow of the device. Experts recommend evaluating perfusion status based on mental status, patient's pallor, extremity perfusion, capillary refill, and Doppler measurements.

- Underestimating the difficulty in managing the airway of pregnant and obese patients. Evidence suggests that respective physiologic and anatomic differences decrease time to oxygen desaturation and make intubation more challenging.

DISCLOSURE

The authors have nothing to disclose.

REFERENCES

1. Cooper MA, Andrews CJ, Holle RL, et al. Lightning-related injuries and safety. Wilderness Medicine. 7th ed. Philadelphia, PA: Elsevier; 2017. p. 60–101.
2. Ritenour AE, Morton MJ, McManus JG, et al. Lightning injury: A review. Burns 2008;34(5):585–94.
3. Gille J, Schmidt T, Dragu A, et al. Electrical injury – a dual center analysis of patient characteristics, therapeutic specifics and outcome predictors. Scand J Trauma Resusc Emerg Med 2018;26(1): 43.
4. Nisar S, Keyloun JW, Kolachana S, et al. Institutional Experience Using a Treatment Algorithm for Electrical Injury. J Burn Care Res 2021;42(3): 351–6.
5. Douillet D, Kalwant S, Amro Y, et al. Use of troponin assay after electrical injuries: a 15-year multicentre retrospective cohort in emergency departments. Scand J Trauma Resusc Emerg Med 2021;29(1): 141.
6. Shaker MS, Wallace DV, Golden DBK, et al. Anaphylaxis-a 2020 practice parameter update, systematic review, and Grading of Recommendations, Assessment, Development and Evaluation (GRADE) analysis. J Allergy Clin Immunol 2020; 145(4):1082–123.
7. Cardona V, Ansotegui IJ, Ebisawa M, et al. World allergy organization anaphylaxis guidance 2020. World Allergy Organ J 2020;13(10):100472.
8. Lieberman P, Camargo CA, Bohlke K, et al. Epidemiology of anaphylaxis: findings of the American College of Allergy, Asthma and Immunology

Epidemiology of Anaphylaxis Working Group. Ann Allergy Asthma Immunol Off Publ Am Coll Allergy Asthma Immunol 2006;97(5):596–602.

9. Brown SGA. Clinical features and severity grading of anaphylaxis. J Allergy Clin Immunol 2004;114(2): 371–6.

10. Murasaka K, Yamashita A, Wato Y, et al. Epidemiology of out-of-hospital cardiac arrests caused by anaphylaxis and factors associated with outcomes: an observational study. BMJ Open 2022;12(8): e062877.

11. Jerschow E, Lin RY, Scaperotti MM, et al. Fatal anaphylaxis in the United States, 1999-2010: temporal patterns and demographic associations. J Allergy Clin Immunol 2014;134(6):1318–28.e7.

12. Lee S, Hess EP, Lohse C, et al. Trends, characteristics, and incidence of anaphylaxis in 2001-2010: A population-based study. J Allergy Clin Immunol 2017;139(1):182–8.e2.

13. Panchal AR, Bartos JA, Cabañas JG, et al. Part 3: Adult Basic and Advanced Life Support: 2020 American Heart Association Guidelines for Cardiopulmonary Resuscitation and Emergency Cardiovascular Care. Circulation 2020;142(16_suppl_2):S366–468.

14. Vanden Hoek TL, Morrison LJ, Shuster M, et al. Part 12: Cardiac Arrest in Special Situations. Circulation 2010;122(18_suppl_3):S829–61.

15. Lott C, Truhlář A, Alfonzo A, et al. European Resuscitation Council Guidelines 2021: Cardiac arrest in special circumstances. Resuscitation 2021;161: 152–219. https://doi.org/10.1016/j.resuscitation. 2021.02.011.

16. Carlson JN, Cook S, Djarv T, et al. Second Dose of Epinephrine for Anaphylaxis in the First Aid Setting: A Scoping Review. Cureus 2020;12(11):e11401.

17. Korenblat P, Lundie MJ, Dankner RE, et al. A retrospective study of epinephrine administration for anaphylaxis: how many doses are needed? Allergy Asthma Proc 1999;20(6):383–6.

18. Brown SGA, Blackman KE, Stenlake V, et al. Insect sting anaphylaxis; prospective evaluation of treatment with intravenous adrenaline and volume resuscitation. Emerg Med J EMJ 2004;21(2):149–54.

19. Molfino NA, Nannini LJ, Martelli AN, et al. Respiratory Arrest in near-Fatal Asthma. N Engl J Med 1991;324(5):285–8.

20. Asthma as the Underlying Cause of Death | CDC. Published September 10, 2019. https://www.cdc. gov/asthma/asthma_stats/asthma_underlying_ death.html. Accessed September 20, 2022.

21. Krishnan V, Diette GB, Rand CS, et al. Mortality in Patients Hospitalized for Asthma Exacerbations in the United States. Am J Respir Crit Care Med 2006;174(6):633–8.

22. Porpodis K, Zarogoulidis P, Spyratos D, et al. Pneumothorax and asthma. J Thorac Dis 2014;6(Suppl 1):S152–61.

23. Jr CAC, Spooner C, Rowe BH. Continuous versus intermittent beta-agonists for acute asthma. Cochrane Database Syst Rev 2003;4. https://doi.org/ 10.1002/14651858.CD001115.

24. Rodrigo GJ, Castro-Rodriguez JA. Anticholinergics in the treatment of children and adults with acute asthma: a systematic review with meta-analysis. Thorax 2005;60(9):740–6.

25. 2020 Focused Updates to the Asthma Management Guidelines: A Report from the National Asthma Education and Prevention Program Coordinating Committee Expert Panel Working Group | NHLBI, NIH. https://www.nhlbi.nih.gov/resources/ 2020-focused-updates-asthma-management- guidelines. Accessed September 20, 2022.

26. Doymaz S, Schneider J, Sagy M. Early administration of terbutaline in severe pediatric asthma may reduce incidence of acute respiratory failure. Ann Allergy Asthma Immunol 2014;112(3):207–10.

27. Adair E, Dibaba D, Fowke JH, et al. The Impact of Terbutaline as Adjuvant Therapy in the Treatment of Severe Asthma in the Pediatric Emergency Department. Pediatr Emerg Care 2022;38(1):e292–4.

28. Travers AA, Jones AP, Kelly KD, et al. Intravenous beta2-agonists for acute asthma in the emergency department. Cochrane Database Syst Rev 2001;1. https://doi.org/10.1002/14651858.CD002988.

29. Jat KR, Chawla D. Ketamine for management of acute exacerbations of asthma in children. Cochrane Database Syst Rev 2012;11:CD009293.

30. Luecke T, Pelosi P. Clinical review: Positive endexpiratory pressure and cardiac output. Crit Care 2005;9(6):607.

31. Leatherman J. Mechanical Ventilation for Severe Asthma. Chest 2015;147(6):1671–80.

32. Brooks R, Cohen-Cymberknoh M, Glicksman C, et al. Manual external chest compression reverses respiratory failure in children with severe air trapping. Pediatr Pulmonol 2021;56(12):3887–90.

33. Althoff MD, Holguin F, Yang F, et al. Noninvasive Ventilation Use in Critically Ill Patients with Acute Asthma Exacerbations. Am J Respir Crit Care Med 2020;202(11):1520–30.

34. Mikkelsen ME, Woo YJ, Sager JS, et al. Outcomes Using Extracorporeal Life Support for Adult Respiratory Failure due to Status Asthmaticus. ASAIO J 2009;55(1):47–52.

35. Drowning Facts | Drowning Prevention | CDC. Published March 10, 2022. https://www.cdc.gov/drowning/ facts/index.html. Accessed September 19, 2022.

36. Szpilman D, Morgan PJ. Management for the Drowning Patient. Chest 2021;159(4):1473–83.

37. Injury Data Visualization Tools | WISQARS | CDC. https://wisqars.cdc.gov/data/non-fatal/home. Accessed October 27, 2022.

38. Clemens T. Persistent Racial/Ethnic Disparities in Fatal Unintentional Drowning Rates Among

Persons Aged ≤29 Years — United States, 1999–2019. MMWR Morb Mortal Wkly Rep 2021;70. https://doi.org/10.15585/mmwr.mm7024a1.

39. Schmidt AC, Sempsrott JR, Hawkins SC, et al. Wilderness Medical Society Clinical Practice Guidelines for the Treatment and Prevention of Drowning: 2019 Update. Wilderness Environ Med 2019;30(4, Supplement):S70–86.

40. Tobin JM, Ramos WD, Pu Y, et al. Bystander CPR is associated with improved neurologically favourable survival in cardiac arrest following drowning. Resuscitation 2017;115:39–43.

41. Claesson A, Lindqvist J, Herlitz J. Cardiac arrest due to drowning—Changes over time and factors of importance for survival. Resuscitation 2014; 85(5):644–8.

42. Dyson K, Morgans A, Bray J, et al. Drowning related out-of-hospital cardiac arrests: Characteristics and outcomes. Resuscitation 2013;84(8):1114–8.

43. Fukuda T, Ohashi-Fukuda N, Hayashida K, et al. Bystander-initiated conventional vs compression-only cardiopulmonary resuscitation and outcomes after out-of-hospital cardiac arrest due to drowning. Resuscitation 2019;145:166–74.

44. Leavy JE, Crawford G, Leaversuch F, et al. A Review of Drowning Prevention Interventions for Children and Young People in High, Low and Middle Income Countries. J Community Health 2016; 41(2):424–41.

45. Szpilman D, de Barros Oliveira R, Mocellin O, et al. Is drowning a mere matter of resuscitation? Resuscitation 2018;129:103–6.

46. Althaus U, Aeberhard P, Schüpbach P, et al. Management of profound accidental hypothermia with cardiorespiratory arrest. Annals of surgery 1982; 195(4):492.

47. Vanden Hoek TL, Morrison LJ, Shuster M, et al. Part 12: cardiac arrest in special situations: 2010 American Heart Association guidelines for cardiopulmonary resuscitation and emergency cardiovascular care. Circulation 2010;122(18_suppl_3):S829–61.

48. Jekich BM, Drake BD, Nacht JY, et al. Avalanche Fatalities in the United States: A Change in Demographics. Wilderness Environ Med 2016;27(1): 46–52.

49. Falk M, Brugger H, Adler-Kastner L. Avalanche survival chances. Nature 1994;368(6466):21.

50. Lott C, Truhlár A. Cardiac arrest in special circumstances. Curr Opin Crit Care 2021;27(6):642–8.

51. Mahoney BA, Smith WA, Lo D, et al. Emergency interventions for hyperkalaemia. Cochrane Database Syst Rev 2005;2005(2):CD003235.

52. Paice B, Gray JM, McBride D, et al. Hyperkalaemia in patients in hospital. Br Med J Clin Res Ed 1983; 286(6372):1189–92.

53. Peacock WF, Rafique Z, Clark CL, et al. Real World Evidence for Treatment of Hyperkalemia in the Emergency Department (REVEAL-ED): A Multicenter, Prospective, Observational Study. J Emerg Med 2018;55(6):741–50.

54. Reid A, Jones G, Isles C. Hypokalaemia: common things occur commonly – a retrospective survey. JRSM Short Rep 2012;3(11):80.

55. Goyal A, Spertus JA, Gosch K, et al. Serum Potassium Levels and Mortality in Acute Myocardial Infarction. JAMA 2012;307(2):157–64.

56. Hansen BA, Ø Bruserud. Hypomagnesemia in critically ill patients. J Intensive Care 2018;6(1):21.

57. Panchal AR, Berg KM, Kudenchuk PJ, et al. American Heart Association Focused Update on Advanced Cardiovascular Life Support Use of Antiarrhythmic Drugs During and Immediately After Cardiac Arrest: An Update to the American Heart Association Guidelines for Cardiopulmonary Resuscitation and Emergency Cardiovascular Care. Circulation 2018;138(23):e740–9.

58. Okumura T, Suzuki K, Fukuda A, et al. The Tokyo Subway Sarin Attack: Disaster Management, Part 2: Hospital Response. Acad Emerg Med 1998; 5(6):618–24.

59. Baker DJ. Exposure to toxic hazards. In: Baker DJ, editor. Toxic trauma: a basic clinical guide. Springer International Publishing; 2016. p. 49–67.

60. De Groot R, Van Zoelen GA, Leenders MEC, et al. Is secondary chemical exposure of hospital personnel of clinical importance? Clin Toxicol 2021;59(4): 269–78.

61. Erickson TB, Thompson TM, Lu JJ. The approach to the patient with an unknown overdose. Emerg Med Clin North Am 2007;25(2):249–81. abstract vii.

62. Manini AF, Nair AP, Vedanthan R, et al. Validation of the Prognostic Utility of the Electrocardiogram for Acute Drug Overdose. J Am Heart Assoc 2017; 6(2):e004320.

63. Manini AF, Hoffman RS, Stimmel B, et al. Clinical Risk Factors for In-hospital Adverse Cardiovascular Events After Acute Drug Overdose. Acad Emerg Med 2015;22(5):499–507.

64. Dezfulian C, Orkin AM, Maron BA, et al. Opioid-Associated Out-of-Hospital Cardiac Arrest: Distinctive Clinical Features and Implications for Health Care and Public Responses: A Scientific Statement From the American Heart Association. Circulation 2021;143(16):e836–70.

65. Mattson CL. Trends and Geographic Patterns in Drug and Synthetic Opioid Overdose Deaths — United States, 2013–2019. MMWR Morb Mortal Wkly Rep 2021;70. https://doi.org/10.15585/mmwr.mm7006a4.

66. Gummin DD, Mowry JB, Beuhler MC, et al. 2020 Annual Report of the American Association of Poison Control Centers' National Poison Data System (NPDS): 38th Annual Report. Clin Toxicol Phila Pa 2021;59(12):1282–501.

67. Seger DL, Loden JK. Naloxone reversal of cloni-dine toxicity: dose, dose, dose. Clin Toxicol 2018; 56(10):873–9.

68. Jang DH, Spyres MB, Fox L, et al. Toxin-induced cardiovascular failure. Emerg Med Clin North Am 2014;32(1):79–102.

69. Rotella JA, Greene SL, Koutsogiannis Z, et al. Treatment for beta-blocker poisoning: a systematic review. Clin Toxicol 2020;58(10):943–83.

70. Smolinske S, Hoffman RS, Villeneuve E, et al. Utilization of lipid emulsion therapy in fatal overdose cases: an observational study. Clin Toxicol 2019; 57(3):197–202. https://doi.org/10.1080/15563650. 2018.1504954.

71. Baud FJ, Barriot P, Toffis V, et al. Elevated Blood Cyanide Concentrations in Victims of Smoke Inhalation. N Engl J Med 1991;325(25):1761–6.

72. Buckley NA, Juurlink DN, Isbister G, et al. Hyperbaric oxygen for carbon monoxide poisoning. Cochrane Database Syst Rev 2011;4:CD002041. pub3.

73. Galvagno SM, Nahmias JT, Young DA. Advanced trauma life support® Update 2019: management and applications for adults and special populations. Anesthesiol Clin 2019;37(1):13–32.

74. Burlew CC, Moore EE, Moore FA, et al. Western Trauma Association critical decisions in trauma: Resuscitative thoracotomy. J Trauma Acute Care Surg 2012;73(6):1359–63.

75. Millin MG, Galvagno SM, Khandker SR, et al, Standards and Clinical Practice Committee of the National Association of EMS Physicians (NAEMSP), & Subcommittee on Emergency Services–Prehospital of the American College of Surgeons' Committee on Trauma (ACSCOT). Withholding and termination of resuscitation of adult cardiopulmonary arrest secondary to trauma: Resource document to the joint NAEMSP-ACSCOT position statements. J Trauma Acute Care Surg 2013; 75(3):459–67.

76. Srinivasan V, Nadkarni VM, Helfaer MA, et al, for the American Heart Association National Registry of Cardiopulmonary Resuscitation Investigators. Childhood Obesity and Survival After In-Hospital Pediatric Cardiopulmonary Resuscitation. Pediatrics 2010;125(3):e481–8.

77. CDC. Obesity is a common, serious, and costly disease. Centers for Disease Control and Prevention; 2022. https://www.cdc.gov/obesity/data/adult. html.

78. Aoki M, Hagiwara S, Oshima K, et al. Obesity was associated with worse neurological outcome among Japanese patients with out-of-hospital cardiac arrest. Intensive Care Med 2018;44(5):665–6.

79. Noheria A, Teodorescu C, Uy-Evanado A, et al. Distinctive profile of sudden cardiac arrest in middle-aged vs. older adults: A community-based study. Int J Cardiol 2013;168(4):3495–9.

80. Jayaraman R, Reinier K, Nair S, et al. Risk Factors of Sudden Cardiac Death in the Young. Circulation 2018;137(15):1561–70.

81. Tellson A, Qin H, Erwin K, et al. Efficacy of acute care health care providers in cardiopulmonary resuscitation compressions in normal and obese adult simulation manikins. Proceedings (Baylor University. Medical Center) 2017;30(4):415–8.

82. Di Giacinto I, Guarnera M, Esposito C, et al. Emergencies in obese patients: a narrative review. J Anesth Analg Crit Care 2021;1(1):13.

83. Dargin J, Medzon R. Emergency Department Management of the Airway in Obese Adults. Ann Emerg Med 2010;56(2):95–104.

84. Parker BK, Manning S, Winters ME. The Crashing Obese Patient. West J Emerg Med 2019;20(2): 323–30.

85. Nanson J, Elcock D, Williams M, et al. Do physiological changes in pregnancy change defibrillation energy requirements? Br J Anaesth 2001;87: 237–9.

86. Tan EK, Tan EL. Alterations in physiology and anatomy during pregnancy. Best Pract Res Clin Obstet Gynaecol 2013;27(6):791–802.

87. Einav S, Kaufman N, Sela HY. Maternal cardiac arrest and perimortem caesarean delivery: evidence or expert-based? Resuscitation 2012;83:1191–200.

88. Lipman S, Cohen S, Einav S, Jeejeebhoy F, Mhyre JM, Morrison LJ, Katz V, Tsen LC, Daniels K, Halamek LP, Suresh MS, Arafeh J, Gauthier D, Carvalho JCA, Druzin M, Carvalho B, Society for Obstetric Anesthesia, Perinatology. The Society for Obstetric Anesthesia and Perinatology consensus statement on the management of cardiac arrest in pregnancy. Anesth Analg 2014; 118(5):1003–16.

89. Jeejeebhoy FM, Zelop CM, Lipman S, et al, & American Heart Association Emergency Cardiovascular Care Committee, Council on Cardiopulmonary, Critical Care, Perioperative and Resuscitation, Council on Cardiovascular Diseases in the Young, and Council on Clinical Cardiology. Cardiac Arrest in Pregnancy: A Scientific Statement From the American Heart Association. Circulation 2015;132(18):1747–73.

90. Givertz MM, DeFilippis EM, Colvin M, et al. HFSA/SAEM/ISHLT clinical expert consensus document on the emergency management of patients with ventricular assist devices. J Heart Lung Transplant 2019;38(7):677–98.

91. Milicic D, Ben Avraham B, Chioncel O, et al. Heart Failure Association of the European Society of Cardiology position paper on the management of left ventricular assist device-supported patients for the non-left ventricular assist device specialist healthcare provider: Part 2: at the emergency department. ESC Heart Fail 2021;8(6):4409–24.

92. Amer S, Shah P, Hassan S. Gastrointestinal bleeding with continuous-flow left ventricular assist devices. Clin J Gastroenterol 2015;8(2):63–7.

93. Peberdy MA, Gluck JA, Ornato JP, et al. Cardiopulmonary Resuscitation in Adults and Children With Mechanical Circulatory Support: A Scientific Statement From the American Heart Association. Circulation 2017;135(24):e1115–34.

94. Brady W, Weigand S, Bergin J. Ventricular assist device in the emergency department: Evaluation and management considerations. Am J Emerg Med 2018;36(7):1295–9.

95. Dalen JE, Alpert JS. Natural history of pulmonary embolism. Prog Cardiovasc Dis 1975;17(4):259–70.

96. Varriale P, Maldonado JM. Echocardiographic observations during in hospital cardiopulmonary resuscitation. Crit Care Med 1997;25(10):1717–20.

97. Courtney DM, Kline JA. Prospective use of a clinical decision rule to identify pulmonary embolism as likely cause of outpatient cardiac arrest. Resuscitation 2005;65(1):57–64.

98. Courtney DM, Kline JA. Identification of prearrest clinical factors associated with outpatient fatal pulmonary embolism. Acad Emerg Med Off J Soc Acad Emerg Med 2001;8(12):1136–42.

99. Wu J-P, Gu D-Y, Wang S, et al. Good neurological recovery after rescue thrombolysis of presumed pulmonary embolism despite prior 100 minutes CPR. J Thorac Dis 2014;6(12):E289–93.

100. Böttiger BW, Arntz HR, Chamberlain DA, et al. Thrombolysis during Resuscitation for Out-of-Hospital Cardiac Arrest. N Engl J Med 2008;359(25):2651–62.

101. Fava M, Loyola S, Bertoni H, et al. Massive Pulmonary Embolism: Percutaneous Mechanical Thrombectomy during Cardiopulmonary Resuscitation. J Vasc Intervent Radiol 2005;16(1):119–23.

102. Hobohm L, Sagoschen I, Habertheuer A, et al. Clinical use and outcome of extracorporeal membrane oxygenation in patients with pulmonary embolism. Resuscitation 2022;170:285–92.

Impact of Coronavirus Disease 2019 Pandemic on Cardiac Arrest and Emergency Care

Murtaza Bharmal, MD[a], Kyle DiGrande, MD[a], Akash Patel, MD[a],
David M. Shavelle, MD[b], Nichole Bosson, MD, MPH, NRP, FAEMS[c,d,e,*]

KEYWORDS

- Cardiac arrest • Emergency care • Out-of-hospital cardiac arrest • In-hospital cardiac arrest
- COVID-19 pandemic

KEY POINTS

- The COVID-19 pandemic has increased the incidence of both out-of-hospital and in-hospital cardiac arrest.
- The increase in the incidence of cardiac arrest seems to be multifactorial and related to the severity of COVID-19 in the community, reduced access to health care, and patient delays in seeking care.
- During the COVID-19 pandemic, patient survival and neurologic outcome after both out-of-hospital and in-hospital cardiac arrest were reduced.
- The worse outcome may be related to a combination of factors including reduction in bystander cardiopulmonary resuscitation rates, delays in emergency medical system response times and transport, higher incidence of nonshockable rhythms, and reduced access to emergency and in-hospital care because of COVID-19-related hospitalizations.
- A better understanding of the mechanisms by which COVID-19 has disrupted the chain of survival can direct further effort to mitigate the negative impacts on cardiac arrest and patient outcome. Understanding how the system response to a pandemic can be modified to increase lives saved is essential.

INTRODUCTION

Cardiac arrest continues to be a major public health concern. In the United States, the incidence of out-of-hospital cardiac arrest (OHCA) and in-hospital cardiac arrest (IHCA) are approximately 350,000 and 200,000 per year, respectively.[1,2] Despite significant advances in other areas of cardiovascular medicine, survival from cardiac arrest remains low.[3] Effective treatment of cardiac arrest includes bystander cardiopulmonary resuscitation (CPR), early activation of emergency medical services (EMS), early defibrillation, advanced cardiovascular life support, and postresuscitation care that includes targeted temperature management and emergency coronary angiography with

This article originally appeared in *Heart Failure Clinics*, Volume 19 Issue 2, April 2023.
^a Department of Cardiology, University of California Irvine Medical Center, 510 E Peltason Drive, Irvine, CA 92697, USA; ^b MemorialCare Heart and Vascular Institute, Long Beach Medical Center, 2801 Atlantic Avenue, Long Beach, CA 90807, USA; ^c Los Angeles County Emergency Medical Services Agency, 10100 Pioneer Boulevard Ste 200, Santa Fe Springs, CA 90670, USA; ^d Department of Emergency Medicine, Harbor-UCLA Medical Center, 1000 W Carson Street, Torrance, CA, 90509, USA; ^e David Geffen School of Medicine at UCLA, 10833 Le Conte Avenue, Los Angeles, CA 90095, USA
* Corresponding author. Los Angeles County EMS Agency, Los Angeles County Emergency Medical Services, 10100 Pioneer Boulevard Ste 200, Santa Fe Springs, CA 90670.
E-mail address: Nbosson@dhs.lacounty.gov

Cardiol Clin 42 (2024) 307–316
https://doi.org/10.1016/j.ccl.2024.02.015

percutaneous coronary intervention in some cases.

Since the emergence of COVID-19 and the global pandemic declared by the World Health Organization on March 11, 2020, there have been more than 230 million confirmed cases around the world with more than 4.8 million deaths.[4] The COVID-19 pandemic has affected the incidence, presentation, care, and outcome of time-sensitive medical conditions including cardiac arrest.[5] Beyond the direct mortality related to the respiratory infection, health care systems have been overwhelmed by COVID-19-related hospitalizations, disruptions to the work force because of infected health care personnel, and logistical challenges related to implementation of strategies to minimize disease transmission. A reduction in elective cardiovascular procedures, shortened length of hospital stay, and longer delays between symptom onset and hospital treatment have also been observed during the COVID-19 pandemic.[6] In this article, the effects of the COVID-19 pandemic on cardiac arrest are presented, considering data from recent clinical studies, with a focus on the contributing factors and implications for improving outcome.

OUT-OF-HOSPITAL CARDIAC ARREST
Incidence

During the COVID-19 pandemic, the incidence of OHCA significantly increased with multiple geographic regions throughout the world reporting similar trends.[7–12] In the United States, various regions noted an increase in OHCA. Rollman and colleagues[7] reported a 21% increase in the incidence of OHCA in Los Angeles County, CA, USA, a diverse population of approximately 10.1 million persons. Matthew and colleagues[9] found a 62% increase in Detroit, MI, USA, using data from the Cardiac Arrest Registry to Enhance Survival (CARES). Lai and colleagues[12] reported an approximately 3-fold higher incidence of OHCA in New York City, NY, USA, a particularly hard-hit area early in the pandemic, which is also among the largest EMS systems in the United States serving a population of approximately 8.4 million (**Fig. 1**). Similarly, in Europe, Baldi and colleagues[10] analyzed data from the Lombardi Cardiac Arrest Registry that included 4 providences in Italy and found a 58% increase in OHCA. Marion and colleagues[8] found a 2-fold increase in OHCA in Paris, France, and the surrounding suburbs. In a meta-analysis of 10 studies with more than 35,000 OHCA events in various geographic regions, Lim and colleagues[13] found a 120% increase in OHCA.

In contrast to the aforementioned studies, several studies found no increase in OHCA.[11,14–16] Huber and colleagues[11] found no significant increase in OHCA within a community in Germany with a low prevalence of COVID-19 infection. Elmer and colleagues[15] also reported no significant increase in OHCA in Pennsylvania, USA, where the prevalence of COVID-19 was low. Chan and colleagues[17] observed communities with different COVID-19 mortality rates and found the incidence of OHCA was higher largely in communities with high COVID-19 mortality. Although these studies in aggregate suggest that the incidence of OHCA is related to the prevalence of COVID-19 infection within the community, it does not follow that patients experiencing OHCA were predominately COVID-19 positive.[18]

Patient and Arrest Characteristics

During the COVID-19 pandemic, there were also notable changes in baseline patient characteristics among those experiencing OHCA. Lai and colleagues[12] found that patients were older, less likely to be white, and more likely to have comorbid conditions, including diabetes mellitus and hypertension, compared with a prepandemic control group. Nonshockable rhythms (asystole and pulseless electrical activity) were also more common. Sultanian and colleagues[19] further evaluated the association between COVID-19 and the initial arrest rhythm; patients with confirmed COVID-19 were less likely to have a shockable rhythm compared with patients who were known to be COVID-19 negative. While Marijon and colleagues[8] did not note significant differences in baseline characteristics, the investigators observed higher rates of OHCA occurring at home, less frequent bystander CPR, and less frequent shockable rhythms. Two systematic reviews, one by Scquizzato and colleagues[20] that included 6 studies and another by Lim and colleagues with many of the same and totaling 10 studies found lower rates of shockable rhythm, lower rates of witnessed arrests, and lower rates of bystander CPR.[21]

Out-of-Hospital Arrest Management

OHCA is a time-critical emergency, with reduced chance of survival for every minute of delay. Multiple studies documented increased EMS response and transport times during the COVID-19 pandemic.[6,8,18,20,22,23] Use of personal protective equipment (PPE) to ensure health care provider safety and reduce transmission of COVID-19 during on-scene resuscitation likely contributed to delays in treatment and transport.[24] Furthermore,

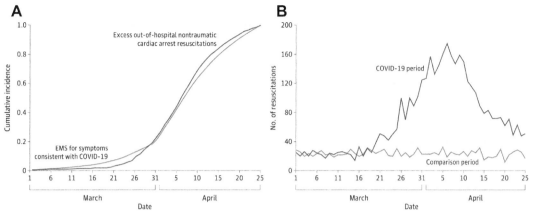

Fig. 1. New York City out-of-hospital nontraumatic cardiac arrest resuscitations, March 1 through April 25, 2020. (*A*) Temporal association between the cumulative percentage of EMS calls for fever, cough, dyspnea, and virallike symptoms consistent with coronavirus disease 2019 (COVID-19) and the number of excess out-of-hospital nontraumatic cardiac arrest resuscitations occurring in New York City in 2020. Excess cases were defined as the daily difference between the number of 2020 and 2019 cases; days with a negative difference were recoded as 0 for graphic presentation. (*B*) The number of daily out-of-hospital nontraumatic cardiac arrest resuscitations. (*From* Lai, P.H., et al., Characteristics Associated With Out-of-Hospital Cardiac Arrests and Resuscitations During the Novel Coronavirus Disease 2019 Pandemic in New York City. JAMA Cardiol, 2020. 5(10): p. 1154-1163.)

workforce reduction due to illness and overwhelmed health care systems leading to longer patient offload times at the hospital resulted in less available resources to respond to time-sensitive emergencies. Changes in resuscitation protocols during the COVID-19 pandemic by various EMS systems in response to resource limitations as well as uncertainties early in the pandemic may have affected prehospital management, response, and transport times.[22,25] Early recommendations, when PPE was scarce, included limiting personnel during the resuscitation, which could have had implications for outcome, and considering the appropriateness of initiation resuscitation.[26] Congruent with the observation of less frequent shockable rhythms, rates of defibrillation were significantly lower during the COVID-19 pandemic.[7] Studies also documented a reduction in attempted resuscitation measures[8]; this was again likely driven by the increase in unfavorable prognostic factors, although a fear of disease transmission by first responders, lack of EMS and hospital resources, and a perception of poor prognosis for COVID-positive patients experiencing OHCA may have contributed.

Outcome

Studies reporting outcome events during the COVID-19 pandemic were consistent and documented lower rates of return of spontaneous circulation (ROSC), less frequent survival to hospital admission, lower survival to hospital discharge, and worse neurologic outcome.[8,9,12,13,20] The

prevalence of COVID-19 infection within the community also seems to be associated with worse outcome for those experiencing OHCA.[17] Chan and colleagues[17] used data from CARES throughout the United States to evaluate the association between OHCA outcomes and the COVID-19 disease burden within geographic areas; whereas ROSC was lower regardless of COVID-19 burden, survival to hospital discharge was primarily lower in communities with moderate to very high COVID-19 mortality rates.

IN-HOSPITAL CARDIAC ARREST
Incidence

Although data are limited, the incidence of IHCA in the United States before the COVID-19 pandemic was estimated at 10 per 1000 admissions.[27] This incidence varies by county and region with reports from the United Kingdom, for example, estimating an incidence of 1.6 per 1000 admissions making comparisons with current pandemic rates challenging.[28] Most recent literature has focused on IHCA occurring among COVID-19-positive patients. The incidence of IHCA seems to have increased during the COVID-19 pandemic, driven by high mortality among patients with COVID-19 and a decrease in hospitalizations for other conditions.[29–33] At the onset of the pandemic, Shao and colleagues[29] reported that 20% experienced IHCA in a consecutive series of patients from Wuhan, China, who required hospitalization for COVID-19 pneumonia. Subsequently, reports from New

York in the United States of hospitalized patients with COVID-19 found IHCA rates of 3% to 7%.[30,31] However, among critically ill patients with COVID-19 in the intensive care unit (ICU), IHCA was more frequent. In a multicenter study from the United States of more than 5000 critically ill patients with COVID-19, 14% suffered IHCA.[32]

The few reports evaluating IHCA rates in non-COVID patients are mixed.[33] In a separate analysis from the aforementioned study, Roedl and colleagues[33] reported a decline in overall hospital admission in Germany during the peak of the pandemic, with an increase in IHCA among all hospitalized patients from the prepandemic era of 4.6% to 6.6% during the pandemic. However, both COVID-positive and COVID-negative patients were included in this study. In a study of only COVID-negative patients in Hong Kong, Tong and colleagues[34] found a decline in IHCA from 1.6 to 1.4 per 1000 admissions before and during the pandemic.

Patient and Arrest Characteristics

Baseline characteristics for patients with IHCA were different during the COVID-19 pandemic compared with the prepandemic era. Studies within the United States found an increased prevalence of IHCA among minorities (black and Hispanic patients) during the COVID-19 pandemic compared with earlier control periods.[30] In addition, studies from multiple geographic regions consistently found a higher prevalence of cardiovascular disease and cardiovascular risk factors in patients with IHCA during the COVID-19 pandemic compared with control periods.[29,31–33] In an evaluation before the pandemic, Andersen and colleagues[28] reported that the underlying cause of arrest was primary cardiac (50%–60%) followed by respiratory. In contrast, the most common cause for arrest in most studies during the pandemic was respiratory and most patients were intubated before the arrest.[29,31,35] Most studies found low rates of a shockable rhythm during the COVID-19 pandemic, ranging from 3% to 18%, similar to prepandemic data.[19,29–32,36] Rates of CPR within the aforementioned studies varied from 50% to 90%.[29,32] In general, time to treatment and resuscitation times were similar during the COVID-19 period compared with prior years.[31,33] When comparing the pandemic period to prepandemic, IHCA more commonly occurred in a general medical ward (as opposed to ICU) in some studies,[29,31] although other studies found higher rates of ICU IHCA during the pandemic.[33] Although location of the arrest has implications for recognition and response time, it may also reflect hospital overcrowding and conversion of non-ICU beds to a semi-ICU setting in some hospital systems and, therefore, would vary by region.

In-Hospital Cardiac Arrest Management

Early in the pandemic, there were little data to inform management. Prone positioning of patients with severe COVID-19, as well as the logistics of maintaining isolation precautions, added further challenges to achieving rapid response and high-quality resuscitation. Several novel treatment approaches were suggested for IHCA during the COVID-19 pandemic, including increased use of mechanical CPR devices, performance of prone CPR, and application of extracorporeal membrane oxygenation (ECMO).[37–39] Each of these presents its own challenges and are not feasible in all health care settings. There are limited data on outcome from prone CPR; however, it has the advantage to reduce delays to initiation of compressions as well as minimizing the complications that could occur from attempting repositioning in the prone patient.[38] ECMO rapidly became a limited resource given the high burden of COVID-19 in many communities and the need for specialty centers with expertise to manage these complicated patients. As such, use of ECMO has been limited to patients with COVID-19 not in cardiac arrest or patients with other causes of IHCA with an overall better prognosis and/or a clear, treatable underlying condition.[37,40]

Outcome

IHCA has a high mortality.[28] Similar to the findings for OHCA, studies reporting outcome events for IHCA during the COVID-19 pandemic were consistent and documented lower rates of ROSC, lower survival to hospital discharge, and worse neurologic outcome.[29,31,32] Survival to hospital discharge ranged from 0% to 14%.[31,32,36] During the peak of the COVID-19 pandemic in Wuhan, China, Shao and colleagues[29] reported 30-day survival of only 2.9%. Hayek and colleagues[32] reported data from a large multicenter registry from the United States and found that survival to hospital discharge was associated with patient age; for those younger than 45 years, survival was 21% compared with only 3% for those older than 80 years. A meta-analysis by Ippolito and colleagues[41] that included 7 studies, with all patients receiving attempted resuscitation, found an in-hospital survival rate of approximately 4%. These low survival rates have led some to question the benefits of performing CPR on patients with COVID-19.[33,42] However, the ability to predict outcome for patients with IHCA is challenging.

The GO-FAR Score (Good Outcome Following Attempted Resuscitation) is a validated scoring system that uses prearrest variables to predict the probability of survival to hospital discharge following IHCA.[43] In the aforementioned study by Aldabagh and colleagues[30] actual survival was compared with the GO-FAR score in 450 patients with IHCA. Unfortunately, COVID-19-positive patients had lower observed survival than predicted by the GO-FAR Score. However, lower survival rates are not entirely consistent across studies; Roedl and colleagues[33] found higher survival in COVID-positive versus COVID-negative patients with IHCA due to respiratory failure, albeit among a small cohort of 43 patients.

The low survival rates for IHCA seems to be multifactorial, related to the presence of the underlying illness at the time of arrest (mechanical ventilation, kidney replacement therapy, or vasopressor support), a high percentage of non-shockable rhythms, lack of therapies to treat the underlying disease process, and potential delays in response time because of isolation procedures, the need to use PPE, and restricted access to COVID-19 units. Improving outcomes of IHCA in patients with COVID-19 will be challenging, because many of the factors associated with poor outcome may not be modifiable. Further investigation into the risks and benefits of performing prolonged CPR in this subset of patients is needed, especially related to the concern for increased aerosolization of viral particles that places health care personnel at increased risk of contracting the infection.

MECHANISM FOR INCREASED CARDIAC ARREST

Multiple different mechanisms have been proposed to explain how the COVID-19 pandemic may have led to the increased incidence and worse outcomes from cardiac arrest. A dichotomy that includes both the direct and indirect effects of COVID-19 is a useful framework to understand this complex interaction[18] (**Table 1**).

Direct Effects of COVID-19

COVID-19 can lead to the occurrence of cardiac arrest throughout multiple pathways. First, the respiratory illness itself with progressive hypoxia from ongoing pneumonia and acute respiratory distress syndrome can trigger cardiac arrest. In addition, particularly in the advanced stages of disease, COVID-19 progresses to a systemic endothelial inflammatory illness with an exaggerated immune response and cytokine storm.[44,45] In patients with preexisting cardiac conditions, this high

Table 1 Direct and indirect effects of coronavirus disease 2019 on cardiac arrest	
Direct Effects	**Indirect Effects**
• Respiratory illness leading to hypoxia • Endothelial inflammatory illness • Exaggerated immune response • Cytokine storm • Vascular thrombosis • Myocarditis • Arrhythmias • Prothrombotic state triggering pulmonary embolism and acute coronary syndrome • Drug treatment causing risk for arrhythmias	• Stringent lockdown measures • Stay-at-home order • Health care reorganization • Reduction in preventive and emergent diagnostic testing and procedures • Overwhelmed EMS and hospital systems • Use of personal protective equipment • Reduction in hospital work force • Delay in patient care • At-risk patients alone more often

Abbreviation: EMS, emergency medical system.

inflammatory burden may induce vascular thrombosis, myocarditis, and cardiac arrhythmias.[46] Even in patients without predisposing conditions, a significant prothrombotic state has been associated with COVID-19 infections with an increased incidence in thromboembolic events including pulmonary embolism and acute coronary syndrome, possibly increasing the risk of cardiac arrest, particularly in the setting of concomitant inflammation.[47,48] Various drug treatments including hydroxychloroquine and azithromycin may further increase the risk of cardiac arrest, particularly in patients with preexisting cardiac conditions.[49]

Indirect Effects of COVID-19

Despite the potential direct effects of COVID-19 on cardiac arrest, the proportion of patients with OHCA with active and/or confirmed COVID-19 infection seems to be relatively low. For example, confirmed and suspected cases of COVID-19 in a French population accounted for only 30% of the observed increase in the incidence of OHCA.[8] Data from the Victorian Ambulance Cardiac Arrest Registry cross-referenced with the Victorian Department of Health and Human Services COVID registry demonstrated less public arrest, less public access defibrillation, lower rates of resuscitation by EMS, longer time to key intervention (defibrillation, epinephrine), and a 50% reduction in survival despite none of the patients in the registry testing positive for COVID-19.[50] These data suggest that the indirect effects may play an equal or even more important role in the increased incidence in and worse outcome from cardiac arrest observed during the COVID-19 pandemic. The potential indirect effects include stringent lockdowns and stay-at-home messaging, health care reorganization, reductions in preventive and emergency procedures, and overwhelmed EMS and hospital systems.

Lockdowns and movement restrictions, along with fear of seeking medical care due to potential exposure to COVID-19, made patients reluctant to seek emergency services, resulting in delayed care and worse outcome. Social restrictions and self-isolation during the pandemic likely caused at-risk patients to be alone more often, thus reducing the occurrence of witnessed arrests and reducing the possibility of bystander CPR[18,51]; this is consistent with a prior study that documented that those living alone were more likely to present with severe complaints and have an increased risk for early mortality.[52] Friedman and Akrenoted a striking increase in overdose-related deaths early in the pandemic, likely due to social isolation leading to both an increased use of substances due to stressors and use of substances while alone.[53]

The COVID-19 pandemic shifted the focus of health care to treatment of those afflicted with the acute respiratory infection while attempting to minimize the spread; this required changes to non-COVID medical care. Health care systems reorganized to accommodate the massive surge of patients with a highly infectious disease. Elective procedures including echocardiograms, cardiovascular stress tests, and coronary angiography were canceled to reallocate resources to COVID-19 treatment, as well as to avoid unnecessary exposure to stable and at-risk patients. During the pandemic, hospitalization rates for congestive heart failure, acute myocardial infarction, and arrhythmias were all lower than those during pre-COVID control periods.[54] Without timely hospitalization and/or prompt medical care, these cardiovascular conditions would be assumed to portend a higher risk for cardiac arrest (**Fig. 2**). Furthermore, early in the pandemic, limitations in PPE and lack of rapid testing availability led to changes to emergency procedures including delaying percutaneous coronary intervention for some patients with ST segment elevation myocardial infarction.[55,56] The psychosocial stress and reluctance to seek care in addition to the limitation of outpatient medical visits and the reduction in elective procedures are all likely contributors to the increased incidence of cardiac arrest.[11,18]

Finally, overwhelmed health care systems experienced challenges in handling the demands of hospitalized patients with COVID-19, in-hospital allocation of resources, and shortages in critical care services, including medical teams, equipment, and ICU bed availability.[6] With less available hospital resources during the pandemic, a higher threshold for hospital admission could have led to more at-risk patients for cardiac arrest being discharged from emergency departments. Response times for EMS were delayed, likely related to an overwhelmed EMS response system, emergency department overcrowding, and the need to use PPE during resuscitation.[12,51] There were also higher rates of nontransport in EMS systems, leaving patients potentially at risk for clinical deterioration.[57]

FUTURE CONSIDERATIONS
Cardiac Arrest Management

Current evidence is uncertain as to whether chest compressions or defibrillation can cause aerosol generalization and increase disease transmission to providers.[58] Airway management is an aerosol-generating procedure most commonly performed by EMS during cardiac arrest resuscitation. Therefore, a careful balance is necessary between the benefits of early resuscitation and the potential for harm to health care providers during resuscitative efforts. Consensus statements from multiple committees agree that chain of survival should be maintained including bystander CPR and public access defibrillation.[58–60] Furthermore, the use of PPE is recommended to ensure the safety of health care professionals during resuscitation, although defibrillation may be considered before donning airborne PPE.

The pandemic has led some to suggest modifications to cardiac arrest care including (1) use of field point-of-care ultrasonography to assess for cardiac standstill as means to supplement prognostication[25]; (2) reduction in the duration of CPR cycle from 2 to 1 minute, given the deterioration in the quality of chest compressions among rescuers wearing PPE[61]; and (3) placement of a towel or mask over the patient's mouth and nose during cardiac resuscitation with compression-only CPR.[60] These modifications may be reasonable as long as they do not interfere with high-quality CPR.

Public Messaging

Particularly early in the pandemic, public health department messaging urged people to stay at home and lockdowns were implemented to reduce movement and potential exposure.

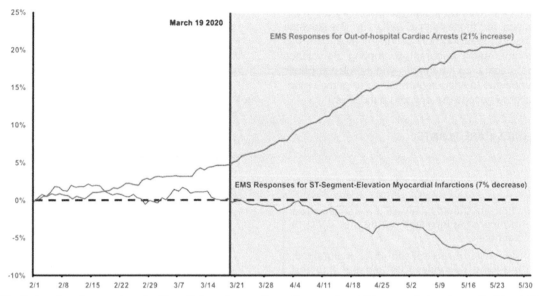

Fig. 2. Los Angeles county out-of-hospital nontraumatic cardiac arrest and ST segment elevation calls, March 19 to May 29, 2020. Significant increase in EMS calls for out-of- hospital cardiac arrest and a significant decrease in EMS call for ST segment elevation myocardial infarction in Los Angeles County, CA, USA. (*From* Rollman, J.E., et al., Emergency Medical Services Responses to Out-of-Hospital Cardiac Arrest and Suspected ST-Segment Elevation Myocardial Infarction During the COVID-19 Pandemic in Los Angeles County. J Am Heart Assoc, 2021. 10(12): p. e019635.)

Although a justifiable and important step to reduce the spread of infection, patients also avoided and minimized visits to outpatient clinics and to hospitals, likely due to this messaging as well as perceived risk of disease contagion. Studies published to date suggest that this resulted in worse outcome for time-sensitive cardiovascular medical conditions including cardiac arrest, ST segment elevation myocardial infarction, and stroke.[7] In response, multiple public messaging campaigns have been initiated.[62] Future messaging should continue to consider the impact on preventative and emergency care and to balance the concern for public and provider safety with the risk of delaying care for time-sensitive emergencies.

System-Level Pandemic Response

Many health care systems became overwhelmed with the surge of patients with acute respiratory illness and when baseline preventative health and emergency services broke down. Delays to both routine and emergency care led to increased severity of illness. Health care systems must consider how to maintain these services while responding to a pandemic surge. Many innovative programs to optimize resources were developed in response to the pandemic and can serve as models for expansion.[63] Building up telemedicine capabilities and mobile-integrated health programs

can help to maintain standard medical care when access to hospital care is limited and/or public concern leads to changes in care-seeking behavior.[64] Dispatch support systems, use of advanced providers for triage, and alternate destinations for transport can optimize deployment of EMS resources to preserve rapid response for time-sensitive emergencies.

SUMMARY

During the COVID-19 pandemic both OHCA and IHCA have increased in incidence while outcomes among patients suffering cardiac arrest are worse. Direct effects of the COVID-19 illness as well as indirect effects of the pandemic on patient's behavior and health care systems have contributed to these changes. Understanding these potential factors offers the opportunity to improve future response and save lives. Fortunately, compared with the first wave of the COVID-19 pandemic, subsequent spikes in COVID-19 incidence seem to show an increase of lesser magnitude of cardiac arrest despite an overall increase in COVID-19 infections. As health care systems have adapted, experience gained from the first wave may have led to better management of patients with COVID-19, allocation of resources, and evaluation of non-COVID medical issues. Efforts at mass vaccination continue and will reduce the severity of disease leading to less severe complications for those with COVID-19. The adverse impact of delaying non-COVID medical care has become readily apparent, prompting the science and medical community to widely release public campaigns to encourage patients to pursue medical care despite the ongoing pandemic.

CLINICS CARE POINTS

- Clinicians should be aware that cardiac arrest incidence has increased during the COVID-19 pandemic.
- The chain of survival should be maintained, including bystander CPR and public access defibrillation.
- Healthcare professionals should use personal protective equipment to reduce risk of exposure during cardiac arrest resuscitation.
- It is important to maintain systems of care during respiratory pandemics in order to reduce harm of delayed access to routine and emergency care.

DISCLOSURE

There are no disclosures from any of the authors.

REFERENCES

1. Virani SS, et al. Heart disease and stroke Statistics-2020 Update: a report from the American heart association. Circulation 2020;141(9):e139–596.
2. Merchant RM, et al. Hospital variation in survival after in-hospital cardiac arrest. J Am Heart Assoc 2014;3(1):e000400.
3. Sasson C, et al. Predictors of survival from out-of-hospital cardiac arrest: a systematic review and meta-analysis. Circ Cardiovasc Qual Outcomes 2010;3(1):63–81.
4. Tracker COVID-19 World Health Organization. 2021. https://covid19.who.int/.
5. Rea T, Kudenchuk PJ. Death by COVID-19: an open investigation. J Am Heart Assoc 2021;10(12):e021764.
6. Kiss P, et al. The impact of the COVID-19 pandemic on the care and management of patients with acute cardiovascular disease: a systematic review. Eur Heart J Qual Care Clin Outcomes 2021;7(1):18–27.
7. Rollman JE, et al. Emergency medical services responses to out-of-hospital cardiac arrest and suspected ST-segment-elevation myocardial infarction during the COVID-19 pandemic in Los Angeles county. J Am Heart Assoc 2021;10(12):e019635.
8. Marijon E, et al. Out-of-hospital cardiac arrest during the COVID-19 pandemic in Paris, France: a population-based, observational study. Lancet Public Health 2020;5(8):e437–43.
9. Mathew S, et al. Effects of the COVID-19 pandemic on out-of-hospital cardiac arrest care in Detroit. Am J Emerg Med 2021;46:90–6.
10. Baldi E, et al. Out-of-Hospital cardiac arrest during the covid-19 outbreak in Italy. N Engl J Med 2020;383(5):496–8.
11. Huber BC, et al. Out-of-hospital cardiac arrest incidence during COVID-19 pandemic in Southern Germany. Resuscitation 2020;157:121–2.
12. Lai PH, et al. Characteristics associated with out-of-hospital cardiac arrests and resuscitations during the novel coronavirus disease 2019 pandemic in New York city. JAMA Cardiol 2020;5(10):1154–63.
13. Lim SL, et al. Incidence and outcomes of out-of-hospital cardiac arrest in Singapore and Victoria: a Collaborative study. J Am Heart Assoc 2020;9(21):e015981.
14. Paoli A, et al. Out-of-hospital cardiac arrest during the COVID-19 pandemic in the Province of Padua, Northeast Italy. Resuscitation 2020;154:47–9.
15. Elmer J, et al. Indirect effects of COVID-19 on OHCA in a low prevalence region. Resuscitation 2020;156:282–3.
16. Sayre MR, et al. Prevalence of COVID-19 in out-of-hospital cardiac arrest: implications for bystander cardiopulmonary resuscitation. Circulation 2020;142(5):507–9.
17. Chan PS, et al. Outcomes for out-of-hospital cardiac arrest in the United States during the coronavirus disease 2019 pandemic. JAMA Cardiol 2021;6(3):296–303.
18. Marijon E, Karam N, Jouven X. Cardiac arrest occurrence during successive waves of the COVID-19 pandemic: direct and indirect consequences. Eur Heart J 2021;42(11):1107–9.
19. Sultanian P, et al. Cardiac arrest in COVID-19: characteristics and outcomes of in- and out-of-hospital cardiac arrest. A report from the Swedish Registry for Cardiopulmonary Resuscitation. Eur Heart J 2021;42(11):1094–106.
20. Scquizzato T, et al. Effects of COVID-19 pandemic on out-of-hospital cardiac arrests: a systematic review. Resuscitation 2020;157:241–7.
21. Lim ZJ, et al. Incidence and outcome of out-of-hospital cardiac arrests in the COVID-19 era: a systematic review and meta-analysis. Resuscitation 2020;157:248–58.
22. Yu JH, et al. Impact of the COVID-19 pandemic on emergency medical service response to out-of-hospital cardiac arrests in Taiwan: a retrospective observational study. Emerg Med J 2021;38(9):679–84.

23. Lim D, et al. The comparison of emergency medical service responses to and outcomes of out-of-hospital cardiac arrest before and during the COVID-19 pandemic in an area of Korea. J Korean Med Sci 2021;36(36):e255.

24. Abrahamson SD, Canzian S, Brunet F. Using simulation for training and to change protocol during the outbreak of severe acute respiratory syndrome. Crit Care 2006;10(1):R3.

25. Ong J, et al. An international perspective of out-of-hospital cardiac arrest and cardiopulmonary resuscitation during the COVID-19 pandemic. Am J Emerg Med 2021;47:192–7.

26. Edelson DP, et al. Interim Guidance for basic and advanced life support in Adults, Children, and Neonates with suspected or confirmed COVID-19: from the emergency cardiovascular care committee and Get with the guidelines-resuscitation adult and Pediatric task forces of the American heart association. Circulation 2020;141(25):e933–43.

27. Morrison LJ, et al. Strategies for improving survival after in-hospital cardiac arrest in the United States: 2013 consensus recommendations: a consensus statement from the American Heart Association. Circulation 2013;127(14):1538–63.

28. Andersen LW, et al. In-hospital cardiac arrest: a review. JAMA 2019;321(12):1200–10.

29. Shao F, et al. In-hospital cardiac arrest outcomes among patients with COVID-19 pneumonia in Wuhan, China. Resuscitation 2020;151:18–23.

30. Aldabagh M, et al. Survival of in-hospital cardiac arrest in COVID-19 infected patients. Healthcare (Basel) 2021;9(10).

31. Miles JA, et al. Characteristics and outcomes of in-hospital cardiac arrest events during the COVID-19 pandemic: a Single-Center experience from a New York city public hospital. Circ Cardiovasc Qual Outcomes 2020;13(11):e007303.

32. Hayek SS, et al. In-hospital cardiac arrest in critically Ill patients with covid-19. multicenter cohort study. BMJ 2020;371:m3513.

33. Roedl K, et al. Effects of COVID-19 on in-hospital cardiac arrest: incidence, causes, and outcome - a retrospective cohort study. Scand J Trauma Resusc Emerg Med 2021;29(1):30.

34. Tong SK, et al. Effect of the COVID-19 pandemic on cardiac arrest resuscitation practices and outcomes in non-COVID-19 patients. J Intensive Care 2021;9(1):55.

35. Chelly J, et al. OHCA (Out-of-Hospital cardiac arrest) and CAHP (cardiac arrest hospital prognosis) scores to predict outcome after in-hospital cardiac arrest: Insight from a multicentric registry. Resuscitation 2020;156:167–73.

36. Thapa SB, et al. Clinical outcomes of in-hospital cardiac arrest in COVID-19. JAMA Intern Med 2021;181(2):279–81.

37. Worku E, et al. Provision of ECPR during COVID-19: evidence, equity, and ethical dilemmas. Crit Care 2020;24(1):462.

38. Douma MJ, Mackenzie E, Brindley PG, et al. A novel and cost-free solution to ensuring adequate chest compressions. Resuscitation 2020;152:93–4.

39. Poole K, et al. Mechanical CPR: who? When? How? Crit Care 2018;22(1):140.

40. Shaefi S, et al. Extracorporeal membrane oxygenation in patients with severe respiratory failure from COVID-19. Intensive Care Med 2021;47(2):208–21.

41. Ippolito M, et al. Mortality after in-hospital cardiac arrest in patients with COVID-19: a systematic review and meta-analysis. Resuscitation 2021;164:122–9.

42. Mahase E, Kmietowicz Z. Covid-19: Doctors are told not to perform CPR on patients in cardiac arrest. BMJ 2020;368:m1282.

43. Rubins JB, Kinzie SD, Rubins DM. Predicting outcomes of in-hospital cardiac arrest: retrospective US validation of the Good outcome following attempted resuscitation Score. J Gen Intern Med 2019;34(11):2530–5.

44. Libby P, Luscher T. COVID-19 is, in the end, an endothelial disease. Eur Heart J 2020;41(32): 3038–44.

45. Fried JA, et al. The variety of cardiovascular presentations of COVID-19. Circulation 2020;141(23): 1930–6.

46. Madjid M, et al. Potential effects of Coronaviruses on the cardiovascular system: a review. JAMA Cardiol 2020;5(7):831–40.

47. Fauvel C, et al. Pulmonary embolism in COVID-19 patients: a French multicentre cohort study. Eur Heart J 2020;41(32):3058–68.

48. Klok FA, et al. Incidence of thrombotic complications in critically ill ICU patients with COVID-19. Thromb Res 2020;191:145–7.

49. Mercuro NJ, et al. Risk of QT interval Prolongation associated with Use of hydroxychloroquine with or without concomitant azithromycin among hospitalized patients testing positive for coronavirus disease 2019 (COVID-19). JAMA Cardiol 2020;5(9):1036–41.

50. Ball J, et al. Collateral damage: Hidden impact of the COVID-19 pandemic on the out-of-hospital cardiac arrest system-of-care. Resuscitation 2020;156: 157–63.

51. Baldi E, et al. COVID-19 kills at home: the close relationship between the epidemic and the increase of out-of-hospital cardiac arrests. Eur Heart J 2020; 41(32):3045–54.

52. Holt-Lunstad J, et al. Loneliness and social isolation as risk factors for mortality: a meta-analytic review. Perspect Psychol Sci 2015;10(2):227–37.

53. Friedman J, Akre S. COVID-19 and the drug overdose Crisis: Uncovering the Deadliest Months in the United States, January-July 2020. Am J Public Health 2021;111(7):1284–91.

54. Gluckman TJ, et al. Case rates, treatment approaches, and outcomes in acute myocardial infarction during the coronavirus disease 2019 pandemic. JAMA Cardiol 2020;5(12):1419–24.

55. Jain V, et al. Management of STEMI during the COVID-19 pandemic: Lessons learned in 2020 to prepare for 2021. Trends Cardiovasc Med 2021; 31(3):135–40.

56. Hakim R, Motreff P, Range G. [COVID-19 and STEMI]. Ann Cardiol Angeiol (Paris) 2020;69(6): 355–9.

57. Harrison NE, et al. Factors associated with Voluntary Refusal of emergency medical system transport for emergency care in Detroit during the early Phase of the COVID-19 pandemic. JAMA Netw Open 2021;4(8):e2120728.

58. Perkins GD, et al. International Liaison Committee on Resuscitation: COVID-19 consensus on science, treatment recommendations and task force insights. Resuscitation 2020;151:145–7.

59. Nolan JP, et al. European Resuscitation Council COVID-19 guidelines executive summary. Resuscitation 2020;153:45–55.

60. Craig S, et al. Management of adult cardiac arrest in the COVID-19 era: consensus statement from the Australasian College for Emergency Medicine. Med J Aust 2020;213(3):126–33.

61. Malysz M, et al. An optimal chest compression technique using personal protective equipment during resuscitation in the COVID-19 pandemic: a randomized crossover simulation study. Kardiol Pol 2020; 78(12):1254–61.

62. Caltabellotta T, et al. Characteristics associated with patient delay during the management of ST-segment elevated myocardial infarction, and the influence of awareness campaigns. Arch Cardiovasc Dis 2021; 114(4):305–15.

63. Monaghesh E, Hajizadeh A. The role of telehealth during COVID-19 outbreak: a systematic review based on current evidence. BMC Public Health 2020;20(1):1193.

64. Demeke HB, et al. Trends in Use of telehealth among health centers during the COVID-19 pandemic - United States, June 26-November 6, 2020. MMWR Morb Mortal Wkly Rep 2021;70(7):240–4.

Out-of-Hospital Cardiac Arrest

Ryan B. Gerecht, MD[a], Jose V. Nable, MD, NRP[b],*

KEYWORDS

- Cardiac arrest • EMS • Prehospital • CPR • Airway management
- Out-of-hospital cardiac arrest (OHCA)

KEY POINTS

- High-quality CPR includes an appropriate compression rate of 100 to 120 bpm, a compression depth of at least 2 inches in adults, minimizing excessive ventilations, allowing for full chest recoil, and a chest compression fraction of at least 80%.
- Pit crew CPR is a highly choreographed approach to OHCA resuscitation, during which specific tasks are preassigned to prehospital providers.
- Immediate endotracheal intubation is deemphasized when resuscitating OHCA, favoring less invasive and easier-to-perform techniques such as supraglottic airway devices.
- Termination of resuscitation protocols empower EMS providers to prioritize their efforts on the scene as opposed to immediate transport, typically resulting in higher quality care by minimizing interruptions in chest compressions.
- When return of spontaneous circulation (ROSC) is achieved, survivors of OHCA continue to require critical care, focused on ensuring adequate cerebral perfusion, as neurologic injury is a significant contributor to either death or poor outcomes following ROSC.

SETTING THE SCENE

Survival from out-of-hospital cardiac arrest (OHCA) is predicated on a community and system-wide approach that includes rapid recognition of cardiac arrest, capable bystander cardiopulmonary resuscitation (CPR), effective basic and advanced life support (BLS and ALS) by EMS providers, and coordinated postresuscitation care. Management of these critically ill patients continues to evolve. This article focuses on the management of OHCA by EMS providers.

CHEST COMPRESSION
High-Performance cardiopulmonary resuscitation

The performance of chest compressions to treat victims of cardiac arrest dates to 1891 when a German Surgeon, Dr Friedrich Maass, described the first successful use of external compressions to achieve the return of spontaneous circulation (ROSC) in 2 young patients who had suffered cardiac arrest in the operating room.[1] Maass noted that direct compression of the heart region at 120 or more compressions per minute resulted in an artificially produced carotid pulse and constriction of the pupils.[1] He was the first to advocate for chest compressions, rather than ventilations alone, to treat those in cardiac arrest. This experience, in addition to experimental animal data, laid the scientific foundation for modern CPR.

Today, the initiation of high-quality or "high-performance" CPR is recognized as the cornerstone of cardiac resuscitation. The most recent American Heart Association (AHA) BLS and ALS guidelines emphasize the importance of immediate

This article originally appeared in *Emergency Medicine Clinics*, Volume 41 Issue 3, August 2023.
a District of Columbia Fire and EMS Department, MedStar Washington Hospital Center, 110 Irving Street Northwest, Washington, DC 20010, USA; b Georgetown University School of Medicine, Georgetown EMS, MedStar Georgetown University Hospital, 3800 Reservoir Road Northwest, Washington, DC 20007, USA
* Corresponding author.
E-mail address: Jose.Nable@georgetown.edu

Cardiol Clin 42 (2024) 317–331
https://doi.org/10.1016/j.ccl.2024.02.014
0733-8651/24/© 2024 Elsevier Inc. All rights reserved.

Box 1
CPR metrics for high-quality resuscitation[2]

Compression rate: 100 to 120/min

Compression depth: at least 2 inches in adults and at least 1/3 the anterior–posterior dimension of the chest in infants and children

Absence of excessive ventilation

Allowing for full chest recoil after each compression

Chest compression fraction greater than 80%

delivery of continuous chest compressions with as few interruptions as possible.[2] In addition, the AHA has identified specific performance metrics that define high-quality CPR (**Box 1**). These CPR metrics have been identified because of their contribution to maximizing blood flow and improving patient outcomes.[3,4] For example, chest compression fraction (CCF) is the proportion of time chest compressions were performed during a cardiac arrest. Data from the Resuscitation Outcomes Consortium Cardiac Arrest Registry (ROCC) indicates that a higher CCF is associated with greater rates of ROSC and survival to hospital discharge.[5,6]

Delivering high-quality CPR in the prehospital environment can be extremely challenging. Chaotic or crowded public scenes, limited personnel or space in which to conduct the resuscitation, provider fatigue, and safety considerations for responders all contribute to the challenges of providing uninterrupted high-quality chest compressions. Numerous publications have highlighted suboptimal CPR performance in the prehospital setting.[7,8]

Pit Crew CPR

To address some of these unique prehospital challenges, many EMS agencies have adopted a so-called pit crew approach to cardiac resuscitation. The name "Pit Crew CPR" comes from the Formula One Racing pit crews that use a highly choreographed, well-defined, and autonomous approach to maximize efficient task completion. In a cardiac arrest resuscitation, this approach assigns each prehospital provider, before arrival on scene, a specific therapeutic task and prespecified location in which to complete this task once patient-side. Examples of these dedicated preassigned tasks include airway management, CPR delivery, monitoring and defibrillation, medication administration, time-keeping, and documentation.

Pit crew CPR is different from a typical team-based approach to resuscitation for at least 3

reasons. The first is that the assignment a provider may assume during the resuscitation is frequently based on when they chronologically arrive on the scene (eg, first paramedic to arrive, second paramedic to arrive, and so forth). The second is that providers are expected to perform their assigned tasks with mastery and autonomy instead of waiting for a team leader to call out or direct the performance of each intervention. The third is the use of choreographed movement between resuscitation positions and the use of standardized communication and commands. EMS protocols for pit crew CPR may differ from agency to agency but the primary goal of utilizing a structured approach to delivering efficient, high-performance CPR in a dynamic environment is the same. The direct effect of a pit crew CPR approach on patient outcomes is difficult to evaluate but has been associated in one large EMS system, as a part of a bundle of best practices, to improve CPR performance metrics, patient survival, and neurologic outcome.[9]

The pit crew approach to CPR does come with notable considerations. The ideal number and/or certification level of EMS providers needed to maximize survival from OHCA is unclear.[10] There may also be an association between the frequency of paramedic exposure to OHCA resuscitation and patient survival. Specifically, a large prehospital study from Australia found patient survival from OHCA significantly increased with the number of OHCAs that responding paramedics had treated in the previous 3 years.[11] In addition, they found that cardiac arrest survival was lower when paramedics had not treated an OHCA during the preceding 6 months. Exposure to either frequent OHCA cases or resuscitation training on a periodic basis is necessary to prevent skill deterioration. Finally, although pit crew CPR emphasizes team members completing tasks with autonomy, the literature suggests that cultivating leadership skills of team leaders via training is associated with improved CPR performance.[12,13] See **Fig. 1** for an example of pit crew resuscitation.

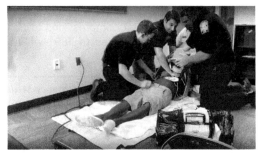

Fig. 1. Example of Pit Crew CPR utilizing preassigned roles (DC Fire and EMS).

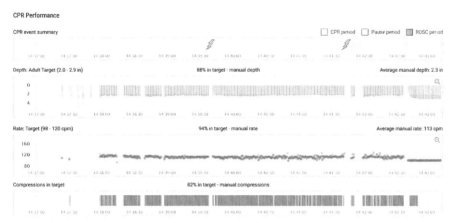

Fig. 2. Sample CPR data collected on modern prehospital monitors (DC Fire and EMS). Adapted from Bystander Use of AEDs Could Double the Number of Survivors. https://www.sca-aware.org/sca-news/bystander-use-of-aeds-could-double-the-number-of-survivors.

Real-Time CPR Feedback

Real-time audio and/or visual feedback on CPR performance is being increasingly used to improve CPR quality during OHCA. Considered one of the more meaningful advances in resuscitation practice in the last 2 decades, cardiac monitors commonly used by EMS providers can integrate with a chest compression sensor or accelerometer to measure the rate, depth, and appropriate release of each compression.[3] The information from the sensor is then analyzed by the monitor and feedback is provided, indicating whether to maintain current performance or increase the rate and/or depth of compressions. Such feedback improves chest compression performance in both human and simulated manikin studies.[14] See **Fig. 2** for an example of CPR data collected on modern monitors. However, the direct effect of audiovisual feedback on patient outcomes is not as clear. A 2020 ICLOR systematic review found that while most studies did not find a significant association between real-time feedback and improved patient outcomes, a few studies did demonstrate clinically important improvement in survival.[2,15,16]

Mechanical CPR

Prolonged, uninterrupted, chest compressions can lead to diminishing performance due to provider fatigue. As such, an increasing number of EMS systems are deploying mechanical chest compression devices. The first mechanical CPR device was introduced in the 1960s and used a pneumatic piston mechanism. Over time, mechanical CPR in the out-of-hospital setting has evolved to include two main devices. The first is the Lund University Cardiopulmonary Assist Device (LUCAS) by Stryker Medical, a battery-powered piston device attached to a suction cup placed on the chest wall. The piston compresses the patient's chest and uses the suction cup to ensure active decompression and chest recoil. The second is the AutoPulse Resuscitation System by Zoll, a battery-powered vest device that uses an electric motor to pull a load-distributing band that encircles the patient's chest, in a rhythmic motion. Regardless of the device used, they both aim to serve a similar function-to deliver continuous compressions at a consistent rate and depth, eliminate responder fatigue, and provide an opportunity to reduce the frequency and length of pauses in compressions.

Studies of mechanical CPR devices have not demonstrated a clear benefit in patient outcomes when compared with high-quality manual CPR. The AHA provides a level 3: no benefit, recommendation for the routine use of mechanical CPR devices.[2] A 2018 Cochrane Systematic Review of 11 trials including 12,944 adult patients concluded that the bulk of evidence from randomized control trials suggests that CPR involving mechanical chest compression devices produce similar clinical outcomes compared to manual CPR.[17]

Despite the clinical equivalency to manual CPR and the significant financial cost of purchasing a mechanical CPR device, many EMS agencies have still adopted this technology. Situations in the out-of-hospital environment whereby providing reliable, high-quality manual compressions is not consistently possible or may pose risk to responders are not uncommon. Examples include scenes with limited personnel, patients requiring prolonged on-scene resuscitation attempts, and performing CPR in the back of a moving ambulance when transport is indicated. These logistical considerations and obstacles to providing high-quality CPR in the out-of-hospital setting led the AHA to provide a 2B recommendation for use of mechanical CPR devices in specific settings when high-quality manual compressions are not possible.[2]

Deployment of mechanical CPR devices during the early phase (first 5 minutes) of resuscitation may be associated with harm due to interruptions in compressions and delaying the defibrillation of shockable rhythms.[18] These devices typically require positioning a back plate under the patient, connecting and adjusting the compression mechanism, and initiating the device in a logistically challenging environment while continuing manual chest compressions, a process often resulting in unacceptably long pauses in compressions.[19,20]

Thus, it is imperative that EMS agencies engage in training that focuses on minimizing pauses in CPR during device deployment. A standardized team approach incorporating a choreographed application of the mechanical CPR device, followed by debriefing can significantly reduce the hands-off chest time. One study found that a quality improvement initiative focused on minimizing pauses during device application decreased compression pauses from a median of 21 to 7 seconds.[21]

Heads up CPR

The basic technique and foundational principles of CPR have not changed significantly since Maass's first description in 1891. However, a new area of active research is the concept of performing CPR with the patient's head elevated. First described in 2014 in a swine model of cardiac arrest, investigators found that a head-up tilt position during CPR significantly increased coronary and cerebral perfusion pressure while decreasing intracranial pressure.[22] A recent meta-analysis of 7 swine studies showed a statistically significant association between heads-up CPR and increased cerebral blood flow, cerebral perfusion pressure, and coronary perfusion pressure compared to conventional CPR.[23]

Although a few EMS agencies have implemented some variation of heads-up CPR, to date outcome data from human trials is limited and many questions remain regarding how to best implement heads-up CPR in a human OHCA population.[24,25] Currently unclear is the optimal head-up CPR height, timing of head elevation during the cardiac arrest, speed of head elevation, head and torso elevation versus whole body elevation, and whether additional specialized resuscitation equipment is needed (eg, impedance threshold device).[23,26] Despite these evolving questions and the need for further human outcome data, heads-up CPR is an exciting and important area of future research.

AIRWAY MANAGEMENT
Timing of Airway Management

Since the 2010 iteration of the AHA guidelines, the premise of immediate endotracheal intubation for patients experiencing cardiac arrest has been challenged.[27] Historically, intubation was considered a paramount goal during resuscitation. The famed mantra of "A-B-C's" (airway-breathing-circulation) has been modified to C-A-B to emphasize circulation because of a deeper and more nuanced understanding of the physiology of cardiac arrest. Resuscitation efforts have thus shifted initial emphasis toward performing high-quality, uninterrupted chest compressions and prompt defibrillation (when necessary) as opposed to immediate invasive airway management. The most recent AHA guidelines continue to deemphasize immediate endotracheal intubation.[2]

Advanced airway management, such as endotracheal intubation, continues to be a challenging manual skill and requires a complex decision-making process, even for the most veteran airway providers.[28] The timing of when (and if) to ultimately perform advanced airway management remains unclear.[29] Advanced techniques can detract providers from focusing on high-quality chest compressions, thereby reducing the survival benefits associated with a high chest compression fraction.[30] Noninvasive techniques are often faster and require less technical expertise, without potentially compromising patient outcomes.[31]

Passive Oxygen Insufflation

Positive pressure ventilation (PPV) via an endotracheal tube, supraglottic airway, or BVM is considered a mainstay of CPR. However, a retrospective study challenged this notion, finding passive insufflation via face mask to be superior to bag-valve-mask (BVM) ventilation in patients with a witnessed arrest.[32] The investigators found passive oxygen insufflation was associated with an increased rate of survival to hospital discharge neurologically intact. The study is limited by its retrospective design, and AHA guidelines do not currently recommend against PPV. However, this study does call attention to the potential risks associated with PPV during OHCA, such as hyperventilation, which can lead to increased intrathoracic pressure and decreased coronary perfusion pressure.[33]

Noninvasive Airway Management

BVM ventilation has been considered foundational through multiple iterations of the AHA guidelines. Since the 2010 guidelines, rescuers have been instructed to start with compressions before initiating rescue breaths.[34] When providing rescue breaths via BVM ventilation, providers should aim for a tidal volume sufficient enough to result in chest rise, typically 500 to 600 mL in adults.[2,35] In unresponsive patients without a gag reflex, it is reasonable to utilize oropharyngeal or nasopharyngeal airways to facilitate ventilation and reduce airway resistance associated with the tongue obstructing the airway.[36] While previously a mainstay in airway management, the use of cricoid pressure to reduce aspiration or improve ventilation is without evidence. Cricoid pressure, in several studies, is paradoxically associated with airway obstruction.[37,38]

Supraglottic airway (SGA) devices can attenuate some of the concerns associated with endotracheal intubation. These devices typically require less training to effectively deploy in the out-of-hospital environment (sometimes even being used by basic life support EMTs). Additionally, the use of an SGA is usually simpler and faster than traditional endotracheal intubation.[39] Lastly, an SGA is easily placed while providing uninterrupted high-quality chest compressions. This contrasts with endotracheal intubation, which can lead to harmful lengthy pauses in CPR, with one study finding an average total duration of intubation-associated interruption of 109.5 seconds.[40]

Indeed, a 2019 AHA focused update on ACLS guidelines stated that the use of SGA devices is reasonable in EMS systems with low endotracheal success rates or few training opportunities for intubation.[41] Even in systems with optimal training opportunities or high success rates, the same guidelines note that either endotracheal intubation or SGA may be used.

Endotracheal Intubation

Endotracheal intubation is an infrequently utilized skill in the prehospital setting. One study of 42 EMS systems found that nearly a third of intubations required more than 1 attempt.[42] Intubation can result in valuable time and resources being diverted from other crucial interventions, such as chest compressions and timely defibrillation. And each attempt increases the likelihood of complications such as hypoxia and airway trauma.

An important US based randomized control trial of OHCA airway management found that a strategy of initial SGA insertion was associated with improved 72-h survival, survival to hospital discharge, and favorable neurologic status at discharge as compared to initial airway management via intubation.[43] Furthermore, a UK-based randomized control trial of OHCA airway management found no difference in the primary outcome of survival to hospital discharge with favorable functional outcomes when comparing an initial SGA versus intubation approach.[31] This suggests that intubation, in nearly all cases of OHCA, should be deemphasized. If endotracheal intubation is performed, the timing of this advanced airway procedure may have crucial implications for the patient's survival. Establishing adequate coronary perfusion pressure through high-quality chest compressions is critical to achieving good outcomes.[44] Therefore, initial resuscitation efforts should not routinely focus on intubation.

It may be appropriate to consider intubation when ventilation cannot be adequately achieved via SGA or BVM. The 2019 ACLS guidelines also note that if advanced airway management might interrupt chest compressions, it is reasonable to defer intubation until after initial CPR efforts have not resulted in immediate ROSC.[41] In systems in which providers perform intubation, frequent retraining on this relatively uncommonly utilized skill is essential.[45] Additionally, video laryngoscopy in the prehospital setting has been shown to increase rates of first-pass success, though with an unclear mortality benefit.[46,47]

VASCULAR ACCESS

While intravenous (IV) access has long been the mainstay for medication delivery, the relatively expedient technique of intraosseous (IO) access has led to its increasing use during cardiac arrest. Particularly in the out-of-hospital environment, the fast and high first-attempt success rate afforded by IO access makes it an appealing method for delivering emergency medication therapy.[48] Therefore, EMS agencies commonly make IO placement their first-line management technique to obtain vascular access.[49]

Recent evidence, however, suggests that the delivery of medications via IV access is associated with better rates of ROSC, survival to hospital discharge, and more favorable neurologic outcome as compared to IO-delivered medications.[50] The quality of this evidence, though, is low. The faster and increased first-pass success of IO placement may balance out the clinical benefits of IV placement. Indeed, depending on the experience of the prehospital provider, focusing on IV access may result in delays to key pharmacologic interventions during cardiac arrest, or distract from more important interventions such as high-quality CPR or rhythm recognition and defibrillation as needed. It, therefore, remains reasonable for EMS systems to continue emphasizing IO access if immediate IV placement is not feasible or unsuccessful.[3]

MEDICATION MANAGEMENT
Epinephrine

The administration of vasopressors during OHCA has long been included in resuscitation algorithms from the AHA. While epinephrine has been commonly used for decades, its effectiveness has also been debated. The α-adrenergic properties of epinephrine have been hypothesized to improve both coronary and cerebral perfusion. However, it is also arrhythmogenic and may increase myocardial oxygen needs.[51]

The most recent iteration of ACLS strengthened the administration of epinephrine to a recommendation from a suggestion.[2] This is primarily due to a large systematic review of the literature which found that epinephrine improves chances of achieving ROSC, survival to hospital discharge, and survival at 3 months postarrest.[52] The review found this improvement to be largest in patients with nonshockable rhythms. It is therefore reasonable to prioritize epinephrine administration in these patients, whereas defibrillation continues to be emphasized as first-line therapy in patients with shockable rhythms.[51]

Antiarrhythmics

Antiarrhythmics, such as lidocaine or amiodarone, have not been demonstrated to be beneficial for overall long-term survival or survival with good neurologic outcomes.[53] These medications, however, do show benefits for achieving ROSC or short-term survival to hospital admission.[54,55] It is therefore not unreasonable to consider antiarrhythmics in shock-resistant ventricular fibrillation (VF) or pulseless ventricular tachycardia (VT).[2] Magnesium is also commonly used for torsades de pointes, though its benefit has mostly been seen in noncontrolled studies.[56]

DEFIBRILLATION

Survival from VF or pulseless VT is highly dependent on prompt defibrillation.[2] Responding providers should also minimize interruptions to CPR in the peri-defibrillation period, as adequate chest compressions are also vital. Nearly half of patients who are defibrillated, however, remain in a shock-refractory rhythm. A recent randomized trial found that double sequential external defibrillation (DSED) or vector-change (VC) defibrillation (in which defibrillator pads are moved to the anterior–posterior position) for OHCA patients with shock-resistant VF are associated with improved survival to hospital discharge as compared to standard defibrillation.[57] DSED was also associated with better neurologic outcomes.

END-TIDAL CO2 MONITORING

Monitoring end-tidal CO2 during cardiac arrest resuscitation provides rescuers with valuable and actionable information. When the partial pressure of CO2 (P_{ETCO2}) remains less than 10 mm Hg despite CPR in intubated patients, achieving ROSC is unlikely.[58,59] This suggests that CO2 monitoring can be used to guide providers with respect to the continuation of resuscitative efforts. Conversely, a sudden increase in P_{ETCO2} to a normal range (35–40 mm Hg) may indicate a return of cardiac output and the presence of ROSC.[60]

RETURN OF SPONTANEOUS CIRCULATION CARE

When ROSC is achieved, survivors of OHCA continue to require critical care crucial to long-term survival with favorable outcomes. Much of this care focuses on ensuring adequate cerebral perfusion, as neurologic injury is a significant contributor to either death or poor outcomes following ROSC.[61] Post-ROSC care also includes ventilatory management, targeted temperature management (when appropriate), and identifying and treating underlying causes of cardiac arrest.

Hemodynamic Support

Hypotension is not uncommon following ROSC, with one large study finding nearly half of the resuscitated patients experience post-ROSC hypotension within an hour of arriving in the ICU.[62] Hypotension, however, is associated with diminished chances of survival and less favorable neurologic outcomes.[63] Hemodynamic support in the post-ROSC period must therefore focus on avoiding low blood pressures, with many studies defining hypotension as SBP less than 90 mm Hg or MAP less than 65 mm Hg. In addition to assessing fluid status, prehospital providers must evaluate the need for vasopressor and/or inotropic support.

Ventilator Management

There is a delicate balance in achieving adequate oxygenation. Hypoxia may result in anoxic brain injury whereas hyperoxia may cause the generation of oxygen free radicals, likewise damaging brain tissue.[64] In one study, post-ROSC hyperoxia (defined as $Pa_{O_2} > 300$ mm Hg) was associated with an increased risk of death.[65] The 2020 AHA guidelines suggest targeting oxygen saturations to a range of 92% to 98%.[2] Just as during the resuscitation phase of cardiac arrest management, post-ROSC care should consider how PPV affects a patient's hemodynamic status. Hyperventilation, for example, may lead to hypotension.

Targeted Temperature Management

Induced hypothermia has been considered a part of post-ROSC care for over a decade, following initial studies demonstrating improved neurologic function.[66,67] The optimal target temperature, however, remains unclear. For example, one randomized prospective trial found no difference in mortality or neurologic outcome in patients targeted to either 33°C or 36°C.[68] Additionally, the initiation of targeted temperature management in the prehospital setting (especially when done via rapid infusion with chilled IV fluids) has been associated with no improvement in outcomes and increased risk of re-arrest.[69–71] Given inconclusive evidence of its benefit in the prehospital setting, it is reasonable for EMS to defer targeted temperature management initiation until the patient arrives at the receiving hospital facility.

TERMINATION OF RESUSCITATION

Given the overall low rates of survival from OHCA, prehospital providers must remain mindful of when resuscitation efforts have become futile. EMS agencies should utilize validated termination of resuscitation (TOR) criteria to determine when resuscitative efforts should be discontinued in the prehospital setting. One of the most studied sets of criteria is the basic life support (BLS) TOR rule.[72] These guidelines suggest that resuscitation efforts can end when all of the following are met: (1) arrest was not witnessed by EMS or first responders, (2) no ROSC achieved before transport, and (3) no shocks delivered.[73] The advanced life support (ALS) TOR rule suggests that resuscitation efforts may cease if all the following criteria are met: (1) arrest was not witnessed by EMS, (2) arrest not witnessed by bystander, (3) bystander CPR not performed, (4) no shock delivered, and (5) no ROSC achieved before transport after ALS care.[74] The duration of resuscitative efforts, however, remains unclear. One retrospective study examining the BLS TOR rule found that 90% of patients who survived to discharge achieved ROSC by 20 minutes, and 99% within 37 minutes.[75] See **Table 1**, comparing the BLS versus ALS TOR rules.

Table 1
Comparing the BLS and ALS TOR criteria[72,75]

BLS Termination of Resuscitation Rules	ALS Termination of Resuscitation Rules
• Arrest not witnessed by EMS • No ROSC achieved before transport • No shocks delivered	• Arrest not witnessed by EMS • Arrest not witnessed by bystander • Bystander CPR not performed • No shock delivered • No ROSC achieved before transport

---

Additionally, transporting patients in cardiac arrest is not without risks. These situations are associated with a higher risk of ambulance crashes, especially as such transports routinely utilize red lights and sirens, potentially harming prehospital providers, their patients, and members of the public.[76,77] Chest compression quality is also worse during ambulance transport.[78] It is also rare for patients to survive OHCA unless ROSC is achieved in the field.[79] TOR protocols thus empower prehospital providers to remain on scene, providing safer and higher quality resuscitation.

In certain scenarios, transportation to the hospital may be appropriate, irrespective of whether ROSC is achieved in the field. For example, the resuscitation of drowning victims even after a prolonged submersion is possible, though not common.[80] It is therefore reasonable to consider transporting drowning victims to the hospital. Additionally, pregnant patients may benefit from immediate transport for the performance of a resuscitative hysterotomy.

When TOR occurs in the prehospital setting, EMS providers become instrumental in the death notification of the decedent's family members. Unfortunately, many prehospital providers report that their training is often inadequate to comfortably perform this task.[81] EMS agencies should therefore develop robust training programs for these situations.

Withholding Resuscitation

Historically, EMS providers have been hesitant to withhold resuscitative efforts when encountering OHCA. The traditional concern has been that deciding not to attempt resuscitation is both a lethal and permanent decision and that an initial attempt at resuscitation can always be stopped later. However, as the practice of EMS medicine has matured, this concern has been challenged.

Today, there are widely accepted situations whereby withholding resuscitative efforts is appropriate given the clinical presentation and/or known patient preferences. The frequency of EMS withholding resuscitation varies significantly by individual agency. In a population-based retrospective study using data from 129 EMS agencies and 86,912 OHCA's in the ROC EPISTRY, the proportion of all OHCA patients not receiving a resuscitation attempt ranged from 0% to 76.1% with an overall withhold rate across all agencies of 45.2%.[82] This is similar to a large cardiac arrest registry database publication from British Columbia, whereby 45% of all OHCA did not receive EMS resuscitation.[83]

The most common situation when EMS withholds resuscitation is due to obvious death. Obvious death is typically defined as the presence of rigor mortis, lividity, body decomposition, decapitation, or burned beyond recognition. In one study, signs of obvious death constituted 80% of the cardiac arrests that did not receive a resuscitation attempt.[83] Local protocols should specify what constitutes medical futility and when EMS providers should and should not initiate resuscitation. In addition, local protocols should detail the specific logistical and administrative tasks that EMS providers must complete after withholding resuscitation (eg, notification of law enforcement and/or the medical examiner).

The second most common situation when EMS withholds resuscitation is due to a do not resuscitate (DNR) order, typically in the form of a state-recognized document such as a Physician Orders for Life-Sustaining Treatment (POLST form). Although the EMS system was designed to respond to emergencies and prevent death, EMS providers must consider the patient's right to autonomy. All 50 states and the District of Columbia authorize some form of out-of-hospital DNR order. However, each EMS jurisdiction may vary in what documentation is required to be present on scene to withhold resuscitation. Traditionally, a fully executed DNR order has been required. When this documentation is lacking or when resuscitation wishes are conveyed by alternative documentation or by verbal request, EMS providers are often mandated to begin resuscitation efforts.[84] This is a potential area for improvement as an unwanted resuscitation attempt violates the patient's right to autonomy, may cause suffering and emotional injury to the patient and the family, is distressing for EMS providers, and unnecessarily expends resources.

Specifically, withholding resuscitation based on verbal requests of family members or caregivers, in the absence of an executed DNR order or the ability of the patient to convey preferences, is not widespread. As many as 50% to 70% of DNR requests to EMS occur verbally without formal written DNR documentation.[85,86] EMS agencies in King County, Washington, the District of Columbia, Los Angeles County, and Southeastern Ontario, among others, now have protocols permitting verbal DNR requests from family and other surrogate decision makers[86–88]

As an example of these protocols, EMS providers in King County, WA are allowed to withhold resuscitation if the patient has a preexisting terminal condition and the patient, family, or caregivers indicate, in writing or verbally, that the patient did not want resuscitation.[86] Implementation of these guidelines was associated with a statistically significant increase in the number of resuscitations withheld. After protocol implementation, honoring verbal DNR requests represented 53% of withheld resuscitations among the participating agencies.[86] The authors of the King County experience found that participating EMS providers had no significant difficulties in making decisions about withholding resuscitation based on a verbal request. Furthermore, the EMS providers reported that there were no complaints or disagreements among family members or other persons on the scene when resuscitation efforts were withheld.[86] A similar level of EMS provider and surrogate decision-maker comfort with withholding resuscitation was also seen in Southern Ontario.[87]

TRANSPORTATION CONSIDERATIONS

When transporting patients who achieve ROSC, careful consideration as to whereby the patient should be transported is appropriate. Similar to the regionalization of care for patients suffering stroke, STEMI, or trauma, there is increasing evidence that transporting patients who have experienced nontraumatic OHCA to specialized cardiac arrest receiving facilities may be associated with improved outcomes including survival with good neurologic function.[89] A 2019 focused AHA update noted the reasonableness of transporting postarrest patients directly to regionalized cardiac arrest centers when the local receiving facility does not offer comprehensive post-ROSC care.[90]

A 12-lead ECG should also be obtained as soon as feasible following ROSC. Patients with STEMI following resuscitation should ideally be transported to PCI-capable facilities as emergent coronary angiography has been associated with a near doubling in the rate of favorable neurologic outcomes.[91]

DC Fire and EMS Pre-Hospital Treatment Protocols

Treatment Protocols - Resuscitation

Refractory VF/VT | 4.4

Goal: < 15 min on scene. Arrive in ED within 30 min of patient collapse	
Criteria	**Yes?**
Witnessed Cardiac Arrest	
Rapid Bystander CPR (within 5 minutes of collapse)	
Initial shockable rhythm (includes shock by AED prior to ALS arrival)	
Refractory VF/pVT unresponsive to at least 3 defibrillations and amiodarone or lidocaine	
No evidence of trauma as the cause for cardiac arrest.	
Not hemorrhaging (e.g., GI bleeding, significant trauma)	
Age 18–70 years old	
Good baseline functional status (living independently- not a long-term care facility resident)	
No prior neurocognitive dysfunction (e.g., dementia)	
No signs of end stage disease • Renal failure with dialysis • Liver Failure • Terminal cancer	
Mechanical CPR device is available on scene for transport	
LUCAS device fits on patient	
$ETCO_2$ > 10 mm/Hg with CPR	
Estimated arrival at ECMO capable ED within 30 minutes of collapse	

If all above criteria are met, patient is a _potential_ ECMO candidate. Notify ECMO capable receiving facility as soon as possible.

Fig. 3. Sample ECPR protocol from DC Fire and EMS.

Extracorporeal CPR (ECPR) via extracorporeal membrane oxygenation (ECMO) has also become increasingly used to manage patients with refractory ventricular fibrillation OHCA.[92] The technique, though, is not without controversy given its cost, heavy resource utilization, and logistical challenges for implementation.[93,94] Selecting the subset of patients who would benefit from ECPR is also unclear.[95] The 2020 AHA guidelines note the lack of sufficient evidence to recommend routine use of EPCR.[2]

There is increasing data in the literature, though, to support this cutting-edge treatment modality. A randomized controlled study at the University of Minnesota was terminated early due to the superiority of an ECMO-based resuscitation being associated with survival to hospital discharge as compared to standard ACLS.[96] Additional studies are needed to identify what types of reversible causes of OHCA and the patient population for which ECPR is most useful. See **Fig. 3** for an example of an ECPR protocol in the District of Columbia for patients with refractory ventricular fibrillation or ventricular tachycardia.

FUTURE IMPROVEMENT

High-performing EMS systems not only focus on the immediate care of individual patients in cardiac arrest but also work to improve future system performance. Two processes utilized by EMS agencies to facilitate improvement are postevent

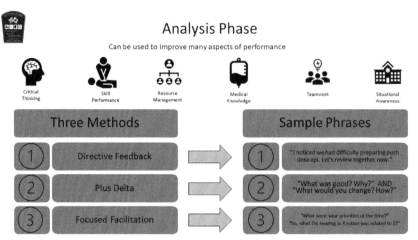

Fig. 4. Sample postresuscitation hot wash tool for debriefing (DC Fire and EMS).

debriefing and engagement in a structured, data-driven, continuous quality improvement (CQI) process.

Postevent Cardiac Arrest Debriefing

Postevent debriefing is defined as a discussion between 2 or more individuals in which aspects of performance are analyzed.[97] During a postevent cardiac arrest debrief, EMS providers discuss the care provided, reflect on teamwork and leadership challenges, review quantitative data collected during the event such as CPR metrics, and ultimately identify opportunities and strategies for improving performance. The debrief should typically be led by the resuscitation team leader and is often greatly enhanced by structuring the discussion using a scripted debriefing framework as well as a checklist.[98]

Debriefs are termed "cold" or "hot" based on when the debriefing occurs relative to the resuscitation attempt. A "hot" debrief occurs immediately after resuscitation is complete, typically after transferring patient care at the hospital or upon return to a firehouse or EMS station. A "cold" debrief occurs sometime after the resuscitation attempt. The performance of structured high-quality "hot" debriefs is of particular importance and interest to busy EMS agencies, whereby logistical constraints often prevent timely or thorough "cold" debriefs. The AHA provides a 2a recommendation for postevent debriefing, noting that a data-informed debriefing has potential benefit for prehospital systems of care.[97] One prospective, observational study demonstrated a significant increase in chest compression fraction as well as a decrease in the duration of longest nonshock pauses after implementing postresuscitation

debriefing and feedback.[99] See **Fig. 4** for a sample hot wash tool utilized for debriefing.

System Continuous Quality Improvement

The foundational principle of CQI involves capturing, analyzing, and regularly reporting data on current performance and then translating this data into actionable opportunities to improve performance.[100] The Resuscitation Academy notes that improvement in the quality of OHCA care is predicated upon a continuous process of "Measure, Improve...Measure, Improve."[101] The use of a systematic CQI approach has been shown to optimize outcomes for patients suffering other time-sensitive conditions such as STEMIs and traumatic injury.[102,103] However, the application of these same improvement techniques to cardiac arrest and CPR quality is not as widespread.[3]

EMS CPR CQI programs should implement processes to acquire and store incident response and CPR performance data from across the entire system. Commonly measured cardiac arrest system quality data includes response time intervals, such as.

- 911 call to response activation
- Dispatch to the arrival of both BLS and ALS providers
- 911 call to first defibrillation

In addition, CPR performance metrics should also be measured and collected. Most common cardiac monitors utilized by EMS providers now permit measurement of chest compression depth and rate, chest recoil, duration of pauses in CPR, and ventilation rates. Furthermore, technology has advanced such that this resuscitation data can now be collected from cardiac monitors wirelessly and aggregated to provide a true system performance review.[104]

Extending CQI beyond local data collection, EMS agencies and receiving hospital facilities are strongly encouraged to contribute to the Cardiac Arrest Registry to Enhance Survival (CARES) database. Established in 2004 by the Centers for Disease Control and Prevention, CARES data is used to help EMS agencies and hospitals benchmark their performance against local, state, and or national metrics. Participation in an OHCA registry enables communities to compare patient populations, interventions, and outcomes with the goal of identifying opportunities to improve the quality of care.[105] Today the CARES database captures standardized data from nearly 150,000 OHCAs annually from 2200 EMS agencies and over 2500 hospitals across a catchment area of approximately 170 million people or 51% of the US population.[106]

Over time, lessons learned from debriefing the performance of individual teams and evaluating system-wide performance can provide valuable and objective feedback to EMS systems. This feedback and knowledge can then be used to identify opportunities for targeted training and resource allocation, thereby potentially improving outcomes from OHCA.

SUMMARY

The management of OHCA is continuously evolving. EMS providers who respond to prehospital resuscitations must focus on providing high-quality CPR. Airway management typically is adequately accomplished with techniques less invasive than endotracheal intubation. Following successful resuscitation, these critically ill patients require a systems-based approach to their care.

CLINICS CARE POINTS

- When managing patients in cardiac arrest, a team-based approach such as pit crew CPR, facilitates a more efficient and standardized resuscitation.
- For most prehospital patients in cardiac arrest, less invasive airway management (such as supraglottic airways) promotes the focus on high-quality and uninterrupted chest compressions.
- After achieving successful ROSC in the prehospital setting, it is reasonable for EMS to defer the initiation of targeted temperature management until arrival at the receiving hospital facility.

DISCLOSURES

The authors have nothing to disclose.

REFERENCES

1. Taw RL. Dr. Friedrich Maass: 100th Anniversary of "New" CPR. Clin Cardiol 1991;14:1000–2.
2. Panchal AR, Bartos JA, Gabanas JG, et al. Part 3: Adult Basic and Advanced Life Support: 2020 American Heart Association Guidelines for Cardiopulmonary Resuscitation and Emergency Cardiovascular Care. Circulation 2020;142(16_suppl_2): S366–468.
3. Meaney PA, Bobrow BJ, Mancini ME, et al. Cardiopulmonary resuscitation quality: [corrected] improving cardiac resuscitation outcomes both inside and outside the hospital: a consensus statement from the American Heart Association. Circulation 2013;128(4):417–35.
4. Talikowska M, Tohira H, Finn J. Cardiopulmonary resuscitation quality and patient survival outcome in cardiac arrest: A systematic review and meta-analysis. Resuscitation 2015;96:66–77.
5. Christenson J, Andrusiek D, Everson-Stewart S, et al. Chest compression fraction determines survival in patients with out-of-hospital ventricular fibrillation. Circulation 2009;120(13):1241–7.
6. Vaillancourt C, Everson-Stewart S, Christenson J, et al. Resuscitation 2011;82(12):1501–7.
7. Wik L, Kramer-Johansen J, Myklebust H, et al. Quality of cardiopulmonary resuscitation during out-of-hospital cardiac arrest. JAMA 2005;293(3): 299–304.
8. Stiell IG, Brown SP, Nichol G, et al. What is the optimal chest compression depth during out-of-hospital cardiac arrest resuscitation of adult patients? Circulation 2014;130(22):1962–70.
9. Hopkins CL, Burk C, Moser S, et al. Implementation of Pit Crew Approach and Cardiopulmonary Resuscitation Metrics for Out-of-Hospital Cardiac Arrest Improves Patient Survival and Neurological Outcome. J Am Heart Assoc 2016;5(1):e002892.
10. Eschmann NM, Pirrallo RG, Aufderheide TP, et al. The association between emergency medical services staffing patterns and out-of-hospital cardiac arrest survival. Prehosp Emerg Care 2010;14(1): 71–7.
11. Dyson K, Bray JE, Smith K, et al. Paramedic Exposure to Out-of-Hospital Cardiac Arrest Resuscitation Is Associated With Patient Survival. Circ Cardiovasc Qual Outcomes 2016;9(2):154–60.
12. Hunziker S, Johansson AC, Tschan F, et al. Teamwork and leadership in cardiopulmonary resuscitation. J Am Coll Cardiol 2011;57(24):2381–8.
13. Yeung JH, Ong GJ, Davies RP, et al. Factors affecting team leadership skills and their

relationship with quality of cardiopulmonary resuscitation. Crit Care Med 2012;40(9):2617–21.

14. Kirkbright S, Finn J, Tohira H, et al. Audiovisual feedback device use by health care professionals during CPR: a systematic review and meta-analysis of randomised and non-randomised trials. Resuscitation 2014;85(4):460–71.

15. Bobrow BJ, Vadeboncoeur TF, Stolz U, et al. The influence of scenario-based training and real-time audiovisual feedback on out-of-hospital cardiopulmonary resuscitation quality and survival from out-of-hospital cardiac arrest. Ann Emerg Med 2013;62(1):47–56.e1.

16. Goharani R, Vahedian-Azimi A, Farzanegan B, et al. Real-time compression feedback for patients with in-hospital cardiac arrest: a multi-center randomized controlled clinical trial. J Intensive Care 2019;7:5.

17. Wang PL, Brooks SC. Mechanical versus manual chest compressions for cardiac arrest. Cochrane Database Syst Rev 2018;8(8):CD007260.

18. Poole K, Couper K, Smyth MA, et al. Mechanical CPR: Who? When? How? Crit Care 2018;22(1):140.

19. Esibov A, Banville I, Chapman FW, et al. Mechanical chest compressions improved aspects of CPR in the LINC trial. Resuscitation 2015;91:116–21.

20. Yost D, Phillips RH, Gonzales L, et al. Assessment of CPR interruptions from transthoracic impedance during use of the LUCAS™ mechanical chest compression system. Resuscitation 2012;83(8):961–5.

21. Levy M, Yost D, Walker RG, et al. A quality improvement initiative to optimize use of a mechanical chest compression device within a high-performance CPR approach to out-of-hospital cardiac arrest resuscitation. Resuscitation 2015;92:32–7.

22. Debaty G, Shin SD, Metzger A, et al. Tilting for perfusion: head-up position during cardiopulmonary resuscitation improves brain flow in a porcine model of cardiac arrest. Resuscitation 2015;87:38–43.

23. Varney J, Motawea KR, Mostafa MR, et al. Efficacy of heads-up CPR compared to supine CPR positions: Systematic review and meta-analysis. Health Sci Rep 2022;5(3):e644.

24. Pepe PE, Scheppke KA, Antevy PM, et al. Confirming the Clinical Safety and Feasibility of a Bundled Methodology to Improve Cardiopulmonary Resuscitation Involving a Head-Up/Torso-Up Chest Compression Technique. Crit Care Med 2019;47(3):449–55.

25. Moore JC, Pepe PE, Scheppke KA, et al. Head and thorax elevation during cardiopulmonary resuscitation using circulatory adjuncts is associated with improved survival. Resuscitation 2022;179:9–17.

26. Huang CC, Chen KC, Lin ZY, et al. The effect of the head-up position on cardiopulmonary resuscitation: a systematic review and meta-analysis. Crit Care 2021;25(1):376.

27. Neumar RW, Otto CW, Link MS, et al. Part 8: Adult advanced cardiac life support: 2010 American Heart Association guidelines for cardiopulmonary resuscitation and emergency cardiac care. Circulation 2010;1222(183):S727–67.

28. Wang HE, Kupas DF, Greenwood MJ, et al. An algorithmic approach to prehospital airway management. Prehosp Emerg Care 2005;9(2):145–55.

29. Wang HE, Benger JR. Endotracheal intubation during out-of-hospital cardiac arrest: New insights from recent clinical trials. J Am Coll Emerg Physicians Open 2019;1(1):24–9.

30. Vaillancourt C, Petersen A, Meier EN, et al. The impact of increased chest compression fraction on survival for out-of-hospital cardiac arrest patients with a non-shockable initial rhythm. Resuscitation 2020;154:93–100.

31. Benger JR, Kirby K, Black S, et al. Effect of a Strategy of a Supraglottic Airway Device vs Tracheal Intubation During Out-of-Hospital Cardiac Arrest on Functional Outcome: The AIRWAYS-2 Randomized Clinical Trial. JAMA 2018;320(8):779–91.

32. Bobrow BJ, Ewy GA, Clark L, et al. Passive oxygen insufflation is superior to bag valve mask ventilation for witnessed fibrillation out of hospital cardiac arrest. Ann Emerg Med 2009;54(5):656–62.

33. Aufderheide TP, Sigurdsson G, Pirrallo RG, et al. Hyperventilation-induced hypotension during cardiopulmonary resuscitation. Circulation 2004;109(16):1960–5.

34. Travers AH, Rea TD, Bobrow BJ, et al. Part 4: CPR overview: 2010 American Heart Association Guidelines for Cardiopulmonary Resuscitation and Emergency Cardiovascular Care. Circulation 2010;122(18 Suppl 3):S676–84.

35. Wenzel V, Keller C, Idris AH, et al. Effects of smaller tidal volumes during basic life support ventilation in patients with respiratory arrest: good ventilation, less risk? Resuscitation 1999;43(1):25–9.

36. Kim HJ, Kim SH, Min JY, et al. Determination of the appropriate oropharyngeal airway size in adults: Assessment using ventilation and an endoscopic view. Am J Emerg Med 2017;35(10):1430–4.

37. Hocking G, Roberts FL, Thew ME. Airway obstruction with cricoid pressure and lateral tilt. Anaesthesia 2001 Sep;56(9):825–8.

38. Hartsilver EL, Vanner RG. Airway obstruction with cricoid pressure. Anaesthesia 2000;55(3):208–11.

39. Kurowski A, Szarpak L, Zasko P, et al. Comparison of direct intubation and Supraglottic Airway Laryngopharyngeal Tube (S.A.L.T.) for endotracheal intubation during cardiopulmonary resuscitation.

Randomized manikin study. Anaesthesiol Intensive Ther 2015;47(3):195–9.

40. Wang HE, Simeone SJ, Weaver MD, et al. Interruptions in cardiopulmonary resuscitation from paramedic endotracheal intubation. Ann Emerg Med 2009;54(5):645–52.e1.

41. Panchal AR, Berg KM, Hirsch KG, et al. American Heart Association focused update on advanced cardiovascular life support: use of advanced airways, vasopressors, and extracorporeal cardiopulmonary resuscitation during cardiac arrest: an update to the American Heart Association guidelines for cardiopulmonary resuscitation and emergency cardiovascular care. Circulation 2019;140:e881–94.

42. Wang HE, Yealy DM. How many attempts are required to accomplish out-of-hospital endotracheal intubation? Acad Emerg Med 2006;13(4):372–7.

43. Wang HE, Schmicker RH, Daya MR, et al. Effect of a Strategy of Initial Laryngeal Tube Insertion vs Endotracheal Intubation on 72-Hour Survival in Adults With Out-of-Hospital Cardiac Arrest: A Randomized Clinical Trial. JAMA 2018;320(8):769–78.

44. Ewy GA, Sanders AB. Alternative approach to improving survival of patients with out-of-hospital primary cardiac arrest. J Am Coll Cardiol 2013;61(2):113–8.

45. Warner KJ, Carlbom D, Cooke CR, et al. Paramedic training for proficient prehospital endotracheal intubation. Prehosp Emerg Care 2010;14(1):103–8.

46. Eberlein CM, Luther IS, Carpenter TA, et al. First-Pass Success Intubations Using Video Laryngoscopy Versus Direct Laryngoscopy: A Retrospective Prehospital Ambulance Service Study. Air Med J 2019;38(5):356–8.

47. Huebinger RM, Stilgenbauer H, Jarvis JL, et al. Video laryngoscopy for out of hospital cardiac arrest. Resuscitation 2021;162:143–8.

48. Reades R, Studnek JR, Vandeventor S, et al. Intraosseous versus intravenous vascular access during out-of-hospital cardiac arrest: a randomized controlled trial. Ann Emerg Med 2011;58(6):509–16.

49. Wampler D, Schwartz D, Shumaker J, et al. Paramedics successfully perform humeral EZ-IO intraosseous access in adult out-of-hospital cardiac arrest patients. Am J Emerg Med 2012;30(7):1095–9.

50. Granfeldt A, Avis SR, Lind PC, et al. Intravenous vs. intraosseous administration of drugs during cardiac arrest: A systematic review. Resuscitation 2020;149:150–7.

51. Bornstein K, Long B, Porta AD, et al. After a century, Epinephrine's role in cardiac arrest resuscitation remains controversial. Am J Emerg Med 2021;39:168–72.

52. Holmberg MJ, Issa MS, Moskowitz A, et al. Vasopressors during adult cardiac arrest: A systematic review and meta-analysis. Resuscitation 2019;139:106–21.

53. Panchal AR, Berg HM, Kudenchuk PJ, et al. American Heart Association Focused Update on Advanced Cardiovascular Life Support Use of Antiarrhythmic Drugs During and Immediately After Cardiac Arrest: An Update to the American Heart Association Guidelines for Cardiopulmonary Resuscitation and Emergency Cardiovascular Care. Circulation 2018;138(23):e740–9.

54. Kudenchuk PJ, Cobb LA, Copass MK, et al. Amiodarone for resuscitation after out-of-hospital cardiac arrest due to ventricular fibrillation. N Engl J Med 1999;341:871–8.

55. Kudenchuk PJ, Brown SP, Daya M, et al. Amiodarone, lidocaine, or placebo in out-of-hospital cardiac arrest. N Engl J Med 2016;374(18):1711–22.

56. Tzivoni D, Banai S, Schuger C, et al. Treatment of torsade de pointes with magnesium sulfate. Circulation 1988;77:392–439.

57. Cheskes S, Verbeek PR, Drennan IR, et al. Defibrillation Strategies for Refractory Ventricular Fibrillation. N Engl J Med 2022 Nov;387(21):1947–56.

58. Grmec S, Kipnik D. Does the Mainz Emergency Evaluation Scoring (MEES) in combination with capnometry (MEESc) help in the prognosis of outcome from cardiopulmonary resuscitation in a prehospital setting? Resuscitation 2003;58(1):89–96.

59. Sandroni C, De Santis P, D'Arrigo S. Capnography during cardiac arrest. Resuscitation 2018;132:73–7.

60. Hartmann SM, Farris RW, Gennaro JL, et al. Systematic Review and Meta-Analysis of End-Tidal Carbon Dioxide Values Associated With Return of Spontaneous Circulation During Cardiopulmonary Resuscitation. J Intensive Care Med 2015;30(7):426–35.

61. Witten L, Gardner R, Holmberg MJ, et al. Reasons for death in patients successfully resuscitated from out-of-hospital and in-hospital cardiac arrest. Resuscitation 2019;136:93–9.

62. Trzeciak S, Jones AE, Kilgannon JH, et al. Significance of arterial hypotension after resuscitation from cardiac arrest. Crit Care Med 2009;37(11):2895–903.

63. Chiu YK, Lui CT, Tsui KL. Impact of hypotension after return of spontaneous circulation on survival in patients of out-of-hospital cardiac arrest. Am J Emerg Med 2018;36(1):79–83.

64. Becker LB. New concepts in reactive oxygen species and cardiovascular reperfusion physiology. Cardiovasc Res 2004;61(3):461–70.

65. Kilgannon JH, Jones AE, Shapiro NI, et al. Association between arterial hyperoxia following

resuscitation from cardiac arrest and in-hospital mortality. JAMA 2010;303(21):2165–71.

66. Ginsberg MD, Sternau LL, GLobus MY, et al. Therapeutic modulation of brain temperature: relevance to ischemic brain injury. Cerebrovasc Brain Metab Rev 1992;4(3):189–225.

67. Colbourne F, Sutherland G, Corbett D. Postischemic hypothermia. A critical appraisal with implications for clinical treatment. Mol Neurobiol 1997; 14(3):171–201.

68. Nielsen N, Wetterslev J, Cronberg T, et al. Targeted temperature management at 33°C versus 36°C after cardiac arrest. N Engl J Med 2013;369(23):2197–206.

69. Kim F, Nichol G, Maynard C, et al. Effect of prehospital induction of mild hypothermia on survival and neurological status among adults with cardiac arrest: a randomized clinical trial. JAMA 2014; 311(1):45–52.

70. Lindsay PJ, Buell D, Scales DC. The efficacy and safety of pre-hospital cooling after out-of-hospital cardiac arrest: a systematic review and meta-analysis. Crit Care 2018;22(1):66.

71. Szarpak L, Filipiak KJ, Mosteller L, et al. Survival, neurological and safety outcomes after out of hospital cardiac arrests treated by using prehospital therapeutic hypothermia: A systematic review and meta-analysis. Am J Emerg Med 2021;42:168–77.

72. Verbeek PR, Vermeulen MJ, Ali FH, et al. Derivation of a termination-of-resuscitation guideline for emergency medical technicians using automated external defibrillators. Acad Emerg Med 2002;9: 671–8.

73. Ebell MH, Vellinga A, Masterson S, et al. Meta-analysis of the accuracy of termination of resuscitation rules for out-of-hospital cardiac arrest. Emerg Med J 2019;36(8):479–84.

74. Morrison LJ, Verbeek PR, Vermeulen MJ, et al. Derivation and evaluation of a termination of resuscitation clinical prediction rule for advanced life support providers. Resuscitation 2007;74(2): 266–75.

75. Drennan IR, Case E, Verbeek PR, et al. A comparison of the universal TOR Guideline to the absence of prehospital ROSC and duration of resuscitation in predicting futility from out-of-hospital cardiac arrest. Resuscitation 2017;111:96–102.

76. Saunders CE, Heye CJ. Ambulance collisions, in an urban environment. Prehosp Disaster Med 1994;9:118–24.

77. Maguire BJ, Hunting KL, Smith GS, et al. Occupational fatalities in emergency medical services: a hidden crisis. Ann Emerg Med 2002;40:625–32.

78. Russi CS, Myers LA, Kolb LK, et al. A Comparison of Chest Compression Quality Delivered During On-Scene and Ground Transport Cardiopulmonary Resuscitation. West J Emerg Med 2016;17(5): 634–9.

79. Wampler DA, Collett LA, Manifold CA, et al. Cardiac arrest survival is rare without prehospital return of spontaneous circulation. Prehosp Emerg Care 2012;16(4):451–5.

80. Szpilman D, Soares M. In-water resuscitation–is it worthwhile? Resuscitation 2004;63(1):25–31.

81. Breyre AM, Benesch T, Glomb NW, et al. EMS Experience Caring and Communicating with Patients and Families with a Life-Limiting-Illness. Prehosp Emerg Care 2022;26(5):708–15.

82. Brooks SC, Schmicker RH, Cheskes S, et al. Variability in the initiation of resuscitation attempts by emergency medical services personnel during out-of-hospital cardiac arrest. Resuscitation 2017; 117:102–8.

83. Yap J, Haines M, Nowroozpoor A, et al. Rationale for withholding professional resuscitation in emergency medical system-attended out-of-hospital cardiac arrest. Resuscitation 2022;170:201–6.

84. Marco CA, Schears RM. Prehospital resuscitation practices: a survey of prehospital providers. J Emerg Med 2003;24:101–6.

85. Guru V, Verbeek PR, Morrison LJ. Response of paramedics to terminally ill patients with cardiac arrest: an ethical dilemma. CMAJ (Can Med Assoc J) 1999;161:1251–4.

86. Feder S, Matheny RL, Loveless RS Jr, et al. Withholding resuscitation: a new approach to prehospital end-of-life decisions. Ann Intern Med 2006;144: 634–40.

87. Mengual RP, Feldman MJ, Jones GR. Implementation of a novel prehospital advance directive protocol in southeastern Ontario. CJEM 2007;9(4):250–9.

88. Grudzen CR, Koenig WJ, Hoffman JR, et al. Potential impact of a verbal prehospital DNR policy. Prehosp Emerg Care 2009;13(2):169–72.

89. Yeung J, Matsuyama T, Bray J, et al. Does care at a cardiac arrest centre improve outcome after out-of-hospital cardiac arrest? - A systematic review. Resuscitation 2019;137:102–15.

90. Panchal AR, Berg KM, Cabañas JG, et al. American Heart Association Focused Update on Systems of Care: Dispatcher-Assisted Cardiopulmonary Resuscitation and Cardiac Arrest Centers: An Update to the American Heart Association Guidelines for Cardiopulmonary Resuscitation and Emergency Cardiovascular Care. Circulation 2019;140(24): e895–903.

91. Dumas F, Bougouin W, Geri G, et al. Emergency Percutaneous Coronary Intervention in Post-Cardiac Arrest Patients Without ST-Segment Elevation Pattern: Insights From the PROCAT II Registry. JACC Cardiovasc Interv 2016;9(10):1011–8.

92. Lamhaut L, Hutin A, Puymirat E, et al. A Pre-Hospital Extracorporeal Cardio Pulmonary Resuscitation (ECPR) strategy for treatment of refractory out hospital cardiac arrest: An observational study and

propensity analysis. Resuscitation 2017;117: 109–17.

93. Alm-Kruse K, Sørensen G, Osbakk SA, et al. Outcome in refractory out-of-hospital cardiac arrest before and after implementation of an ECPR proto-col. Resuscitation 2021;162:35–42.

94. Hsu CH, Meurer WJ, Domeier R, et al. Extracorpo-real Cardiopulmonary Resuscitation for Refractory Out-of-Hospital Cardiac Arrest (EROCA): Results of a Randomized Feasibility Trial of Expedited Out-of-Hospital Transport. Ann Emerg Med 2021; 78(1):92–101.

95. Kim SJ, Kim HJ, Lee HY, et al. Comparing extracor-poreal cardiopulmonary resuscitation with conven-tional cardiopulmonary resuscitation: A meta-analysis. Resuscitation 2016;103:106–16.

96. Yannopoulos D, Bartos J, Raveendran G, et al. Advanced reperfusion strategies for patients with out-of-hospital cardiac arrest and refractory ven-tricular fibrillation (ARREST): a phase 2, single centre, open-label, randomised controlled trial. Lancet 2020;396(10265):1807–16.

97. Cheng A, Eppich W, Grant V, et al. Debriefing for technology-enhanced simulation: a systematic re-view and meta-analysis. Med Educ 2014;48: 657–66.

98. Berg KM, Cheng A, Panchal AR, et al. Part 7: Sys-tems of Care: 2020 American Heart Association Guidelines for Cardiopulmonary Resuscitation and Emergency Cardiovascular Care. Circulation 2020;142(16_suppl_2):S580–604.

99. Bleijenberg E, Koster RW, de Vries H, et al. The impact of post-resuscitation feedback for paramedics on the quality of cardiopulmonary resuscitation. Resuscitation 2017;110:1–5.

100. Institute of Medicine. Resuscitation Research and Continuous Quality Improvement. In: Strategies to improve cardiac arrest survival: a time to Act. Washington, DC: The National Academies Press; 2015. p. 315–62.

101. Resuscitation Academy. A Few Words of Wisdom - The Seven Mantras. In: Ten Steps for improving survival from sudden cardiac arrest. 2020. Avail-able at: https://www.resuscitationacademy.org/ ebooks 2020. Accessed October 17, 2022.

102. Jollis JG, Granger CB, Henry TD, et al. Systems of care for ST-segment-elevation myocardial infarc-tion: a report from the American Heart Association's Mission: Lifeline. Circ Cardiovasc Qual Outcomes 2012;5:423–8.

103. Santana MJ, Stelfox HT. Quality indicators used by trauma centers for performance measurement. J Trauma Acute Care Surg 2012;72:1298–302.

104. Semark B, Årestedt K, Israelsson J, et al. Quality of chest compressions by healthcare professionals using real-time audiovisual feedback during in-hospital cardiopulmonary resuscitation. Eur J Car-diovasc Nurs 2017;16(5):453–7.

105. McNally B, Stokes A, Crouch A, et al. CARES Sur-veillance Group. CARES: Cardiac Arrest Registry to Enhance Survival. Ann Emerg Med 2009;54(5): 674–83.e2.

106. Cardiac Arrest Registry to Enhance Survival. The CARES. In: 2021 CARES Annual Report. 2021. Available at: https://mycares.net/sitepages/uploads/ 2022/2021_flipbook/index.html?page=1. Accessed October 17, 2022.

Moving?

Make sure your subscription moves with you!

To notify us of your new address, find your **Clinics Account Number** (located on your mailing label above your name), and contact customer service at:

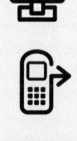

Email: journalscustomerservice-usa@elsevier.com

800-654-2452 (subscribers in the U.S. & Canada)
314-447-8871 (subscribers outside of the U.S. & Canada)

Fax number: 314-447-8029

Elsevier Health Sciences Division
Subscription Customer Service
3251 Riverport Lane
Maryland Heights, MO 63043

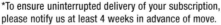

*To ensure uninterrupted delivery of your subscription, please notify us at least 4 weeks in advance of move.

ELSEVIER

Printed and bound by CPI Group (UK) Ltd, Croydon, CR0 4YY

03/10/2024

01040367-0018